Xuē Jǐ's 薛己

# 女科撮要

## Outline of Female Medicine

*Nǚ Kē Cuò Yào*

Lorraine Wilcox, L.Ac.

The Chinese Medicine Database
www.cm-db.com
*Portland, Oregon*

# Outline of Female Medicine

# 女科撮要

## *Nǚ Kē Cuò Yào*

Lorraine Wilcox



1017 SW Morrison #306
Portland, OR 97205 USA

COMP designation original Chinese work and English translation

Cover Design by Jonathan Schell L.Ac.
Library of Congress Cataloging-in-Publication Data:

Xuē Jǐ, fl. 1487 - 1559
[Outline of Female Medicine. English]
Nü Ke Cuo Yao = Outline of Female Medicine.
/ translation Lorraine Wilcox
p. cm.
Includes Index.
ISBN 978-0-9906029-1-0 (alk. paper)
Medicine, Chinese I. Wilcox, Lorraine. II. Title: Outline of Female Medicine.



International Standard Book Number (ISBN): 978-0-9906029-1-0
Printed in the United States of America

# Contents

## Attached Formulas and Notes for Volume 1

## Attached Formulas and Notes for Volume 2

## Appendices

## Unlisted Formulas

## Formulas that Xuē Jǐ said were Mistakenly Used



## Indices

# Translator's Introduction to *Nǚ Kē Cuò Yào* (Outline of Female Medicine)

*Nǚ Kē Cuò Yào* was written by Xuē Jǐ during the *Míng* dynasty (薛己《 女科撮要 》明). A summary of information regarding Xuē Jǐ and this book is given in the table below.

| **Xuē Jǐ 薛己, the Author** | |
|---|---|
| family name | Xuē 薛 |
| *míng*-name* | Jǐ 己 |
| *zì*-name | Xīnfǔ 新甫 |
| *hào*-name | Lìzhāi 立齋 |
| dynasty | Míng 明 |
| born | 1487 |
| died | 1559 |
| Xuē Jǐ's age at death | 72 |
| Xuē Jǐ's age when this book was published | 60 |
| year this book was published | 1548 |
| hometown | Wújùn 吳郡 (Sūzhōu region) |

*Chinese males traditionally took a number of names over the course of their lives. To an outsider, this can be very confusing. The *míng*-name (名) is given by parents shortly after the child is born. The *zì*-name (字) is sometimes called a *courtesy name*. This was used by peers on formal occasions and in writing. A *hào*-name (號) is a self-selected pen name.

## An Outline of Xuē Jǐ's Life and Achievements

Xuē's father, Xuē Kǎi 薛鎧, was a doctor and had been a medical officer of the Imperial Academy of Medicine. Xuē Jǐ studied medicine from his childhood onward. He not only inherited a family lineage, but also studied the important medical texts and rose through the ranks of the Imperial Academy of Medicine.

During the first year of Emperor Zhèngdé's reign (1506), Xuē Jǐ, like his father, became an imperial medical officer. In 1515, at the age of 28, Xuē himself treated Emperor

Zhèngdé. In 1520, he became an Administrative Assistant (second in command) at the Nánjīng Imperial Academy of Medicine. In the ninth year of Emperor Jiājìng's reign (1530), Xuē became Grand Master for Governance (a prestige title) and Commissioner of the Nánjīng Imperial Academy of Medicine. He soon resigned from office (although he was able to retain his titles) and returned to his hometown to practice medicine and write.

Xuē Jǐ wrote prolifically. He authored or edited and annotated at least sixteen books. Some were officially published in his government capacity and others were published after he retired. Xuē was interested in a broad array of topics, including internal medicine, external medicine, diseases of the mouth and teeth, female disorders, and pediatrics. Xuē Jǐ added an extensive number of his own case studies to the various books he wrote and annotated.

| **Books authored by Xuē Jǐ** | | | |
|---|---|---|---|
| *Běn Cǎo Yuē Yán* | 《本草約言》 | Brief Words on Materia Medica | 1520 |
| *Wài Kē Fā Huī* | 《外科發揮》 | Elucidation of External Medicine | 1528 |
| *Wài Kē Xīn Fǎ* | 《外科心法》 | The Heart Method of External Medicine | 1528 |
| *Wài Kē Jīng Yàn Fāng* | 《外科經驗方》 | Experiential Formulas of External Medicine | 1528 |
| *Kǒu Chǐ Lèi Yào* | 《口齒類要》 | Categorized Essentials of the Mouth and Teeth | 1528 |
| *Nèi Kē Zhāi Yào* | 《內科摘要》 | Summary of Internal Medicine | 1529 |
| *Zhèng Tǐ Lèi Yào* | 《正體類要》 | Categorized Essentials of Correcting the Body | 1529 |
| *Lì Yáng Jī Yào* | 《癘瘍機要》 | Key Essentials of Epidemic Sores | 1529 |
| *Nǚ Kē Cuò Yào* | 《女科撮要》 | Outline of Female Medicine | 1548 |
| *Wài Kē Shū Yào* | 《外科樞要》 | Pivotal Essentials for External Medicine | 1571 |
| *Bǎo Yīng Jīn Jìng Lù* | 《保嬰金鏡錄》 | Golden Mirror Record for the Care of Infants | |

| **Xuē Jǐ edited, annotated, and added case histories to the following** | |
|---|---|
| **original author** | **title** |
| Chén Zìmíng 陳自明 | *Fù Rén Dà Quán Liáng Fāng*《婦人大全良方》(All Inclusive Fine Formulas for Women) (1547), originally published in 1238 (Northern Sòng) |
| Wáng Lún 王綸 | *Míng Yī Zá Zhù*《明醫雜著》(Miscellaneous Works of Physicians in Ming Dynasty) (1549) |
| Chén Wénzhōng 陳文中 | *Xiǎo Ér Dòu Zhěn Fāng Lùn*《小兒痘疹方論》(Discussion of Formulas for Pediatric Pox) (1550) |

| | |
|---|---|
| Qián Yǐ 錢乙 | *Xiǎo Ér Yào Zhèng Zhí Jué* 《小兒藥證直訣》(Key to Therapeutics for Children's Diseases) (1551) |
| Xuē Kǎi 薛鎧 (Xuē Jǐ's father) | *Bǎo Yīng Cuò Yào* 《保嬰撮要》(Outline of Infant Care) (1555) |

## Xuē's Relationship with the Royal Family

Xuē Jǐ himself was one of the doctors to treat the royal family. In 1518, Emperor Zhèngdé appointed Xuē Jǐ to attend to the heir to the throne, Zhū Yòuyuán.[1] Xuē Jǐ then went to Ānlù Prefecture in Húguǎng[2] to become part of the heir's household. In 1521, the year Emperor Zhèngdé died, Xuē Jǐ accompanied Zhū Hòucōng (who became Emperor Jiājìng) to Běijīng.[3]

In 1528, the Empress Dowager Lady Jiǎng suffered wasting thirst.[4] Xuē Jǐ prescribed a formula for her containing *kǔ guā, shān yào, yù zhú,* and *gé gēn.*[5] She took them as a decoction and it was extremely effective. Emperor Jiājìng was quite pleased. The people of Ānlù Prefecture were then encouraged to plant *kǔ guā, gé gēn,* and the other ingredients of the formula.

1. Zhū Yòuyuán 朱祐杬 was a cousin of Emperor Zhèngdé. He died before Zhèngdé so Zhū Yòuyuán's son, Zhū Hòucōng 朱厚熜, then became the heir.
2. Ānlù Prefecture in Húguǎng 湖廣安陸州: This is in today's city of Zhōngxiáng 鍾祥市 in Húběi Province. Húguǎng was a province of China during the *Yuán* and *Míng* dynasties. It was divided into Húběi and Húnán during the *Qīng* dynasty. Together, these are also sometimes known as Liǎnghú.
3. Zhèngdé had no surviving children. His cousin and adopted son Zhū Hòucōng became Emperor Jiājìng 嘉靖. Zhū Hòucōng was the biological son of Zhū Yòuyuán, whom Xuē Jǐ had been attending for the previous three years.
4. Lady Jiǎng was Emperor Jiājìng's mother. Wasting thirst (*xiāo kě*) is more or less parallel to diabetes.
5. 苦瓜、山藥、玉竹、葛根。

## The School of Warm Supplementation

The School of Warm Supplementation[6] favored strengthening the patient with warming herbs, since yáng is life. There were many contributors to the School of Warm Supplementation. Besides Xuē Jǐ, some identify Lǐ Dōngyuán,[7] Zhāng Jièbīn, Zhào Xiànkě, Sūn Yīkuí, and Lǐ Zhōngzǐ[8] as belonging to this school of thought. This school was not as standardized as some of the earlier intellectual traditions that had only one founder. Each doctor emphasized different aspects. Some favored supplementing and regulating the spleen and stomach, others emphasized kidney yáng and *mìng mén* fire. Others, such as Xuē, emphasized both the spleen and kidneys.

## Xuē Jǐ's Practice Style

Zhū Dānxī's theories remained popular in the *Míng* dynasty and Xuē lived in the same general region as Zhū. Because Zhū generally advocated using cooling herbs to nourish yīn and descending herbs to counter excessive minister fire, these had become popular methods. While appropriate in some patients, Xuē worried that this could damage yáng qì and harm the spleen and kidneys if routinely used. Xuē also generally avoided attacking formulas whenever possible. Because of this, Xuē preferred the theories of Lǐ Dōngyuán on the importance of the spleen and stomach. He also saw value in strengthening the water and fire of the kidneys. In this, Wáng Bīng[9] and Qián Yǐ[10] influenced his thought.

Xuē's most commonly used formulas (including variations) are:

| | | |
|---|---|---|
| *Bǔ Zhōng Yì Qì Tāng* | 補中益氣湯* | F2-5 |
| *Liù Wèi Dì Huáng Wán* | 六味地黃丸 | F2-16 |

6. *Wēn bǔ xué pài* 溫補學派.
7. Lǐ lived a few hundred years earlier and was the founder of the Supplement Earth School, but some say he also originated the school of warm supplementation.
8. 李東源、張介賓、趙獻可、孫一奎、李中梓。
9. Wáng Bīng edited and annotated *Sù Wèn* during the *Táng* dynasty.
10. Qián Yǐ was a famous pediatric doctor of the *Sòng* dynasty who emphasized the kidneys. He was the original author of *Liù Wèi Dì Huáng Wán*. Xuē Jǐ's father, Xuē Kǎi, practiced pediatrics so it is likely that Xuē Jǐ was exposed to Qián Yǐ quite a bit.

| | | |
|---|---|---|
| *Bā Wèi Wán* | 八味丸 | F2-17 |
| *Sì Jūn Zǐ Tāng* | 四君子湯 | F2-26 |
| *Liù Jūn Zǐ Tāng* | 六君子湯 | F2-6 |
| *Bā Zhēn Tāng* | 八珍湯 | F2-8 |
| *Shí Quán Dà Bǔ Tāng* | 十全大補湯 | F2-7 |
| *Xiǎo Chái Hú Tāng* | 小柴胡湯 | F2-12 |

* For a description of the indexing numbers for the formulas, see the *For the Reader* section, in the Translator's Introduction below.

Because this book discusses the treatment women,[11] we can add:

| | | |
|---|---|---|
| *Guī Pí Tāng* | 歸脾湯 | F2-3 |
| *Sì Wù Tāng* | 四物湯 | F2-51 |
| *Xiāo Yáo Sǎn* | 逍遙散 | F2-2 |

One can easily see from this list that Xuē favored supplementation of the spleen and kidneys. These formulas are all still popular today, so reading Xuē's cases can guide us in our modern clinical practice. They can expand our understanding of formulas we already use. While some of the other formulas Xuē used may be inappropriate today due to the inclusion of endangered species or toxic ingredients, much of his medicine is still appropriate for the modern clinic. He often used common ingredients, and fewer animal, mineral substances, or rare and expensive ingredients than some of his contemporaries. This is surprising as he would not have been limited by rarity or expense in his role as an imperial medical officer.

Since Xuē Jǐ favored supplementation (especially warm supplementation), he was disinclined to see a condition as excess; if an excess was acknowledged, it was usually viewed as the branch, with deficiency as the root. He therefore rarely used purely draining formulas and never used attacking formulas. Even in conditions that appear like excess, Xuē preferred to use supplementing formulas, adding draining herbs to them as needed.

As an extension of the same idea, Xuē Jǐ favored using mild herbs over a longer period of time. He felt drastic (violent-acting) herbs and quick fixes only caused harm in the long run. Xuē frequently warned against drastic herbs. Quite a few of his case studies describe the damage done by looking for a quick remedy to fix a condition. Here is an example:

11. Xuē also used these formulas quite a bit in his trauma patients. See *Zhèng Tǐ Lèi Yào* (Categorized Essentials of Correcting the Body), for example.

**1-8-6** 一室女年十七，瘰久不愈，天癸未通，發熱咳嗽，飲食少思；或欲用通經丸 。余曰：此症潮熱，經候不調者，不治，所喜脈不澀，且不潮熱，尚可治 。但養氣血，益津液，其經自行 。惑於速效，仍用之 。余曰：非其治也，此乃慓悍之劑，大助陽火，陰血得之則妄行，脾胃得之則愈虛 。經果通而不止，飲食愈少，更加潮熱，遂致不救 。

A seventeen year old unmarried girl had scrofula for a long time without recovering. Her *tiān guǐ* had never flowed. She had fever, cough, and little thought of food or drink. Someone wanted her to use *Tōng Jīng Wán* UFx-2. I said: "This disease of tidal fever and out of tune menstrual timing cannot be treated [that way]. I am pleased that the pulse is not rough and there are no tidal fevers at this time, so it is still treatable. We must only nourish qì and blood and boost jīnyè-fluids. Then menstruation will move on its own."[12] She was mislead by [the promise of] quick results and used *Tōng Jīng Wán* UFx-2 anyway. I said: "This is not the [proper] treatment. This prescription is swift and fierce and will strongly aid yáng fire. When yīn blood receives it, it will move recklessly. When the spleen and stomach receive it, they will become more deficient." As a result [of her taking *Tōng Jīng Wán*], her menstruation flowed and did not stop. Her eating and drinking decreased even more, it further increased her tidal fevers, and subsequently she could not be saved.

Since his prescriptions were milder than those of some of the other doctors, they needed to be taken for a longer period of time in order to affect complete recovery. Xuē often wrote 'after more than a hundred doses...' or 'the patient recovered after more than a year.' This may seem like a long time, but if his cases are truthfully reported, Xuē cured serious diseases without causing side effects or damaging other aspects of the patient's qì or body. His philosophy was that if the patient's original qì is strong, he or she can recover from any illness. Therefore, he avoided any quick fixes that could cause harm, but the treatment was slower acting.

Another special characteristic of Xuē Jǐ's style was the administration of different formulas at different times of the day. In this book, such a method is explicitly described in thirteen cases. There may have been many more, because the author often wrote that he

12. Throughout the cases, Xuē Jǐ frequently writes "I said:..." What follows is usually his clinical impressions. Sometimes, it is clearly dialogue with someone else. Other times, perhaps he said the words to himself. It may also simply be a literary device for introducing the diagnosis after the history and symptoms are described.

prescribed a patient several formulas in one day. However, he did not always mention the time each formula was to be taken. One technique was to use herbs to supplement the spleen, qì, or yáng in the morning and herbs to supplement the kidneys, blood, or yīn in the evening. The reasoning in some of the other cases was sometimes less apparent.

> **1-2-5**一婦人素勤苦，因喪子飲食少思，忽吐血甚多而自止，此後每勞則吐數口，瘵症已具，形體甚倦，午前以補中益氣，午後以歸脾湯送地黃丸而愈。
>
> A woman was usually hard-working. Because she mourned her child, she had little thought of food and drink. She suddenly vomited of a lot of blood and then it stopped without intervention. After this, she vomited several mouthfuls every time she was taxed, and when an episode of this disease was finished, her body was extremely weary. Before noon I had her take *Bŭ Zhōng Yì Qì Tāng* F2-5; after noon she used *Guī Pí Tāng* F2-3 to swallow *Dì Huáng Wán* F2-16 and she recovered.

As seen in the above case, Xuē often had a patient use a decoction of one formula to swallow a pill of another formula.

Xuē Jĭ included many case histories to illustrate his treatments: his books are filled with his own cases. This book contains 183 cases. Case studies are important because we can see the doctor's clinical thought in action. Essays on a topic often provide insight to a theory, but when case after case is provided, the application of the theory becomes clear.

## Later Criticisms of Xuē Jǐ's Work

Later doctors frequently criticize earlier ones. Xú Dàchūn (1693-1771, *Qīng*) was always very hard to please. He was not afraid to use strong words of criticism and Xuē was no exception. In *Yī Xué Yuán Liú Lùn*,[13] Xú wrote:

> 薛立齋尤浮泛荒謬，猶聖賢之學，變而為腐爛時文。
>
> Xuē Lìzhāi (Xuē Jǐ) was especially superficial and absurd; it is as if the learning of the sages and worthies mutated into a putrid and festering contemporary style of writing.

Xú Dàchūn's main problem with Xuē, as for most other doctors, was that he incorporated later schools of medical thought, rather than sticking to the classics.

Just as Xuē felt doctors such as Zhū Dānxī placed too much emphasis on cooling herbs, some later doctors felt the school of warm supplementation (including its proponents like Xuē) relied too heavily on the use of warm and hot herbs and excessive supplementation. The preface to *Wài Kē Shū Yào*[14] explains that Xuē died of a disease with sores. Since external medicine was one of his specialties, there were those at that time who took it as a failure of Xuē's style of medicine and spoke ill of the doctor. Xuē's biography in *Sì Kù Quán Shū*[15] also implied that Xuē Jǐ hastened his own death by excessive use of supplementing formulas. However Xuē Jǐ was 72 years old when he passed, which was not considered young at the time

Others felt that Xuē was a jack of all trades, master of none. From the list of Xuē's books above, it can be seen that he tackled many departments of medicine. External medicine was the topic on which he most focused, but Xuē wrote books on gynecology, pediatrics, internal medicine, and so forth. Xuē was more of an eclectic than an innovator, as

13. *Yī Xué Yuán Liú Lùn*《醫學源流論》(Discussion on the Origins and Development of Medicine) by Xú Dàchūn 徐大椿, published in 1757. Xú was a classicist who was not fond of many post-Hàn teachings.
14. The preface was written by one of Xuē's followers, Shěn Qǐyuán 沈啟原, and was dated 1571. Xuē Jǐ died in 1559.
15. *Sì Kù Quán Shū*《四庫全書》(The Complete Library in Four Sections) was a *Qīng* dynasty encyclopedic collection of works commissioned by Emperor Qiánlóng. It was completed in 1782.

this passage from *Zhōng Guó Yī Xué Yuán Liú Lùn* (Discussion of the Source and Course of Chinese Medicine, published in 1935) by Xiè Lìhéng[16] shows:

> Xuē Jǐ adopted the theories of Zhāng Zhòngjǐng 張仲景 (ca. 150-219) for *wàigǎn* 外感 (external afflictions), Dōngyuán 東垣 (i.e., Lǐ Gǎo 李杲, 1180-1251) for *nèishāng* 內傷 (internal damage), the Hé 河 medical lineage (i.e., Liú Wánsù 劉完素, 1120-1200) for febrile illnesses, and Dānxī 丹溪 (Zhū Zhènhēng 朱震亨, 1281-1358) for miscellaneous illnesses.[17]

Because of this, some felt his grasp of the medicine was rather superficial.

## About This Book, *Nǚ Kē Cuò Yào*

It should be noted that while *Nǚ Kē Cuò Yào* discusses the treatment of women, it is not strictly an obstetrics and gynecology text. The emphasis is on reproductive disorders, but a number of sections are on non-reproductive conditions that women tend to suffer, including urinary problems, painful joints, scrofula, and skin conditions. In addition, many of the postpartum conditions would not be considered gynecological today. Surprisingly, infertility, abdominal lumps, and symptoms of menopause do not have their own entries, but are occasionally discussed in other sections.[18]

*Nǚ Kē Cuò Yào* was written in an outline format. There is no overall discussion of the reproductive physiology of women. Diseases commonly suffered by women are broken into thirty headings. Each entry gives a list of general signs and symptoms accompanying the chief complaint, the pattern diagnosis, and the formula to treat it. Occasionally the author included passages from earlier books or provided his own short comments on the topic. After the breakdown of patterns and their formulas, Xuē Jǐ gave one or more cases from his own practice. A few are testimonials from the husband (or other male relative) of the patient.

16. 謝利恆《中國醫學源流論》. Xiè Lìhéng was a respected medical historian,
17. Translated by Margaret Wee Siang Ng and from her dissertation: Male Brushstrokes and Female Touch: Medical Writings on Childbirth in Imperial China, unpublished dissertation, Department of History, Faculty of Arts, McGill University, Montreal, 2013.
18. For a discussion of why menopause was not addressed as a separate condition in older Chinese medicine, see Not Very Traditional, Nor Exactly Chinese, So What Kind of Medicine is It? by Volker Scheid from the *Journal of Chinese Medicine*, Number 82, 2006.

The reader should note that Xuē did not always repeat the chief complaint in each case. For example, if a case is under the heading of abnormal vaginal discharge, one should assume that the patient suffered a discharge, even if it is not mentioned.

*Nǚ Kē Cuò Yào* has two volumes. The first discusses women who are not pregnant. The second is about diseases of pregnancy and postpartum conditions. At the end of each volume, Xuē included the recipes for formulas he used. The reasoning for order of the formulas and their placement in Volume 1 or Volume 2 is unclear. Formulas mentioned in Volume 1 are often found at the end of Volume 2, and formulas never used in Volume 1 may be found at the end of Volume 1. Neither are they consistently grouped by category or symptom. For the reader's convenience, all the formulas have been placed at the end of the book in this translation. The original order of the formulas has been retained and the numbering system used by the translator identifies the volume in which a formula was placed by Xuē.

*Nǚ Kē Cuò Yào* was written for the practitioner who already has an understanding of Chinese anatomy, physiology, pattern diagnosis, individual herbs, and formulas. It was meant to be a clinical guide and to illustrate the critical thinking of the author in clinic. Certainly Xuē also wanted to show the effectiveness of his personal style. Besides giving clinical guidance for treatment, the cases were used as proof that his theories were valid. In a number of them, he highlights the mistaken treatment of other practitioners, often with disastrous results.

In a book about treating women, one can observe something of the social interactions and attitudes between men and women. Xuē Jǐ's interactions with women and female practitioners seem more enlightened than some of his contemporaries. In some cases he discussed treatment with midwives, and included some tips he learned from them. He described some manual techniques that would be used by midwives during childbirth. Many other doctors only reviled midwives and would not discuss manual techniques, including acupuncture or moxibustion, as these were considered below the dignity of a scholar-physician. One of Xuē's other areas of interest, external medicine, was also often looked down upon because it involved manual techniques such as lancing sores. It seems then, that even though Xuē had treated the imperial family himself, he had the virtue of humility.

## For the Reader

The recipes for formulas that were found at the end of Volume 1 in the original text have been moved. They are now located before the formulas for Volume 2 so that all formulas are given in the same section of our translation.

Indexing and numbering makes a book such as this much more usable. Each of the thirty disease categories is numbered as follows:

| Examples | Volume Number | Topic number in the Volume | Meaning |
|---|---|---|---|
| 1-3 | 1 | 3 | The third topic in Volume 1 (Immovable Menstrual Block) |
| 2-5 | 2 | 5 | The fifth topic in Volume 2 (Retention of Placenta) |

Each case has its own number as well:

| Examples | Volume Number | Topic number in the volume | Case Number | Meaning |
|---|---|---|---|---|
| 1-3-4 | 1 | 3 | 4 | The fourth case under the third topic in Volume 1 |
| 2-5-1 | 2 | 5 | 1 | The first case under the fifth topic in Volume 2 |

Finally, the formulas are indexed as follows:

| Examples | Letter | Volume Number | Formula Number | Meaning |
|---|---|---|---|---|
| F1-3 | F = Formula | 1 | 3 | The third recipe originally given in the end of Volume 1 (*Zuǒ Jīn Wán* F1-3) |
| F2-27 | F = Formula | 2 | 27 | The twenty-seventh recipe originally given in the end of in Volume 2 (*Yì Gōng Sǎn* F2-27) |
| UF-6 | UF = Unlisted Formula that the author used but did not give the recipe | not included | 6 | The sixth recipe given in the translator's appendix of unlisted formulas at the end of the book (*Huó Mìng Yǐn* UF-6) |

| UFx-8 | UFx = Unlisted Formula that the author did not use (taken by the patient without being prescribed by the author) | not included | 8 | The eighth recipe given in the translators appendix of unlisted and unused formulas at the end of the book (*Jiǎn Hóng Wán* UFx-8) |
|---|---|---|---|---|

As for the formulas, note that the indications listed are often focused on the topic of the book – women's diseases. A formula often has many more indications than are listed here, but Xuē limited his description of uses to the ones that were relevant.

## A Few Terms

I will not make an extensive glossary here, but a few terms warrant discussion. Some years ago I stuck closely to the terminology developed by Nigel Wiseman. As my understanding grows, I now sometimes deviate from it. One reason is that terms have been used differently in different time periods and by different authors. The terms below do not have a good English equivalent or Xuē Jǐ used them in his own way.

**Descending** (*xià* 下): This word is used in many ways in general speech and in medical contexts. Its meanings include down, below, under, lower, to descend, to move downward, to swallow, to come out from below, the lower body, and so forth. In this text it is used in many different ways and is translated differently according to the context. The problem comes when discussing the treatment principle of *xià* 下. This is often translated as *purge* (which means to cleanse, not to descend). Wiseman uses *precipitate* (precipitation descends from above, but English speakers have difficulty seeing the connection). Bensky discusses *downward-draining* herbs (probably the best rendering but cumbersome). There is no perfect translation.

While the treatment principle of descending (*xià*) tends to result in a bowel movement, the emphasis is on descending something unwanted and letting it out through the lower orifices. It is also used for blood stasis in the uterus, inducing labor, retention of placenta, and so forth. Especially since this book discusses female issues, a more inclusive understanding of descending (*xià*) is necessary.

**Attune** (*tiáo* 調): This is another word that has a lot of different meanings when translated to English: attune, harmonize, blend, regulate, well-adjusted, to be in accord with, to have rapport, and so forth. It is used for tuning a musical instrument. It is often used in regard to menstruation. *Yuè jīng bù tiáo* 月經不調 is usually translated as irregular (*bù tiáo* 不調) menstruation (*yuè jīng* 月經). However, in English *irregular menstruation* usually connotes a problem in timing, most likely sometimes early and sometimes late. In this book I prefer to translate *tiáo* 調 using words related to attune. In disease, various aspects can be out of tune (*bù tiáo* 不調) and in treatment, the principle is to attune (*tiáo* 調) whatever is out of tune. This is used in the same sense as tuning a musical instrument – the strings should not be too tight or too loose. Besides this, Xuē Jǐ often tells us that the patient attuned herself, meaning that she adjusted her lifestyle to make it more suitable.

**Channel** (*jīng* 經): The author often attributed a symptom to a problem in a channel, even though it seems organ-related to the modern practitioner. He used this term in the same way as entering channels for herbs. An herb that enters the spleen channel may actually treat the spleen organ.

**Original qì** (*yuán qì* 元氣): While pronounced the same, do not confuse it with source qì (*yuán qì* 原氣). Original qì is used more or less as a synonym for right qì (*zhèng qì* 正氣), the sum of everything that promotes health in the body. Xuē Jǐ considered that supporting original qì was far more important than dispersing evils.

## Finally

One more item to discuss is that in this book, qì or blood deficiency could result in fevers or heat conditions. In modern times we tend to think of these as contributing to cold conditions, or at least not making heat. To understand the older view, please refer to the writings of Lǐ Dōngyuán 李東垣 and Zhū Dānxī 朱丹溪, much of which have been translated into English.

**Warning:** Please note that some of the formulas in this book are not appropriate for use today. They may contain herbs that are now considered toxic or unclean. They may contain herbs from endangered species. In the sections that give the recipes for the formulas, the translator has tried to footnote all instances of herbs that can no longer be used. However, it is possible that some herbs to be avoided have been missed. While most of the formulas in this book are still quite clinically relevant, it is the practitioner's responsibility to determine whether they are appropriate for use in a specific case, or if they are appropriate for use at all in the modern world.

## Acknowledgements

As always, Yue Lu helped me with the difficult passages regarding medicine. Without her, this book would only be a draft. Jerome Jiang helped me with the cultural and historical details in the introduction and some of the testimonials or cases. Jonathan Schell did his magic to turn the manuscript into a book. Stephanie Tyiska gave many useful suggestions for making this a better read; because of her there are quite a few more footnotes explaining less well-known terms and I have discussed additional topics in the introduction. Beyond this, her enthusiasm for Xuē Jǐ's cases has given me confidence that the reader will also find this book clinically useful.

# 前序
## Preface

余聞軒岐事業遐哉邈矣，其言說流布，至今未盡泯也 。然傳者或效或否，豈其書不可盡信耶，是存乎人焉耳 。語曰醫不通儒，不可以言醫，其以是歟！

I have heard that the achievements of Xuān [Huángdì] and Qí Bó are long lasting and profound. Their words and theories have been disseminated up until today and have not died out. Although they have been passed down, they are sometimes effective and sometimes not. How is it that their writings cannot be trusted? This is due to the human aspect. A proverb says that a doctor who does not become a scholar cannot be called a doctor. It is because of this!

太醫院使薛君立齋雅近於儒，其以醫名世也固宜 。君嘗以日所施活者，述其病原，詳其脈候，著其方，驗有所得，輒錄之，積匯成帙，標曰:《 家居醫錄 》。他日呈於大司馬中丞約庵翁，翁覽而善之，授余以鋟諸梓 、且命申其說 。

The Commissioner of the Imperial Academy of Medicine is Master Xuē Lìzhāi. He is refined enough to appear as a scholar and his medical skills are certainly famous among his contemporaries. Master Xuē has used his experience from his daily work of saving people, described the etiology, detailed the pulse conditions, wrote down the formulas, and recorded whatever has been effective. He then gathered it into a book entitled *Household Medical Records* (jiā jū yī lù).[1] Later on he presented it to the Minister of War and Vice Censor-in-Chief, an Honored Old Man named Yuē Ān. The Honored Old Man looked at it and approved. He instructed me to have all the wood blocks for printing carved and further commanded me to explain his theories.

1. It seems that no book was ever published with this name. Perhaps it was a working title that was never used when Xuē's books were published. Or maybe Xuē used it as a name for the body of his own work.

余曰:噫!是仁者之心哉！或曰：何謂也?夫醫，術也，而心術觀焉。世之醫者，得一方輒以自秘，取一效即以自多；人病在身，而渠病在心，且弗之藥，是尚可以言醫！薛君以名醫致身，不自秘而以示人，將欲致人人於名醫。

I say: Ah! This is a heart of benevolence! Perhaps you might say: What do you mean by that? Medicine is skill, but heart skills may also be displayed. For generations, whenever a doctor obtained a formula, he always kept it as his own secret. If he found even one effective formula, he became conceited. People are sick in their bodies, but the larger disease is in the heart-mind; in the same way, someone who does not give herbal medicine can still be called a doctor![2] Master Xuē is seen as a famous doctor who has dedicated his life; he has not kept his own secrets but has instead instructed people, so he is about to make everyone into famous doctors [by publishing all these effective formulas].

中丞翁撫綏畿輔，振衰剔弊，既登斯民仁壽之域，復布其醫書，欲壽斯民於無窮，玆非仁者之事哉！是宜梓之，以訓於世，觀者毋徒執其方而求得其心焉，則是錄也，其可傳矣。

The Honored Old Man, the Vice Censor-in-Chief, fosters the people around the capital. He braces up the weak and weeds out their maladies. He has already ascended into the domain of promoting benevolence and long life for the common people. On top of that, he has disseminated Xuē's medical books, endlessly wishing longevity for the common people. Isn't this putting benevolence into action! So it is appropriate to carve the printing blocks to teach the world. The reader must not simply follow these formulas, but must also seek to obtain Xuē's heart-mind. Then his record can be passed on.

嘉靖戊申春正月吉劍江存所範慶書

In spring, on the first day of the first month of the *wù shēn* year of Jiājìng's reign (1548), in Jiànjiāng, written by Fàn Qìng

2. This passage is difficult. It seems to say that some doctors are so selfish they are hardly practicing medicine. But those who perform benevolent acts, such as publishing this book, are actually performing medicine of the heart-mind.

# 《女科撮要·卷上·經候不調》

## 1-1 Menstrual Timing Out of Tune[3]

經曰:飲食入胃，遊溢精氣，上輸於脾，脾氣散精，上歸於肺，通調水道，下輸膀胱，水精四布，五經並行。故心脾平和，則經候如常。

The Classic says[4]: "Food and drink enter into the stomach. Their essence and qì float up and brim over, transported upward by the spleen. Spleen qì distributes the essence and above it is offered to the lungs which regulate the waterways. They transport it down to the urinary bladder. Water and essence spread in all directions, flowing in the five channels at the same time." Thus when the heart and spleen are harmonious, the timing of menstruation is normal.

苟或七情內傷，六淫外侵，飲食失節，起居失宜，脾胃虛損，則月經不調矣。若先期而至者，有因脾經血燥，有因脾經鬱滯，有因肝經怒火，有因血分有熱，有因勞役火動。其過期而至者，有因脾經血虛，有因肝經血少，有因氣虛血弱。

If the seven emotions cause internal damage or the six excesses invade the exterior; if one fails to regulate food and drink or rising and dwelling [lifestyle] become inappropriate, the spleen and stomach become deficient and then the monthly flow falls out of tune.

- If menstruation arrives early, the reason is blood dryness of the spleen channel,[5] or

3. The translator has numbered each chapter to make it easier to navigate or refer to other passages. The first number is the volume of the book; the number after the hyphen is the chapter number within that volume. For example, 1-2 is the second chapter in Volume 1. Below, the author's case histories are also numbered by adding a hyphen and a digit to the end of the chapter number. 2-4-3 is the third case in the fourth section of Volume 2.
4. In *Sù Wèn*, Chapter 21.
5. The author often attributed a symptom to a problem in a channel, even though it seems organ-related to a modern practitioner. He used this term in the same way as *entering channels* for herbs. An herb may enter the spleen channel but it actually treats the spleen organ.

constraint and stagnation of the spleen channel, or fiery anger of the liver channel, or heat of the blood division,[6] or taxation stirring up fire.

- If its arrival is overdue, the reason is blood deficiency of the spleen channel, or scant blood of the liver channel, or qì deficiency and blood weakness.

主治之法：脾經血燥者，加味逍遙散；脾經鬱滯者，歸脾湯；肝經怒火者，加味小柴胡湯；血分有熱者，加味四物湯；勞役火動者，補中益氣湯；脾經血虛者，人參養榮湯；肝經血少者，六味地黃丸；氣虛血弱者，八珍湯 。

The governing treatment method:

- Use *Jiā Wèi Xiāo Yáo Sǎn* F2-1 for blood dryness of the spleen channel.[7]
- Use *Guī Pí Tāng* F2-3 for constraint and stagnation of the spleen channel.
- Use *Jiā Wèi Xiǎo Chái Hú Tāng* F2-13 for fiery anger of the liver channel.
- Use *Jiā Wèi Sì Wù Tāng* F2-52 for heat of the blood division.
- Use *Bǔ Zhōng Yì Qì Tāng* F2-5 for taxation that stirs up fire.
- Use *Rén shēn Yǎng Róng Tāng* F1-28 for blood deficiency of the spleen channel.
- Use *Liù Wèi Dì Huáng Wán* F2-16 for scant blood of the liver channel.
- Use *Bā Zhēn Tāng* F2-8 for qì deficiency and blood weakness.

蓋血生於脾土，故云脾統血 。凡血病當用苦甘之劑，以助其陽氣而生陰血，俱屬不足 。大凡肝脾血燥，四物為主；肝脾血弱，補中益氣為主；肝脾鬱結，歸脾湯為主；肝經怒火，加味逍遙為主 。

Since blood is engendered by spleen earth, we say that the spleen unites blood. Whenever there is blood-related pain, use bitter and sweet prescriptions to aid yáng qì and engender yīn blood; both aspects belong to insufficiency. Generally speaking:

6. Blood division: While Yè Tiānshì 葉天士 (1667-1746, *Qīng*) is given credit for developing the four divisions or four levels of warm disease (*wēn bìng* 溫病) theory, one can see he did not develop it in a vacuum. The four divisions are *wèi*, qì, *yíng*, and *xuè* ( 衛氣營血) . The blood division (*xuè fēn* 血分) is the final division and means that heat has entered the blood. Here, *blood division* also refers to heat in the blood, although it is not in the context of the four divisions – that was not developed until about two hundred years later.

7. The author gave the indications, ingredients, method of preparation, and mode of administration for most of the herbal formulas he mentioned. He put some formulas at the end of Volume 1 and others at the end of Volume 2.

- *Sì Wù Tāng* F2-51 governs blood dryness of the liver and spleen.
- *Bǔ Zhōng Yì Qì Tāng* F2-5 governs blood deficiency of the liver and spleen.
- *Guī Pí Tāng* F2-3 governs binding constraint of the liver and spleen.
- *Jiā Wèi Xiāo Yáo Sǎn* F2-1 governs fiery anger of the liver channel.

## 治驗（肝經怒火、風、熱，等症附）
## Treatment Experience (conditions such as fiery anger of the liver channel, wind, and heat are appended)

**1-1-1**一婦人內熱作渴，飲食少思，腹內近左初如雞卵，漸大四寸許，經水三月一至，肢體消瘦，齒頰似瘡，脈洪數而虛，左關尤甚；此肝脾鬱結之症。外貼阿魏膏，午前用補中益氣湯，午後以加味歸脾湯。兩月許，肝火少退，脾土少健，仍與前湯送六味地黃丸，午後又用逍遙散送歸脾丸。又月餘，日用蘆薈丸二服，空心以逍遙散下，日晡以歸脾湯下。喜其謹疾，調理年餘而愈。

A woman had internal heat that made her thirsty, with little thought of food and drink. There was [a lump] inside her abdomen on the left that was initially the size of a chicken egg and gradually enlarged to about four *cùn* (about twelve or thirteen centimeters). Her menstruation arrived once in three months. Her body became emaciated and her teeth and jaws looked like wounds. Her pulse was surging and rapid but deficient; the left guān was especially so. These were symptoms of binding constraint of the liver and spleen. Externally I applied *Ā Wèi Gāo* F1-18 [to the lump]. I used *Bǔ Zhōng Yì Qì Tāng* F2-5 before noon and *Jiā Wèi Guī Pí Tāng* F2-4 after noon. In about two months, the liver fire decreased and receded while her spleen earth became a little stronger. I had her swallow *Liù Wèi Dì Huáng Wán* F2-16 with the previous decoctions. After noon she also used *Xiāo Yáo Sǎn* F2-2 to swallow *Guī Pí Wán* F2-3.(8) Then for more than a month, she used two doses of *Lú Huì Wán* F1-19 per day, swallowed on an empty stomach with *Xiāo Yáo Sǎn* F2-2; at sunset she swallowed it with *Guī Pí Tāng* F2-3. Happily, she took care of her disease by attuning and rectifying herself for more than a year, so she recovered.

8. The traditional method for cooking is to boil *Xiāo Yáo Sǎn* F2-2 (a powder) in water. It is then strained and the liquid is swallowed. So even though it is named a powder (*sǎn*), it becomes a liquid and can be used to swallow pills.

**1-1-2**一婦人腹內一塊，不時上攻；或痛作聲，吞酸痞悶，月經不調，小便不利，二年餘矣。面色青黃相兼。余作肝脾氣滯，以六君子加芎、歸、柴胡、炒連、木香、吳茱各少許二劑，卻與歸脾湯下蘆薈丸。三月餘，肝脾和而諸症退，又與調中益氣加茯苓、丹皮，中氣健而經自調。

A woman had a lump inside her abdomen that would attack upward at no particular time; sometimes it was so painful it made her cry out. She had sour swallowing and *pǐ*-glomus[9] with oppression. Her menstruation was out of tune and her urination was inhibited. This went on for more than two years. Her complexion was *qīng*-green and yellow at the same time. I took this as qì stagnation of the liver and spleen and used two doses of *Liù Jūn Zǐ Tāng* F2-6 adding a little each of *chuān xiōng, dāng guī, chái hú,* stir-fried *huáng lián, mù xiāng,* and *wú zhū yú;* I further gave her *Lú Huì Wán* F1-19 to be swallowed with *Guī Pí Tāng* F2-3. After more than three months, her liver and spleen became harmonious and all the symptoms receded. I again gave her *Tiáo Zhōng Yì Qì Tāng* F1-21 adding *fú líng* and *mǔ dān pí;* her center qì strengthened and her menstruation attuned itself.

**1-1-3**一婦人發熱口乾，月經不調，兩腿無力，服祛風滲濕之劑，腿痛體倦，二膝浮腫，經事不通。余作肝脾腎三經血虛火燥症，名鶴膝風，用六味、八味二丸兼服，兩月形體漸健，飲食漸進，膝腫漸消，不半載而痊。

A woman had fever with dry mouth, her menstruation was out of tune, and both legs were feeble. She took a prescription to eliminate wind and percolate dampness, but her legs became painful and her body became tired. She developed superficial swelling of both knees and her menstruation did not flow. I took this as symptoms of blood deficiency with fire and dryness of the three channels: liver, spleen, and kidneys. This is named crane's knee wind (*hè xī fēng*). I had her take *Liù Wèi Wán* F2-16 and *Bā Wèi Wán* F2-17 at the same time. In two months her body gradually grew stronger, she gradually began eating and drinking again, and the swelling in her knees gradually dispersed. She recovered in less than half a year.

前症若脾腎虛寒，腿足軟痛；或足膝枯細，用八味丸。若飲食過多，腿足或臀內酸脹；或浮腫作痛，用補中益氣加茯苓、半夏主之。

9. *Pǐ*-glomus (痞) is a subjective feeling of fullness and obstruction in the abdomen or chest. Nothing is found upon palpation.

- If the above symptoms are due to deficient cold spleen and kidneys with weak painful legs and feet, or withered, thin feet and knees, use *Bā Wèi Wán* F2-17.
- If eating and drinking are excessive and there is aching and distention of the legs and feet or within the buttocks, or if superficial swelling causes pain, it is governed by *Bǔ Zhōng Yì Qì Tāng* F2-5 with the addition of *fú líng* and *bàn xià*.

**1-1-4**一婦人性沉靜，勤於女工，善怒，小腹內結一塊，或作痛，或痞悶，月經不調。恪服伐肝之劑，內熱寒熱，胸膈不利，飲食不甘，形體日瘦，牙齦蝕爛。此脾土不能生肺金，肺金不能生腎水，腎水不能生肝木，當滋化源，用補中益氣、六味地黃，至仲春而愈。

A woman's temperament was deep and quiet; she was diligent in her needlework but tended to get angry. The inside of her lower abdomen was bound up with a lump that was sometimes painful; sometimes there was *pǐ*-glomus with oppression. Her menstruation was out of tune. She scrupulously took prescriptions to attack the liver, and then developed internal heat, [sensations of] cold and heat, and inhibited chest and diaphragm. Her food and drink did not taste sweet, her body became thinner day by day, and her teeth were eroded and rotten. This was inability of spleen earth to engender lung metal. Lung metal was unable to engender kidney water and kidney water was unable to engender liver wood. She should nourish and transform the source so I used *Bǔ Zhōng Yì Qì Tāng* F2-5 and *Liù Wèi Dì Huáng Wán* F2-16. She recovered by the middle month of spring.

**1-1-5**松江太守何恭人，性善怒，腹聚一塊，年餘，形體骨立，倏熱往來，腭蝕透腮。或泥春旺木剋土，仍行伐肝。時季冬，肝脈洪數，按之弦緊，餘脈微弱。余曰：洪數弦緊，肝經真氣虛而邪氣實也，自保不及，何能剋土?況面色青中隱白，乃腎水不足，肝木虧損，肺金剋制，惟慮至春木不能發生耳。勉用壯脾胃滋腎水之劑，肝脈悉退。後大怒，耳內出血，肝脈仍大，按之如無，煩躁作渴。此無根之火，以前藥加肉桂二劑，肝脈仍斂，熱渴頓退。復因大怒，以致飲食不進，果卒於季冬辛巳日。此木衰弱而金刑剋，信夫。

Mr. Hé was the prefect of Sōngjiāng [near Shànghǎi]. His wife had an irascible temperament. A lump gathered in her abdomen for over a year and she became skin and bones.

Sudden fevers came and went and her palate eroded through to the cheek. Perhaps stubborn wood was at peak strength in spring and controlled earth,[10] so [her doctors] repeatedly acted to chop down the liver. During the last month of winter,[11] her liver pulse was surging and rapid but bowstring and tight when pressed. The rest of her pulses were faint and weak. I said: Surging, rapid, bowstring, and tight means true qì of the liver channel is deficient, but evil qì is excessive. [The liver's] self-protection was inadequate; how could it control earth? Moreover her facial color had white hidden within *qīng*-green, so kidney water was insufficient and liver wood was feeble, while lung metal controlled and restrained them. My sole worry was that wood would be unable to expand and engender until spring arrived. We did our best using prescriptions to strengthen the spleen-stomach and to enrich kidney water; the liver pulse completely receded. Later she became quite angry and blood came out of her ears. The liver pulse was still large, but it felt like nothing was there when pressed. Vexation and agitation made her thirsty. This was unrooted fire. I used two doses of the previous herbs adding *ròu guì*. The liver pulse was then reigned in and the heat and thirst immediately receded. She relapsed again due to strong anger. The result was that she could not eat or drink so she died during the last month of winter on a *xīn sì* day.[12] This was debilitated wood with metal punishing and controlling it. Believe it!

**1-1-6**一婦人經候過期，發熱倦怠；或用四物、黃連之類，反兩月一度，且少而成塊；又用峻藥通之，兩目如帛所蔽。余曰:脾為諸陰之首，目為血脈之宗，此脾傷五臟，皆為失所，不能歸於目矣。遂用補中益氣、《濟生》歸脾二湯，專主脾胃，年餘尋愈。

A woman had late menstruation with fever and fatigue. She sometimes used medicine such as *Sì Wù Tāng* F2-51 with *huáng lián*, but contrary to expectations she had one period in two months; furthermore the quantity was scant and there were clots. Then she used drastic herbs to make it flow. Both eyes looked like they were covered with silk. I said: The spleen is the leader of all yīn and the eyes are the ancestor of the blood vessels. This is spleen damage with all five *zàng*-organs becoming homeless and unable to return

10. Her tendency toward anger made the wood element so strong that its assault on earth (the mouth and the flesh) eroded the palate through to the cheek.
11. The last month of each season belongs to earth element.
12. *Xīn sì* day 辛巳日: *Xīn* is the heavenly stem associated with yīn metal. *Sì* is the earthly branch associated with yīn fire. The metal of *xīn* controlled wood of liver while the fire of *sì* burned the wood of liver. Since she was extremely ill and weak, the elemental nature of this day did not let her pass through.

[nourishment] to the eyes.[13] I then used two decoctions, *Bǔ Zhōng Yì Qì Tāng* F2-5 and *Jì Shēng Guī Pí Tāng* F2-3. I focused on governing the spleen and stomach and she recovered after more than a year.

**1-1-7**一婦人兩眉棱痛，後及太陽，面青喜怒。余作膽經風熱，用選奇湯合逍遙散，加山梔、天麻、黃耆、半夏、黃芩而愈。此症失治，多致傷目，或兩耳，出膿則危矣。

A woman had pain at the ridge of her eyebrows that later reached Tài Yáng. Her face was *qīng*-green and she tended to get angry. I took this as wind heat of the gallbladder channel and used *Xuǎn Qí Tāng* F2-69 combined with *Xiāo Yáo Sǎn* F2-2 adding *zhī zǐ*,[14] *tiān má, huáng qí, bàn xià,* and *huáng qín*. She recovered. If the treatment for this condition is missed, it often causes damage to the eyes or ears; it is dangerous when pus comes out.

**1-1-8**一婦人耳鳴內熱，經行不調，肢體倦怠，飲食無味。余以為肝脾虛熱，用四君加柴胡、山梔、丹皮、甘草而愈。

A woman had tinnitus with internal heat and her menstruation moved out of tune. Her body was fatigued and food had no flavor. I took this as deficiency heat of the liver and spleen and used *Sì Jūn Zǐ Tāng* F2-26 plus *chái hú, zhī zǐ, mǔ dān pí,* and *gān cǎo*. She recovered.

**1-1-9**一婦人素勤苦，冬初患咳嗽發熱，久而吐血盜汗，經水兩三月一至，遍身作痛。或用化痰降火，口噤筋攣，謂余曰:何也?余曰:此血虛而藥益損耳。遂用加減八味丸及補中益氣加麥門、五味、山藥治之，年餘而痊。

13. Since the spleen makes post-heaven qì, when it is deficient, the other organs do not receive nourishment. While the eyes correspond to the liver according to five element theory, all five *zàng*-organs have a relationship with them. The spleen corresponds to the eyelids, the heart to the canthii, the lungs to the whites (sclera), the liver to the iris, and the kidneys to the pupils. In this case, the author thought that because the spleen was deficient, each of the organs was unable to take care of its corresponding region of the eyes.

14. The author used the name *shān zhī* 山梔, but most English readers are more familiar with *zhī zǐ* 梔子. Both refer to the same herb. I have used the more familiar terms in the English text for a number of herbs. For example, the author wrote *dān pí* 丹皮 but I changed it to *mǔ dān pí* 牡丹皮. I did not make these changes in the Chinese characters.

A woman was habitually hard-working. At the beginning of winter she suffered cough and fever. After a long time she began coughing up blood and had night sweating. Her menstrual periods arrived once in two or three months and her entire body was painful. Someone used herbs to transform phlegm and descend fire but then she got lockjaw and spasms of the sinews. They asked me why. I said: This is blood deficiency and those herbs increased the harm. I then treated her using *Jiā Jiǎn Bā Wèi Wán* F2-18 and *Bǔ Zhōng Yì Qì Tāng* F2-5 adding *mài mén dōng, wǔ wèi zǐ,* and *shān yào*. She recovered after more than a year.

**1-1-10**一婦人耳內或耳後項側作痛，寒熱口苦，月經不調。余以為肝火氣滯而血凝，用小柴胡加山梔、川芎、丹皮治之，諸症悉退。

A woman had pain inside her ear or sometimes behind her ear on the side of her nape, with [sensations of] cold and heat and bitter mouth. Her menstruation was out of tune. I took this as liver fire with qì stagnation and congealed blood. I treated her using *Xiǎo Chái Hú Tāng* F2-12 adding *zhī zǐ, chuān xiōng,* and *mǔ dān pí*. All of her symptoms receded.

**1-1-11**一婦人年四十，素性急，先因飲食難化，月經不調，服理氣化痰藥，反肚腹膨脹，大便泄瀉；又加烏藥、蓬朮，肚腹腫脹，小便不利；加豬苓、澤瀉，痰喘氣急，手足厥冷，頭面肢體腫脹，指按成窟，脈沉細，右寸為甚。余曰:此脾肺之氣虛寒，不能通調水道，下輸膀胱，滲泄之令不行，生化之氣不運。即東垣所云:水飲留積，若土之在雨中，則為泥矣；得和風暖日，水濕去而陽化自然，萬物生長。喜其脈相應，遂與《金匱》加減腎氣丸料服之，小便即通，數劑腫脹消半，四肢漸溫，自能轉側；又與六君加木香、肉桂、炮薑，治之痊愈。後不戒七情飲食，即為泄瀉，仍用前藥，加附子五分而安。

A forty year old woman was impatient by temperament. At first, because she had difficulty transforming food and drink and her menstruation was out of tune, she took herbs to rectify qì and transform phlegm. Contrary to expectations, her belly became inflated and distended, and she got diarrhea. Then *wū yào* and *péng zhú* were added to her formula but her belly became swollen and distended, and her urination was inhibited. They added *zhū líng* and *zé xiè*, which resulted in phlegm panting, rapid breathing, and reversal cold of the hands and feet. Her head, face, limbs, and body became swollen and distended; pressing with a finger left a cavity. Her pulse was sunken and fine, extremely so in the right *cùn*. I said: This is deficiency cold of spleen and lung qì with inability to regulate the waterways and transport [fluids] downward to the urinary bladder. It does not allow the movement of percolating and discharging [fluids through the urine], qì is not transporting [fluids] to engender and transform them. This is what Lǐ Dōngyuán meant when he said[15]: Watery rheum lingers and accumulates; if earth is out in the rain, it becomes muddy; if it can catch a gentle breeze on a warm day, water and damp are removed and yáng spontaneously transforms; the ten-thousand things will engender and grow. I was pleased that the pulses corresponded. I then gave her a batch of *Jīn Guì Jiā Jiǎn Shèn Qì Wán* F2-17 to take. Her urine flowed freely so after several doses, the swelling and distention dispersed by half, her four limbs gradually warmed up, and she was able to move about on her own. I next treated her with *Liù Jūn Zǐ Tāng* F2-6 adding *mù xiāng, ròu guì,* and *pào jiāng* and she completely recovered. Later she did not avoid the seven emotions and [regulate her intake of] food and drink, so she developed diarrhea. I used the same herbs as before adding five *fēn* (1.85 grams) of *fù zǐ* and she become peaceful.

**1-1-12**一婦人飲食每用碗許，稍加，非大便不實，必吞酸噯腐。或以為胃火，用二陳、黃連、枳實，加內熱作嘔。余曰:此未傳寒中，故噯氣吞酸，脹滿痞悶。不信，仍作火治虛症，並至月經不止，始信。余以六君加炮薑、木香數劑，元氣漸復，飲食漸進。又以補中益氣加炮薑、木香、茯苓、半夏，數劑痊愈。後因飲食勞倦，兼之怒氣，飲食頓少，元氣頓怯，用前藥更加發熱，誠似實火，脈洪大，按之而虛，兩尺如無。此命門火衰，用補中益氣加薑、桂及八味丸，兼服兩月餘，諸症悉愈。

A woman could only ingest about a bowlful each of food and drink; if she ate a little more, she had unformed stool, sour swallowing, and rotten belching. Someone took this as stomach fire and used *Èr Chén Tāng* F2-42 with *huáng lián* and *zhǐ shí*. This increased internal heat and made her vomit. I said: This is not transmission of cold strike, thus there is belching, sour swallowing, distention, fullness, and *pǐ*-glomus with oppression. They did not believe me and still took it as fire in their treatment of this deficiency condition. Eventually, her menstrual period would not stop, so they began to believe me. I used several doses of *Liù Jūn Zǐ Tāng* F2-6 adding *pào jiāng* and *mù xiāng*; her original qì gradually returned. She gradually began eating and drinking again. I then used several doses of *Bǔ Zhōng Yì Qì Tāng* F2-5 adding *pào jiāng, mù xiāng, fú líng,* and *bàn xià,* and she completely recovered. Later due to [indiscretions of] food and drink, taxation fatigue,

15. The source of this quotation is elusive.

and furthermore anger, her eating and drinking suddenly decreased and her original qì suddenly started shrinking. I used the previous herbs but they further increased the fever. It indeed seemed like excess fire. The pulse was surging and large, but it was deficient when pressed, and both *chǐ* felt like nothing was there. This was debility of mìng mén fire. I used *Bǔ Zhōng Yì Qì Tāng* F2-5 adding ginger and cinnamon, as well as *Bā Wèi Wán* F2-17. They were taken together for more than two months. All her symptoms completely recovered.

此症若因中氣虛弱者，用人參理中湯或六君子加木香、炮薑；不應，用左金丸，或越鞠丸；虛寒者，加附子，或附子理中湯，無有不愈。

If these sympromﾠs are due to deficient weak central qì, use *Rén shēn Lǐ Zhōng Tāng* F2-24 or *Liù Jūn Zǐ Tāng* F2-6 adding *mù xiāng* and *pào jiāng*.

- If she does not respond, use *Zuǒ Jīn Wán* F1-3 or *Yuè Jū Wán* F1-2;
- For deficiency coldness, add *fù zǐ* or use *Fù Zǐ Lǐ Zhōng Tān* F2-25.

No one will fail to recover.

**1-1-13**一婦人素有頭暈，不時而作，月經遲而少。余以為中氣虛，不能上升而頭暈，不能下化而經少，用補中益氣湯而愈。後因勞而仆，月經如湧，此勞傷火動，用前湯加五味子一劑，服之即愈。前症雖云亡血過多，氣無所附，實因脾氣虧損耳。

A woman was often dizzy; it came on at no particular time. Her menstrual period came late and was scant. I took this as central qì deficiency with inability to ascend leading to dizziness, and inability to descend and transform leading to scant menstrual periods. I used *Bǔ Zhōng Yì Qì Tāng* F2-5 and she recovered. Later, she collapsed [fell down] due to taxation and her menstruation gushed out; this was taxation damage with fire stirring. I used a dose of the previous decoction adding *wǔ wèi zǐ*; she took it and then recovered. Although the above pattern was said to be collapse of blood with excessive bleeding, qì had nowhere to attach itself. In reality it was due to debility of spleen qì.

**1-1-14**一婦人年四十，勞則足跟熱痛。余以為陰血虛極，急用聖愈湯而痊。後遍身瘙癢，誤服風藥，發熱抽搐，肝脈洪數。此乃肝家血虛火盛而生風。以天竺、膽星為丸，用四物、麥門、五味、芩、連、炙草、山梔、柴胡，煎送而愈。

When a forty year old woman was taxed, her heels became hot and painful. I took this as extreme yīn and blood deficiency. I quickly used *Shèng Yù Tāng* F1-11 and she recovered. Later when she had itching of her entire body, she mistakenly took herbs for wind and developed fever and convulsions; her liver pulse was surging and rapid. This was the blood deficiency of the liver household with fire flourishing so wind was generated. I made pills of tiān zhú and dǎn xīng, and boiled *Sì Wù Tāng* F2-51 with *mài mén dōng, wǔ wèi zǐ, huáng qín, huáng lián, zhì gān cǎo, zhī zǐ,* and *chái hú.* She [used the decoction] to swallow [the pills] and recovered.

**1-1-15**一婦人兩足發熱，日晡益甚，小便自遺，或時不利。余以為肝熱陰挺，不能約制。午前用白朮、茯苓、丹皮、澤瀉各五分，乾山藥、山茱、麥門各一錢，熟地四錢，酒炒黑黄柏七分，知母五分，不數劑而諸症悉愈。若用分利之劑，愈損真陰，必致不起。

Both feet of a woman felt feverish; this increased a lot at sunset with spontaneous incontinence of urine, or sometimes urination was inhibited. I took this as liver heat with vaginal protrusion with inability [of the vagina] to stay within its bounds. Before noon she used five *fēn* (1.85 grams) each of *bái zhú, fú líng, mǔ dān pí,* and *zé xiè*; one *qián* (3.73 grams) each of dried *shān yào, shān zhū yú,* and *mài mén dōng*; four *qián* (14.92 grams) of *shú dì huáng*; seven *fēn* (2.59 grams) of *huáng bǎi* which was liquor-fried until black; and five *fēn* (1.85 grams) of *zhī mǔ*. She had not taken many doses when all the symptoms completely recovered. If I had used prescriptions to divide and disinhibit [urination], there would be more harm to true yīn and this would cause her to die.

**1-1-16**一婦人月事未期而至，發熱自汗，服清熱止汗之劑，反作渴頭痛，手掉身麻。此因肝經風熱，用柴胡、炒芩連、炒山梔、歸、芍、生地、丹皮各一錢，參、耆、苓、朮各一錢五分，川芎七分，甘草五分，二劑其汗全止，更以補中益氣而愈。凡發熱久者，陽氣亦自病，須調補之。

A woman's menstrual period arrived when it was not the time, with fever and spontaneous sweating. She took a prescription to clear heat and stop sweating, but contrary to expectations it gave her thirst and headache. Her hands shook and her body become numb. This was due to wind heat in the liver channel. I used two doses of the following: one *qián* (3.73 grams) each of *chái hú,* stir-fried *huáng qín* and *huáng lián,* stir-fried *zhī zǐ, dāng guī, sháo yào, shēng dì huáng,* and *mǔ dān pí*; 1.5 *qián* (5.6 grams) each of *rén shēn, huáng qí, fú líng,* and *bái zhú;* seven *fēn* (2.59 grams) of *chuān xiōng;* and five *fēn* (1.85 grams) of *gān cǎo.* The sweating completely stopped. I further used *Bǔ Zhōng Yì Qì Tāng* F2-5 and she recovered. Whenever there is fever for a long time, yáng qì also automatically becomes diseased, so you must attune and supplement it.

**1-1-17**一婦人經行後，勞役失調，忽然昏憒，面赤吐痰。此元氣虛火妄動，急飲童便，神思漸爽；更用參、耆各五錢，芎、歸各三錢，玄參、柴胡、山梔、炙草各一錢，一劑；又用逍遙散加五味、麥門，稍定。但體倦面黃，此脾土真虛之色也，又以十全大補加五味、麥門，治之而愈。若投以發散之劑，禍在反掌，慎之。

After a woman's menstruation flowed, she became taxed and imbalanced, and she suddenly became muddleheaded. Her face was red and she spit out phlegm. This was original qì deficiency with reckless stirring of fire. I quickly had her drink child's urine[16] and her mental state gradually brightened. I further used one dose of five *qián* (18.65 grams) each of *rén shēn* and *huáng qí;* three *qián* (11.19 grams) each of *chuān xiōng* and *dāng guī;* and one *qián* (3.73 grams) each of *xuán shēn, chái hú, zhī zǐ,* and *zhì gān cǎo.* In another treatment I used *Xiāo Yáo Sǎn* F2-2 adding *wǔ wèi zǐ* and *mài mén dōng,* and she stabilized a little. However her body was tired and her face was yellow; this color showed true [qì] deficiency of spleen earth. Then I treated her with *Shí Quán Dà Bǔ Tāng* F2-7 adding *wǔ wèi zǐ* and *mài mén dōng* and she recovered. If I had given her dispersing prescriptions, misfortune would come as easily as flipping over one's hand; be careful of this.

**1-1-18**西賓錢思習子室年三十，尚無嗣，月經淋瀝無期，夫婦異處者幾年矣，思習欲為娶妾，以謀諸餘。余曰：此鬱怒傷肝，脾虛火動，而血不歸經，乃肝不能藏，脾不能攝也，當清肝火，補脾氣。遂與加味歸脾、逍遙二藥四劑，送至其家，仍告其姑曰：服此病自愈，而當受胎，妾可無娶也。果病愈，次年生子。

The wife of Private Tutor Qián Sīxí was thirty years old but they still had no heir. Her periods trickled at no particular time. Husband and wife dwelled separately for several years [he was a live-in tutor] and Sīxí wanted to take on a concubine, planning all the de-

16. Child's urine (*tóng biàn* 童便): This is the urine of a boy who is ten years old or younger. The best is the first urine of the day taken in the morning of the day before the full moon. It is salty and cold in nature. Child's urine nourishes yīn, descends fire, cools blood, and scatters stasis. In the past it was used to treat cough, vomiting blood, nosebleeds, postpartum dizziness, and so forth.

tails. I said, "This is constrained anger damaging the liver with spleen deficiency and fire stirring. Blood cannot return to its channels; it is inability of the liver to store and inability of the spleen to contain. We should clear liver fire and supplement spleen qì." Then I gave four doses of two formulas, *Jiā Wèi Guī Pí Tāng* F2-4 and *Xiāo Yáo Sǎn* F2-2. He took them home and explained to the wife saying, "If you take them, the disease will recover on its own and you should become pregnant. Then I won't need to take on a concubine." Consequently the disease recovered and the next year she gave birth to a son.

**1-1-19**一婦人多怒，經行或數日，或半月即止，三年後淋瀝無期，肌體倦瘦，口乾內熱，盜汗如洗，日晡熱甚。余用參、耆、歸、朮、茯神、遠志、棗仁、麥門、五味、丹皮、龍眼肉、炙草、柴胡、升麻，治之獲痊。此症先因怒動肝火，血熱妄行，後乃脾氣下陷，不能攝血歸源，故用前藥。

A woman had a lot of anger. When menstruation moved, it might last several days or half a month before it stopped. After three years it trickled at irregular times. Her muscles and body were tired and thin. She had dry mouth, internal heat, night sweating as if she had taken a bath, and high fever at sunset. I treated it with *rén shēn, huáng qí, dāng guī, bái zhú, fú shén, yuǎn zhì, suān zǎo rén, mài mén dōng, wǔ wèi zǐ, mǔ dān pí, long yǎn ròu, zhì gān cǎo, chái hú,* and *shēng má* and she was able to recover. This disease was first due to anger stirring up liver fire with reckless movement of hot blood; later it was spleen qì sinking downward with inability to contain the blood and return it to the source, so I used the above herbs.

若胃熱亡津液，而經不行，宜清胃；若心火亢甚者，宜清心；若服燥藥過多者，宜養血；若病久氣血衰，宜健脾胃。

- If stomach heat makes *jīnyè*-fluids collapse and menstruation does not move, it is appropriate to clear heat from the stomach.
- If heart fire is extremely hyperactive, it is appropriate to clear heat from the heart.
- If someone takes too many drying herbs, it is appropriate to nourish blood.
- If the disease lasts a long time and qì and blood are debilitated, it is appropriate to strengthen the spleen and stomach.

**1-1-20**一婦人年五十，內熱晡熱，經水兩三月一來，此血虛而有熱。用逍遙散加山茱治之而愈。

A fifty year old woman suffered internal heat with late afternoon fever; her menstrual flow came once in two or three months. This was blood deficiency with heat. I treated her with *Xiāo Yáo Sǎn* F2-2 adding *shān zhū yú* and she recovered.

若兼有痰作渴；或小便不調；或頭暈白帶，宜用腎氣丸。

- If phlegm made thirst at the same time, or urination was out of tune, or if there was dizziness with white vaginal discharge, it is appropriate to use *Shèn Qì Wán* F2-17.

**1-1-21**一婦人氣血素虛，經行不調，飲食少思，日晡熱甚。用十全大補加山茱、山藥、丹皮、麥門、五味而愈。次年秋患寒熱，或用清脾飲，而元氣愈弱。余仍以前藥而愈。

A woman usually had qì and blood deficiency and her menstruation was out of tune. She had little thought of food and drink and had high fever at sunset. I used *Shí Quán Dà Bǔ Tāng* F2-7 adding *shān zhū yú, shān yào, mǔ dān pí, mài mén dōng,* and *wǔ wèi zǐ* and she recovered. In autumn of the next year she suffered [sensations of] cold and heat and someone used *Qīng pí Yǐn* UFx-1,[17] but her original qì became weaker. I still used the previous herbal medicine and she recovered.

**1-1-22**一婦人生七胎矣，月經不調，兩足發熱，年餘而身亦熱，勞則足酸痛。又年許，唇腫裂痛。又半年，唇裂見血，形體瘦倦，飲食無味，月水不通，唇下腫如黑棗。或用通經丸等藥而死。

A woman had given birth seven times; her menstruation was out of tune and both feet felt feverish. For more than a year, her body also felt hot. When she was taxed, her feet were achy and painful. Also for about a year, her lips were swollen, cracked, and painful. In addition, for a half a year, her cracked lips bled, her body became emaciated and tired,

17. Formula index numbers that begin with UF were not listed (unlisted) by the author in the formulas at the end of each volume. Some of these formulas he recommended for patients but for some reason they were not included. Those that begin with UFx were never used by the author in this book. In many cases he expressed his opinion that these were too drastic to use. There is an appendix with the information on these formulas.

food and drink had no flavor, her menstruation did not flow, and there was a swelling below her lips that looked like a black *zǎo*-date. Someone used herbs such as *Tōng Jīng Wán* UFx-2 and she died.

**1-1-23**一婦人善怒，經不調，唇腫裂，服消毒藥，唇脹出血，年餘矣。余曰：當培養脾胃，以滋化源。不信，仍服前藥，及追蝕狀如翻花瘤而死。

A woman with out of tune menstruation tended to be angry. Her lips were swollen and split. She took herbs to disperse toxins, but her lips became distended and bled. This went on for more than a year. I said: We should bank up and nourish the spleen and stomach by enriching and transforming the source. She did not believe me. She continued using the previous herbs until it eroded into a tumor that was shaped like an inverted flower,[18] and then she died.

**1-1-24**一膏粱之婦，產後月經不調，唇裂內熱；每焮作，服寒涼之劑。後不時出水。余用加味清胃散而愈。後值春令，兼怒，唇口腫脹，寒熱作嘔痰甚少食。用小柴胡加山梔、茯苓、桔梗，諸症頓愈。但內熱仍作，乃以加味逍遙散，調理而安。

After giving birth, a woman who was accustomed to eating rich food suffered menstruation that was out of tune. She had cracked lips and internal heat. Every time it flared up, she took cold and cooling prescriptions. Afterwards it discharged water at no particular time. I used *Jiā Wèi Qīng Wèi Sǎn* F2-11 and she recovered. Later she became angry during the spring. Her lips and mouth became swollen and distended, with [sensations of] cold and heat, vomiting a lot of phlegm, and eating little. I used *Xiǎo Chái Hú Tāng* F2-12 adding *zhī zǐ*, *fú líng*, and *jié gěng*. All her symptoms immediately recovered. However the internal heat was still there. I then used *Jiā Wèi Xiāo Yáo Sǎn* F2-1 to attune and rectify her and she became peaceful.

**1-1-25**一婦人性善怒，產後唇腫內熱，用清熱敗毒；唇口腫脹，日晡熱甚，月水不調，用降火化痰；食少作嘔，大便不實，唇出血水，用理氣消導；胸膈痞滿，頭目不清，唇腫經閉，用清胃行血；肢體倦怠，發熱煩躁，涎水湧出，欲用通經之劑。

18. The term inverted flower (*fān huā* 翻花) or reverse flower (*fān huā* 反花) is used for different abnormalities on the surface of the body such as sores, tumors, or hemorrhoids. They are fleshy growths that spread outward and appear in the shap of a flower.

A woman was irascible by temperament. After giving birth, her lips were swollen and she had internal heat so she used herbs to clear heat and conquer toxins. Her lips and mouth became swollen and distended, she had high fever at sunset, and her menstruation was out of tune. She used herbs to descend fire and transform phlegm but then she vomited whenever she ate a small amount, had unformed stool, and her lips bled and watered. She used herbs to rectify qì and disperse and lead out [food accumulations] but then she developed *pǐ*-glomus and fullness of her chest and diaphragm, her head and eyes were not clear, her lips were swollen, and her menstruation was blocked. She used herbs to clear heat from the stomach and move blood but then her limbs and body were weary, she had fever, vexation and agitation, and saliva gushed out. She was about to use a prescription to free menstruation.

余曰:病本七情，肝脾虧損，數行攻伐，元氣益虛故耳。法當補陰益陽，遂以加味歸脾湯、加味逍遙散、補中益氣湯;如法調治，元氣漸復，唇瘡亦愈。

I said: The root of the disease is the seven emotions. The liver and spleen are feeble since they have been attacked several times [with all the previous herbal medicine]. Original qì is increasingly deficient. The treatment method should be to supplement yīn and boost yáng. I then used *Jiā Wèi Guī Pí Tāng* F2-4, *Jiā Wèi Xiāo Yáo Sǎn* F2-1, and *Bǔ Zhōng Yì Qì Tāng* F2-5. This method attuned her and made order. Her original qì gradually returned and the sores on the lips also recovered.

後因怒，寒熱耳痛，胸膈脹悶，唇焮腫甚。此是怒動肝火而血傷，遂用四物合小柴胡加山梔頓愈。

Later due to anger, she had [sensations of] cold and heat, earache, and distention and oppression of the chest and diaphragm. Her lips flared up and became extremely swollen. This was anger stirring up liver fire with damage to blood. I then used *Sì Wù Tāng* F2-51 combined with *Xiǎo Chái Hú Tāng* F2-12 adding *zhī zǐ* and she immediately recovered.

後又怒，脅乳作脹，肚腹作痛，嘔吐酸涎，飲食不入，小水不利。此是怒動肝木剋脾土，乃用補脾氣、養脾血而愈。

Later she got angry again, with distended rib-sides and breasts, bellyache, vomiting sour saliva, not eating or drinking, and inhibited urination. This was anger stirring up liver wood to control spleen earth. I then used herbs to supplement spleen qì and nourish spleen blood and she recovered.

又因勞役怒氣，飲食失時，發熱喘渴，體倦不食，去血如崩，唇腫熾甚。此是肝經有火，脾經氣虛，遂用補中益氣加炒黑山梔、芍藥、丹皮而愈。此症每見，但治其瘡，不固其本，而死者多矣。

Again due to taxation and anger, and eating at the wrong times, she had fever, panting, thirst, and tired body. She did not eat and had bleeding that was like bēng-flooding. Her lips were swollen and blazing hot. This was fire of the liver channel and qì deficiency of the spleen channel. I then used *Bǔ Zhōng Yì Qì Tāng* F2-5 adding *zhī zǐ* that was stir-fried until black, *sháo yào*, and *mǔ dān pí*, and she recovered. In cases where this condition is seen, many will die if you simply treat the sores and do not secure the root.

## 《女科撮要·卷上·經漏不止》
## 1-2 Incessant Menstrual Spotting

經云:陰虛陽搏，謂之崩。又云:陽絡傷血外溢，陰絡傷血內溢。又云:脾統血，肝藏血；

The Classic says[19]: "When yīn is deficient and yáng wrestles with it, it is called *bēng*-flooding." It also says[20]: "When the yáng *luò*-networks are damaged, blood overflows on the outside; when the yīn *luò*-networks are damaged, blood overflows on the inside." It also says[21]: The spleen controls blood while the liver stores blood.

其為患：因脾胃虛損，不能攝血歸源；或因肝經有火，血得熱而下行；或因肝經有風，血得風而妄行；或因怒動肝火，血熱而沸騰；或因脾經鬱結，血傷而不歸經；或因悲哀太過，胞絡傷而下崩。

19. In *Sù Wèn*, Chapter 7.
20. In *Líng Shū*, Chapter 66.
21. "The spleen controls blood" is not found in *Sù Wèn* or *Líng Shū* although the concept may be stated using other words. "The liver stores blood" is found in *Sù Wèn*, Chapter 62 and *Líng Shū*, Chapter 8.

When these things lead to the disease [of spotting or flooding]:

- Inability to contain the blood and return it to the source is due to spleen and stomach deficiency.
- Or blood becomes hot and moves downward due to fire in the liver channel.
- Or blood receives wind and moves recklessly due to wind in the liver channel.
- Or blood becomes hot and boils over due to anger stirring up liver fire.
- Or blood is damaged and does not return to its channel due to binding constraint of the spleen channel.
- Or the uterine *luò*-networks (*bāo luò*) are damaged and flood downward due to excessive grief and sorrow.

治療之法:脾胃虛弱者，六君子湯加當歸、川芎、柴胡；脾胃虛陷者，補中益氣湯加酒炒芍藥、山梔；肝經血熱者，四物湯加柴胡、山梔、苓、朮；肝經怒火者，小柴胡湯加山梔、芍藥、丹皮；脾經鬱火者，歸脾湯加山梔、柴胡、丹皮；哀傷胞絡者，四君子湯加柴胡、升麻、山梔。

The treatment methods:

- For deficient weak spleen and stomach, use *Liù Jūn Zǐ Tāng* F2-6 adding *dāng guī, chuān xiōng,* and *chái hú.*
- For spleen and stomach deficiency with sinking, use *Bǔ Zhōng Yì Qì Tāng* F2-5 adding *sháo yào* that was stir-fried in liquor and *zhī zǐ.*
- For heat in the blood of the liver channel, use *Sì Wù Tāng* F2-51 adding *chái hú, zhī zǐ, fú líng,* and *bái zhú.*
- For fiery anger of the liver channel, use *Xiǎo Chái Hú Tāng* F2-12 adding *zhī zǐ, sháo yào,* and *mǔ dān pí.*
- For constrained fire of the spleen channel, use *Guī Pí Tāng* F2-3 adding *zhī zǐ, chái hú,* and *mǔ dān pí.*
- For grief damaging the uterine *luò*-networks (*bāo luò*), use *Sì Jūn Zǐ Tāng* F2-26 adding *chái hú, shēng má,* and *zhī zǐ.*

故東垣、丹溪諸先生云:凡下血症，須用四君子以收功，斯言厥有旨哉。若大吐血後，毋以脈診，當急用獨參湯救之。其發熱潮熱，咳嗽脈數，乃是元氣虛弱，假熱之脈也，尤當用人參之類。此等症候，無不由脾胃先損而患，故脈洪大，察其中有胃氣受補可救。設用寒涼之藥，復傷脾胃生氣，使血反不歸源也。

Thus both doctors, Lǐ Dōngyuán and Zhū Dānxī, said that whenever there is the symptom of bleeding below, you must use *Sì Jūn Zǐ Tāng* F2-26 to receive results. These words are significant. If it occurs after vomiting a lot of blood, do not [bother to take the time to] use pulse diagnosis; you should quickly use *Dú Shēn Tāng* F1-9 to rescue her. Her fevers, tidal fevers, cough, and rapid pulse are from deficient weak original qì; her pulse shows false heat. One should especially use herbs similar to *rén shēn*. The symptoms suffered in this kind of disease always come primarily from harm to the spleen and stomach, so when the pulse is surging and large, observe if there is stomach qì within it; if so, the patient can receive supplementation and can be rescued. If you use cold and cool herbs, you repeatedly damage [the ability of] the spleen and stomach to engender qì, and contrary to expectations, blood is not allowed to return to its source.

## 治驗（吐血等症附）
## Treatment Experience
## (patterns such as vomiting blood are appended)

**1-2-1**一婦人年將七十，素有肝脾之症，每作則飲食不進；或胸膈不利；或中脘作痛；或大便作瀉；或小便不利。余用逍遙散加山梔、茯神、遠志、木香而愈。後憂女孀居，不時吐紫血，每作先倦怠煩熱，以前藥加炒黑黃連三分，吳茱二分，頓愈。復因怒，吐赤血甚多，躁渴垂死。此血脫也，法當補氣，乃用人參一兩，苓、朮、當歸各三錢，陳皮、炮黑乾薑各二錢，炙草、木香各一錢，一劑頓止。信藥有回生之功，不可委於天命也。

A woman was about to turn seventy. She usually had liver and spleen symptoms; every time they occurred she could not eat and drink, or her chest and diaphragm would be inhibited, or Zhōng Wǎn [the region of Rèn 12] was painful, or she would get diarrhea, or she would have inhibited urination. I used *Xiāo Yáo Sǎn* F2-2 adding *zhī zǐ*, *fú shén*, *yuǎn zhì*, and *mù xiāng* and she recovered. Later she worried when her daughter became a widow. She vomited purple blood at no particular time; before each episode she was weary with vexation heat. I used the previous herbs adding three *fēn* (1.12 grams) of *huáng lián* that was stir-fried until black and two *fēn* (0.74 grams) of *wú zhū yú*, and she immediately recovered. She relapsed due to anger and vomited quite a lot of red blood. She was agitated and thirsty and was dying. This was blood desertion. The treatment method should be to supplement qì. I then used one *liǎng* (37.3 grams) of *rén shēn*; three *qián* (11.19 grams) each of *fú líng, bái zhú,* and *dāng guī*; two *qián* (7.46 grams) each of *chén pí* and *gān jiāng* that was blast-fried until black; and one *qián* (3.73 grams) each of *zhì gān cǎo* and *mù xiāng*. The vomiting immediately stopped after one dose. Trust that the medicine has the effect of returning life; one cannot have faith in fate (*tiān mìng*).

**1-2-2**一婦人年六十有四，久鬱怒，頭痛寒熱，春間乳內時痛，服流氣飲之類益甚，不時有血如經行。又大驚恐，飲食不進，夜寐不寧，乳腫及兩脅焮痛如炙，午後色赤。余以為肝脾鬱火血燥，先以逍遙散加酒炒黑龍膽一錢、山梔一錢五分，二劑腫痛頓退，又二劑而全消。再用歸脾加炒梔、貝母，諸症悉愈。

A sixty-four year old woman had constrained anger for a long time with headache and [sensations of] cold and heat. In spring she sometimes had pain inside of her breasts. She took herbs in the category of *Liú Qì Yǐn Zǐ* F1-29 but the symptoms increased a lot. She bled as if she were menstruating but at no particular time. She was also greatly frightened and did not eat or drink. Her sleep was not peaceful at night. Her breasts were swollen, both rib-sides flared up with pain as if they were roasting, and her complexion was red in the afternoons. I took this as constrained fire of the liver and spleen with blood dryness. I first used two doses of *Xiāo Yáo Sǎn* F2-2 adding one *qián* (3.73 grams) of *lóng dǎn cǎo* that was stir-fried with liquor until black and 1.5 *qián* (5.6 grams) of *zhī zǐ*; the swelling and pain immediately receded. After two more doses, it had completely dispersed. I then used *Guī Pí Tāng* F2-3 adding stir-fried *zhī zǐ* and *bèi mǔ*, and all her symptoms completely recovered.

**1-2-3**一婦人久患血崩，肢體消瘦，飲食到口但聞腥臊，口出津液，強食少許，腹中作脹。此血枯之症，肺肝脾胃虧損之患；用八珍湯、烏賊魚骨圓，兼服兩月而經行，百餘劑而康寧如舊矣。

A woman suffered bēng-flooding for a long time and her body became emaciated. When food and drink reached her mouth it smelled bad and *jīnyè*-fluids came out of her mouth; she had to force herself to eat a little and then she would have abdominal distention. These were symptoms of blood dryness with debility of the lungs, liver, spleen, and stomach. I used *Bā Zhēn Tāng* F2-8 and *Wū Zéi Yú Gǔ Yuán* F1-14. She took them together for two months and her menstruation flowed [properly]; after more than a hundred doses she was in good health like before.

**1-2-4**一婦人性躁急，瘰癧後吐血發熱，兩脅脹痛，日晡為甚。余以為怒氣傷肝，氣血俱虛，遂朝用逍遙散倍加炒黑山梔、黃柏、貝母、桔梗、麥門、五味，夕以歸脾湯送地黃丸，諸症並愈。

A woman's temperament was restless and impatient. After developing scrofula, she began vomiting blood, with fever and distending pain of both rib-sides. This became severe at sunset. I took it as anger damaging the liver and deficiency of both qì and blood. I then used *Xiāo Yáo Sǎn* F2-2 in the mornings adding double the *zhī zǐ* which was stir-fried until black, *huáng bǎi, bèi mǔ, jié gěng, mài mén dōng,* and *wǔ wèi zǐ*. In the evening she used *Guī Pí Tāng* F2-3 to swallow *Dì Huáng Wán* F2-16. All her symptoms equally recovered.

**1-2-5**一婦人素勤苦，因喪子飲食少思，忽吐血甚多而自止，此後每勞則吐數口，瘵症已具，形體甚倦，午前以補中益氣，午後以歸脾湯送地黃丸而愈。

A woman was usually hard-working. Because she mourned her child, she had little thought of food and drink. She suddenly vomited of a lot of blood and then it stopped without any intervention. After this, she vomited several mouthfuls every time she was taxed. After an episode of this disease, her body was extremely weary. I had her take *Bǔ Zhōng Yì Qì Tāng* F2-5 before noon; after noon she used *Guī Pí Tāng* F2-3 to swallow *Dì Huáng Wán* F2-16 and she recovered.

**1-2-6**一女子素鬱結，胸滿食少，吐血面赤，用地黃丸及歸脾加山梔、貝母、芍藥而愈。

A girl[22] usually had binding constraint with chest fullness, decreased food intake, vomiting blood, and red face. I used *Dì Huáng Wán* F2-16 along with *Guī Pí Tāng* F2-3 adding *zhī zǐ, bèi mǔ,* and *sháo yào,* and she recovered.

**1-2-7**一婦人面黃或赤，時覺腰間或臍下作痛，四肢困倦，煩熱不安，其經若行，先發寒熱，兩肋如束，其血如崩。此脾胃虧損，元氣下陷，與相火濕熱所致，用補中益氣加防風、芍藥、炒黑黃柏，間以歸脾湯調補化源，血自歸經矣。

22. It is likely that 'girl' here not only meant a younger female, but also that she was unmarried at the time.

The face of a woman was yellow or red. At times she felt pain around her waist or below her umbilicus. Her four limbs were tired, she had vexation heat, and was not peaceful. When her menstruation flowed, at first there were fever and chills, both ribs felt like they were bound up, and the bleeding was like *bēng*-flooding. This was caused by debility of the spleen and stomach, original qì sinking downward, and damp heat from minister fire. I used *Bǔ Zhōng Yì Qì Tāng* F2-5 adding *fáng fēng, sháo yào,* and *huáng bǎi* that was stir-fried until black. After an interval I used *Guī Pí Tāng* F2-3 to attune, supplement, and transform the source; her blood spontaneously returned to its channel.

**1-2-8**一婦人因怒崩血，久不已，面青黃而或赤，此肝木製脾土，而血虛也，用小柴胡合四物，以清肝火生肝血，又用歸脾、補中二湯，以益脾氣生肝血而瘥。

A woman was *bēng*-flooding due to anger. It didn't stop for a long time. Her face was *qīng*-green, yellow and sometimes red. This was liver wood controlling spleen earth with blood deficiency. I used *Xiǎo Chái Hú Tāng* F2-12 combined with *Sì Wù Tāng* F2-51 to clear liver fire and engender liver blood. I also used two decoctions, *Guī Pí Tāng* F2-3 and *Bǔ Zhōng Yì Qì Tāng* F2-5 to boost spleen qì and engender liver blood. She recovered.

此症若因肝經有風熱，而血不寧者，用防風一味為丸，以兼症之藥煎送；或肝經火動而血不寧者，用條芩炒為丸，以兼症之藥煎送，無有不效。

- If this disease is due to wind heat of the liver channel and blood is not peaceful, make *fáng fēng* alone into pills and swallow them with a compatible decoction for the disease.
- Or if fire stirs in the liver channel and blood is not peaceful, make stir-fried tiáo qín into pills and swallow them with with a compatible decoction for the disease.

This will never fail to be effective.

**1-2-9**一婦人性急，每怒非太陽、耳、項、喉、齒、胸、乳作痛，則胸滿吞酸，吐瀉少食，經行不止。此皆肝火之症，肝自病則外症見，土受剋則內症作。若自病見，用四物加白朮、茯苓、柴胡、炒梔、炒龍膽；若內症作，用四君加柴胡、芍藥、神曲、吳茱、炒過黃連，諸症漸愈。惟月經不止，是血分有熱，脾氣尚虛，以逍遙散倍用白朮、茯苓、陳皮，又以補中益氣加酒炒芍藥，兼服而調。

A woman was impatient by temperament. Every time she got angry, if she did not have pain in Tài Yáng, the ears, nape, throat, teeth, chest, and breasts, then she would have chest fullness, sour swallowing, vomiting, diarrhea, reduced food intake, and her menstruation would flow incessantly. These were all symptoms of liver fire. When the liver itself was sick, an external pattern was seen [pain in the regions listed above]; when earth received control, an internal pattern was made [the second set of symptoms listed]. When self-disease appeared,[23] I used *Sì Wù Tāng* F2-51 adding *bái zhú, fú líng, chái hú,* stir-fried *zhī zǐ,* and stir-fried *lóng dǎn cǎo.* If interior disease occurred, I used *Sì Jūn Zǐ Tāng* F2-26 adding *chái hú, sháo yào, shén qū, wú zhū yú,* and thoroughly stir-fried *huáng lián.* All patterns gradually recovered. Only her menstruation did not stop; this was heat in the blood division and spleen qì was still deficient. I used *Xiāo Yáo Sǎn* F2-2 adding double *bái zhú, fú líng,* and *chén pí.* I then used *Bǔ Zhōng Yì Qì Tāng* F2-5 adding *sháo yào* that was stir-fried in liquor. She took both at the same time and became attuned.

**1-2-10**乾內錢氏，年五十歲，辛丑患崩，諸藥罔效；壬寅八月，身熱肢痛，頭暈涕出，吐痰少食。眾作火治，轉熾絕粒，數日淹淹伏枕，僅存呼吸。兄方浙歸診之，謂脾胃虛寒，用八味丸料一劑，使急煎服。然胃虛久，始下咽，翌早遂索粥數匙。再劑，食倍，熱減痛止，兼服八味丸良愈。

In the *xīn chǒu* year [1541] when Fāng Qián's wife, nee Qián, was fifty years old[24] she suffered bēng-flooding; various medicines were ineffective. In the eighth lunar month of *rén yín* [1542], she felt feverish, with painful limbs, dizziness, running nose, spitting phlegm, and reduced food intake. The common doctors treated this as fire, but it began blazing.

23. Self-disease: In other words, in the liver alone. Liver fire made the liver sick. This case also mentions the liver making the spleen sick, which would not be self-disease.
24. This case, the next one, and 1-12-14 are letters from the husbands of patients expressing gratitude to Xuē Jǐ for his medical care. This first one is from a brother (or perhaps a cousin) of Xuē Jǐ whose wife was ill. She was treated by Xuē. In the first line, the brother refers to himself in the third person. There are a few other testimonials like this throughout the book.

She totally stopped eating and for several days she simply lay on her pillow doing nothing more than breathing. My older brother [Xuē Jǐ] had just returned to Zhèjiāng and he examined her. He said it was deficiency cold of the spleen and stomach and quickly boiled the ingredients of one dose of *Bā Wèi Wán* F2-17 and had her take it. Although her stomach deficiency had lasted for a long time, she began to swallow the medicine and the next morning she demanded several spoonfuls of rice porridge. She had another dose and then ate twice as much. The fever decreased and the pain stopped. She continued to take *Bā Wèi Wán* F2-17 and recovered quite a bit.

癸卯秋，因勞役憂怒，甲辰春夏崩復作，六月二十日，胸飽發熱，脊痛，腰不可轉，神氣怫鬱；或作內傷；或作中暑，崩水沸騰，兼以便血，煩渴引飲，粒米不進，至七月十三日，晝夜暈憒，時作時止，計無所出。仍屈兄診之，脈洪無倫，按之微弱，此無根之火，內真寒而外假熱也。以十全大補加附子一劑，暈止，食粥三四匙，崩血漸減，日服八味丸，始得痊愈。

Due to taxation, worry, and anger during autumn of the *guǐ mǎo* [1543] year, her *bēng*-flooding relapsed in the spring and summer of the *jiǎ chén* year [1544]. On the twentieth day of the sixth lunar month, she suffered chest fullness as if she had eaten too much, fever, pain of the spine, inability to turn at the waist, and the qì of her *shén*-spirit was anxious and depressed. Perhaps it was internal damage or perhaps it was summerheat stroke. She had *bēng*-flooding like water boiling over and at the same time blood in the stool. She suffered vexation thirst and the desire to drink, but she would not swallow even one grain of rice. This lasted until the thirteenth day of the seventh month. She was dizzy and muddleheaded off and on, day and night. We were unable to think of a way [to help her]. She again yielded to my older brother examining her. Her pulse was surging and lacked coherence, but fine and weak when pressed. This was unrooted fire; the inside had true cold and the outside had false heat. He used one dose of *Shí Quán Dà Bǔ Tāng* F2-7 adding *fù zǐ* and the dizziness stopped. She ate three or four spoonfuls of porridge and the flooding of blood gradually decreased. Every day she took *Bā Wèi Wán* F2-17 and she began to obtain complete recovery.

乾山妻兩構危疾，命懸須臾，荷兄遠救，誠解倒懸之急。處方神良，知無出此。野人懷恩，姑俟後日玉環之報云爾。

My wife twice suffered a dangerous disease. Her fate was suspended for a while. I am grateful to my older brother who came from afar to save her. He indeed resolved her urgent and severe suffering. His prescriptions have magical benefits; no knowledge can surpass his. I cherish his kindness, so we will wait for the future when Yùhuán [the wife] can repay him.

嘉靖甲辰季秋表弟方乾頓首拜書

In the last month of autumn of the *jiă chén* year of Jiājìng's reign [1544], younger brother of a different surname, Fāng Qián, bows and respectfully writes this

**1-2-11**大化內患月事不期，崩血昏憒，發熱不寐。或謂血熱妄行，投以寒劑益甚；或謂胎成受傷，投以止血，亦不效，乃敬延先生診之。曰:此脾氣虛弱，無以統攝故耳，法當補脾，而血自止矣。用補中益氣加炮薑，不數劑而驗。惟終夜少睡驚悸，另服八物湯，更不效。叩諸先生，曰雜矣。乃與歸脾湯加炮薑以補心脾，遂如初。謹敘其梗概以附醫案，俾後之患者，得有所取法云。

I am Guī Dàhuà; my wife suffered menstruation that was out of tune with flooding of blood. She was muddleheaded and had fever and insomnia. Someone said it was heat in the blood with reckless movement and gave her a cold prescription but it increased a lot. Someone said it was injury to the fetus during pregnancy and gave her herbs to stop bleeding but this was also ineffective. Then I respectfully sent for the doctor (Xuē Jǐ) to examine her. He said: This is deficient weak spleen qì that is unable to control [the blood]. The method should be to supplement the spleen and then the bleeding will spontaneously stop. He used *Bŭ Zhōng Yì Qì* F2-5 adding *pào jiāng*. It was effective after not many doses. Only reduced sleep for the whole night and fright palpitations remained, so another [doctor] gave her *Bā Wù Tāng*[25] but it was still ineffective. I asked [Xuē Jǐ] about the various doctors and he said: [Their treatments were] random.[26] We then gave her *Guī Pí Tāng* F2-3 adding *pào jiāng* to supplement the heart and spleen, and then she was like before [all this happened]. I carefully recount the broad outline and append it to the medical cases so that the sufferers who come later have a model to follow.

嘉靖甲辰孟冬晚生歸大化頓首拜書

In the first month of winter of the *jiă chén* year of Jiājìng's reign [1544], Guī Dàhuà bows and respectfully writes this

25. *Bā Wù Tāng* is another name for *Bā Zhēn Tāng* F2-8 or possibly *Fù Zĭ Bā Wù Tāng* F2-77.

26. The treatments of other doctors were inconsistent and not appropriate, according to Xuē Jĭ.

# 《女科撮要·卷上·經閉不行》
## 1-3 Immovable Menstrual Block

夫經水陰血也，屬衝任二脈，主上為乳汁，下為月水 。其為患：

Menstrual water is yīn blood. It belongs to both the *chōng* and *rèn* vessels which govern milk above and menstrual fluids below. When these things lead to the disease [of menstrual block]:

有因脾虛而不能生血者；有因脾鬱傷而血耗損者；有因胃火而血消爍者；有因脾胃損而血少者；有因勞傷心而血少者；有因怒傷肝而血少者；有因腎水不能生肝而血少者；有因肺氣虛不能行血而閉者 。

- There are cases due to spleen deficiency with inability to engender blood.
- There are cases due to constraint damaging the spleen and consuming the blood.
- There are cases due to stomach fire dispersing and searing the blood.
- There are cases due to harm to the spleen and stomach decreasing the blood.
- There are cases due to taxation damaging the heart and decreasing the blood.
- There are cases due to anger damaging the liver and decreasing the blood.
- There are cases due to inability of kidney water to engender the liver decreasing the blood.
- There are cases due to lung qì deficiency with inability to move blood causing the block.

治療之法:若脾虛而不行者，調而補之；脾鬱而不行者，解而補之；胃火而不行者，清而補之；脾胃損而不行者，調而補之；勞傷心血而不行者，靜而補之；怒傷肝而不行者，和而補之；肺氣虛而不行者，補脾胃；腎虛而不行者，補脾肺 。

The treatment method:
- If the spleen is deficient and there is no movement [of menstruation], attune and supplement.
- If the spleen is constrained and there is no movement, resolve and supplement.

- If there is stomach fire and no movement, clear and supplement.
- If the spleen and stomach are harmed and there is no movement, attune and supplement.
- If taxation damages heart blood and there is no movement, quiet and supplement.
- If anger damages the liver and there is no movement, harmonize and supplement.
- If there is lung qì deficiency and no movement, supplement the spleen and stomach.
- If there is kidney deficiency and no movement, supplement the spleen and lungs.

經云：損其肺者益其氣，損其心者調其榮衛，損其脾者調其飲食，適其寒溫，損其肝者緩其中，損其腎者益其精。審而治之，庶無誤矣。

The Classic says[27]: "For harm to the lungs, boost the patient's qì; for harm to the heart, attune the patient's *yíng* and wèi; for harm to the spleen, attune the patient's food and drink and make the cold-heat [balance] appropriate; for harm to the liver, relax the patient's center; for harm to the kidneys, boost the patient's *jīng*-essence." If you examine this and treat according to it, you will not make mistakes.

## 治驗
## Treatment Experience

**1-3-1**一婦人停食，飽悶發熱，或用人參養胃湯益甚；再用木香檳榔丸，泄瀉吐痰，腹中成塊，飲食少思；又用二陳、黃連、濃樸之類，前症益甚，腹脹不食，月經不至。余以為中氣虧損，用補中益氣加茯苓、半夏，三十餘劑，脾胃健而諸症愈；又二十餘劑，而經自行。

A woman had food retention and oppression when she ate too much, with fever. She sometimes used *Rén Shēn Yǎng Wèi Tāng* F2-73 but the symptoms increased a lot. She also used *Mù Xiāng Bīng Láng Wán* UFx-3, but she got diarrhea and vomited phlegm. She developed a lump in her abdomen and had little thought of food and drink. She then used

27. In *Nán Jīng*, Difficulty 14《十四難》.

*Èr Chén Tāng* F2-42 adding *huáng lián, nóng pǔ*[28] and the like, but the previous symptoms increased a lot. She had abdominal distention, did not eat, and her menstrual period did not arrive. I took this as enfeebled central qì and used more than thirty doses of *Bǔ Zhōng Yì Qì Tāng* F2-5 adding *fú líng* and *bàn xià*. Her spleen and stomach grew stronger and all her symptoms recovered. Her menstruation moved on its own again after I gave her another twenty-plus doses.

前症若脾虛不能消化飲食者，宜用六君子湯，補而消之；虛寒者，加砂仁、木香、炮薑，溫而補之；其食積成形者，以前藥煎送保和丸。大抵食積痞塊，症為有形，所謂邪氣勝則實，真氣奪則虛，惟當養正辟邪，而積自除矣。雖然堅者削之，客者除之，胃氣未虛，或可少用；若病久虛乏者，則不宜用。

For the above symptoms:

- If there is spleen deficiency with inability to disperse and transform food and drink, it is appropriate to use *Liù Jūn Zǐ Tāng* F2-6 to supplement and disperse.
    - For deficiency cold, add *shā rén, mù xiāng,* and *pào jiāng* to warm and supplement.
    - If the food accumulation becomes substantial, boil the above herbs and use them to swallow *Bǎo Hé Wán* F1-1.

Generally speaking, with food accumulations and *pǐ*-glomus lumps, the pattern is substantial; this is what is called 'there is excess when the evil qì is victorious; there is deficiency when true qì is captured.' One should only nourish the right and ward off evils, and then the accumulation will eliminate itself. One can 'pare away what is hard and eliminate the guest' when stomach qì is not deficient; perhaps we can use this infrequently. However, if disease has lasted a long time and there is deficiency, it is not appropriate to use this.

**1-3-2**一婦人飲食後，或腹脹，或吞酸，服枳朮丸，吞酸益甚，飲食日少，胸膈痞滿，腿內酸痛，畏見風寒；又服養胃湯一劑，腿內作痛；又二劑，腿浮腫，月經不行。余以為鬱結所傷，脾虛濕熱下注，侵晨用四君、芎、歸、二陳，午後以前湯送越鞠丸，飲食漸進，諸症漸愈。又用歸脾、八珍二湯，兼服兩月餘而經行。

28. *Nóng pǔ* 濃樸 is an alternate name for *hòu pǔ* 厚朴.

After eating and drinking a woman sometimes had abdominal distention or sour swallowing. She took *Zhǐ Zhú Wán* [UFx-4], but the sour swallowing increased a lot. Every day her eating and drinking decreased. She also suffered *pǐ*-glomus and fullness of the chest and diaphragm and achy pain on the inside of her legs. She feared the appearance of wind and cold. She then took one dose of *Yǎng Wèi Tāng* [F2-73] and the inside of her legs became painful. She took two more doses, and then her legs developed superficial swelling and her menstruation did not move. I took this as damage from binding constraint and spleen deficiency with damp heat pouring downward. Toward dawn I used *Sì Jūn Zǐ Tāng* [F2-26] with *chuān xiōng, dāng guī,* and *Èr Chén Tāng* [F2-42]. After noon she used the above decoctions to swallow *Yuè Jū Wán* [F1-2]. She gradually began eating and drinking and all symptoms gradually recovered. I then used both *Guī Pí Tāng* [F2-3] and *Bā Zhēn Tāng* [F2-8]. She took them together for more than two months and her menstruation moved.

**1-3-3**一婦人性沉多慮，月經不行，胸滿少食，或作脹，或吞酸。余以為中氣虛寒，用補中益氣加砂仁、香附、煨薑二劑，胸膈和而飲食進；更以六君加芎、歸、貝母、桔梗、生薑、大棗數劑，脾胃健而經自調矣。

A woman was serious by temperament and worried a lot. Her menstruation did not move. She had chest fullness, decreased food intake, sometimes distention, and sometimes sour swallowing. I took this as deficient cold central qì and used two doses of *Bǔ Zhōng Yì Qì Tāng* [F2-5] adding *shā rén, xiāng fù,* and *wēi jiāng*. Her chest and diaphragm became harmonious and she began eating and drinking again. I further used several doses of *Liù Jūn Zǐ Tāng* [F2-6] adding *chuān xiōng, dāng guī, bèi mǔ, jié gěng, shēng jiāng,* and *dà zǎo*. Her spleen and stomach grew stronger and her menstruation attuned itself.

**1-3-4**一婦人素有胃火，服清胃散而安。後因勞役，躁渴內熱，肌肉消瘦，月經不行。此胃火消爍陰血，用逍遙散加丹皮、炒梔，以清胃熱；用八珍湯加茯苓、遠志，以養脾血，而經自行矣。

A woman usually had stomach fire. She took *Qīng Wèi Sǎn* [F2-10] and became peaceful. Later due to taxation, she had agitation, thirst, and internal heat. Her muscles and flesh became emaciated and menstruation did not move. This was stomach fire dispersing and searing yīn blood. I used *Xiāo Yáo Sǎn* [F2-2] adding *mǔ dān pí* and stir-fried *zhī zǐ* to clear stomach heat. I used *Bā Zhēn Tāng* [F2-8] adding *fú líng* and *yuǎn zhì* to nourish spleen blood and her menstruation moved by itself.

**1-3-5**一婦人久患瘧，形體怯弱，內熱晡熱，自汗盜汗，飲食少思，月事不行，服通經丸，虛症悉具。此因虛而致瘧疾，因瘧而致經閉，用補中益氣及六味地黃丸，各百餘劑，瘧愈而經自行。

A woman suffered *nüè*-malaria for a long time. Her body was physically weak, with internal heat, late afternoon fever, spontaneous sweating, night sweating, and little thought of food and drink. Her menstruation did not move so she took *Tōng Jīng Wán* UFx-2, and then deficiency symptoms manifested all over. This deficiency led to [more episodes of] *nüè*-malarial disease and the *nüè*-malaria led to menstrual block. I used more than a hundred doses each of *Bǔ Zhōng Yì Qì Tāng* F2-5 and *Liù Wèi Dì Huáng Wán* F2-16. The *nüè*-malaria recovered and her menstruation moved by itself.

**1-3-6**一婦人久患瘧，瘧作則經不行，形虛脈大，頭痛懶食，大便泄瀉，小便淋漓，口乾唇裂，內熱腹膨。皆元氣下陷，相火合病，用補中益氣湯治之尋愈。惟不時頭痛，乃加蔓荊子而痛止。又兼用六味地黃丸而經行。

A woman suffered *nüè*-malaria for a long time. During episodes of *nüè*-malaria, menstruation did not move. Her physical form was deficient but her pulse was large. She suffered headaches, lazy eating, diarrhea, dribbling urination, dry mouth, cracked lips, internal heat, and inflated abdomen. All this was a combination disease of original qì sinking downward and minister fire [flaring upward]. I used *Bǔ Zhōng Yì Qì Tāng* F2-5 to treat her and she recovered soon after. Only headaches that occurred at no particular time remained so I then added *màn jīng zǐ* and the pain stopped. Then I used *Liù Wèi Dì Huáng Wán* F2-16 at the same time and her menstruation moved.

**1-3-7**一婦人因勞，耳鳴頭痛體倦，此元氣不足，用補中益氣加麥門、五味而痊。三年後得子，因飲食勞倦，前症益甚，月經不行，晡熱內熱，自汗盜汗，用六味地黃丸、補中益氣湯頓愈。

Due to taxation, a woman had tinnitus, headaches, and weariness of the body. This was insufficient original qì. I used *Bǔ Zhōng Yì Qì Tāng* F2-5 adding *mài mén dōng* and *wǔ wèi zǐ* and she recovered. Three years later she had a son. Due to [inappropriate] food and drink and taxation fatigue, the previous pattern increased a lot. Her menstruation did not move, and she had late afternoon fever, internal heat, spontaneous sweating, and night sweating. I used *Liù Wèi Dì Huáng Wán* F2-16 and *Bǔ Zhōng Yì Qì Tāng* F2-5 and she immediately recovered.

前症若因血虛有火，用四物加山梔、柴胡；不應，八珍加前藥。若氣虛弱，用四君子。若怒耳便聾或鳴者，實也小柴胡加芎、歸、山梔；虛用補中益氣加山梔。若午前甚作火，治用小柴胡加炒連、炒梔；氣虛用補中益氣。午後甚作血虛，用四物加白朮、茯苓。若陰虛火動；或兼痰甚作渴，必用地黃丸以壯水之主。

For the above symptoms:

- If they are due to blood deficiency with fire, use *Sì Wù Tāng* F2-51 adding *zhī zǐ* and *chái hú*.
    - If she does not respond, use *Bā Zhēn Tāng* F2-8 adding the above herbs.
- If there is deficient weak qì, use *Sì Jūn Zǐ Tāng* F2-26.
- When anger makes deafness or ringing in the ears:
    - If it is due to excess; use *Xiǎo Chái Hú Tāng* F2-12 adding *chuān xiōng, dāng guī*, and *zhī zǐ*.
    - For deficiency use *Bǔ Zhōng Yì Qì* F2-5 adding *zhī zǐ*.
- If the symptoms are severe before noon and become fire, treat with *Xiǎo Chái Hú Tāng* F2-12 adding stir-fried *huáng lián* and stir-fried *zhī zǐ*.
    - For qì deficiency use *Bǔ Zhōng Yì Qì Tāng* F2-5.
- If it is severe in the afternoon and it becomes blood deficiency, use *Sì Wù Tāng* F2-51 adding *bái zhú* and *fú líng*.
- If it is due yīn deficiency with fire stirring, or if there is a lot of phlegm making thirst at the same time, you must use *Dì Huáng Wán* F2-16 to invigorate the governor of water.

經云：頭痛耳鳴，九竅不利，腸胃之所生也。脾胃一虛，耳目九竅皆為之病。

The Classic[29] says: "With headaches and ringing in the ears, the nine orifices are inhibited; this is engendered by the intestines and stomach." When the spleen and stomach are both deficient, the ears, eyes, and nine orifices all become ill.

**1-3-8**一婦人胃氣素弱，為哭母吐血咳嗽，發熱盜汗，經水三月不行。余以為悲則傷肺，思則傷脾，遂朝服補中益氣加桔梗、貝母、知母，夕用歸脾湯送地黃丸而愈。

29. *Sù Wèn*, Chapter 28.

A woman usually had weak stomach qì. Because of crying for her mother she vomited blood, and had cough, fever, and night sweating. Her menstruation did not move for three months. I took this as grief damaging the lungs and as thought damaging the spleen. Then she took *Bǔ Zhōng Yì Qì Tāng* F2-5 adding *jié gěng, bèi mǔ,* and *zhī mǔ* in the mornings; she used *Guī Pí Tāng* F2-3 to swallow *Dì Huáng Wán* F2-16 in the evenings and she recovered.

## 《女科撮要·卷上·帶下》
## 1-4 Abnormal Vaginal Discharge (*dài xià*)

或因六淫七情；或因醉飽房勞；或因膏粱濃味；或服燥劑所致，脾胃虧損，陽氣下陷；或濕痰下注，蘊積而成，故言帶也。

This may be due to the six excesses [external evils] and seven emotions; or due to drunkenness, overeating, or bedroom taxation; or due to rich food with concentrated flavors; or caused by taking drying prescriptions. These lead to debility of the spleen and stomach with yáng qì sinking downward or lead to dampness and phlegm pouring downward. They accumulate and become this, so it is said to be *discharge.*[30]

凡此皆當壯脾胃、升陽氣為主，佐以各經見症之藥。若屬肝則青，小柴胡加山梔；或濕熱壅滯，小便赤澀，龍膽瀉肝湯；屬心則赤，小柴胡加黃連、山梔、當歸；屬肺則白，補中益氣加山梔；屬脾則黃，六君子加山梔、柴胡，不應，歸脾湯；屬腎則黑，六味地黃丸；若氣血俱虛，八珍湯；陽氣下陷，補中益氣湯；濕痰下注，前湯加茯苓、半夏、蒼朮、黃柏；氣虛痰飲下注，四七湯送腎氣丸。

Whenever it occurs, all instances should be governed by invigorating the spleen and stomach and ascending yáng qì. Use assisting herbs for each channel where a pattern appears.

30. *Dài* 帶 literally means a belt or girdle. It is the name of one of the eight extraordinary vessels – the one that goes around the waist like a belt. *Dài* is also used in the term *dài xià* 帶下. This can refer to women's diseases in a general sense (diseases below the belt), but usually refers specifically to abnormal vaginal discharge. *Dài* can be an apreviation for *dài xià* as seems to be the case here.

- If it belongs to the liver, the discharge is *qīng*-green; use *Xiǎo Chái Hú Tāng* F2-12 adding *zhī zǐ*.
- If it is damp heat obstructing and stagnating with rough red urine, use *Lóng Dǎn Xiè Gān Tāng* F1-13.
- If it belongs to the heart, it is red; use *Xiǎo Chái Hú Tāng* F2-12 adding *huáng lián, zhī zǐ*, and *dāng guī*.
- If it belongs to the lungs, it is white; use *Bǔ Zhōng Yì Qì Tāng* F2-5 adding *zhī zǐ*.
- If it belongs to the spleen, it is yellow; use *Liù Jūn Zǐ Tāng* F2-6 adding *zhī zǐ* and *chái hú*.
    - If she does not respond, use *Guī Pí Tāng* F2-3.
- If it belongs to the kidneys, it is black; use *Liù Wèi Dì Huáng Wán* F2-16.
- If it is deficiency of both qì and blood, use *Bā Zhēn Tāng* F2-8.
- If it is yáng qì sinking downward, use *Bǔ Zhōng Yì Qì Tāng* F2-5.
- If it is dampness and phlegm pouring downward, use the previous formula adding *fú líng, bàn xià, cāng zhú*, and *huáng bǎi*.
- If it is qì deficiency with phlegm-rheum pouring downward, swallow *Shèn Qì Wán* F2-17 with *Sì Qī Tāng* F1-16.

## 治驗
## Treatment Experience

**1-4-1** 一婦人年逾六十，內熱口乾，勞則頭暈，吐痰帶下。或用化痰行氣，前症益甚，飲食愈少，肢體或麻，恪服祛風化痰，肢體常麻，手足或冷或熱，日漸消瘦。余曰：症屬脾氣虛弱而不能生肺，祛風之劑，復損諸經也，當滋化源。遂用補中益氣加茯苓、半夏、炮薑，二十餘劑，脾氣漸復，飲食漸加，諸症頓愈。

A woman who was more than sixty years old had internal heat with dry mouth. When taxed, she had dizziness, spit phlegm, and had abnormal vaginal discharge. Sometimes she used herbs to transform phlegm and move qì but the previous symptoms increased a lot, while her eating and drinking decreased and her body was sometimes numb. She diligently took herbs to dispel wind and transform phlegm, but her body became numb all the time, her hands and feet were sometimes cold and sometimes hot, and she gradually became more emaciated each day. I said: "Her symptoms belong to deficient weak spleen qì that is unable to engender the lungs. The prescription to dispel wind again harmed the various channels. We should enrich and transform the source." I then used more than twenty doses of *Bǔ Zhōng Yì Qì Tāng* F2-5 adding *fú líng, bàn xià,* and *pào jiāng.* Her spleen qì gradually returned, eating and drinking gradually increased, and all the symptoms immediately recovered.

**1-4-2** 一孀婦腹脹脅痛，內熱晡熱，月經不調，肢體酸麻，不時吐痰。或用清氣化痰，喉間不利，帶下青黃，腹脅膨脹；用行氣之劑，胸膈不利，肢體時麻。此鬱怒傷損肝脾，前藥益甚也。朝用歸脾湯以解脾鬱生脾氣，夕用加味逍遙散以生肝血清肝火，兼服百餘劑，而諸症愈。

A widow had abdominal distention, rib-side pain, internal heat, late afternoon fever, menstruation that was out of tune, aching and numbness of her body, and she spit phlegm at no particular time. Perhaps she used herbs to clear qì and transform phlegm, but then she suffered inhibited throat, *qīng*-green and yellow vaginal discharge, inflated abdomen and distended rib-sides. She used prescriptions to move qì, but her chest and diaphragm became inhibited and sometimes her body was numb. This was constrained anger damaging the liver and spleen. The previous herbs increased it a lot. In the mornings I used *Guī Pí Tāng* F2-3 to resolve constraint of the spleen and engender spleen qì; in the evenings I used *Jiā Wèi Xiāo Yáo Sǎn* F2-1 to engender liver blood and clear liver fire. She took more than a hundred doses of both concurrently and all her symptoms recovered.

**1-4-3** 一婦人瘧久，兼之帶下，發後口乾倦甚。余用七味白朮散加麥門、五味，作大劑，煎與恣飲，再發稍可，乃用補中益氣加茯苓、半夏，十餘劑而愈。

A woman suffered *nüè*-malaria at the same time as abnormal vaginal discharge. After episodes, she had dry mouth and weariness of the body. I used *Qī Wèi Bái Zhú Sǎn* F2-68 adding *mài mén dōng* and *wǔ wèi zǐ*; a large dose was boiled for her to drink at will. She relapsed but it was slightly better. I then used more than ten doses of *Bǔ Zhōng Yì Qì Tāng* F2-5 adding *fú líng* and *bàn xià,* and she recovered.

凡截瘧，余常以參、朮各一兩，生薑四兩，煨熟煎服即止；或以大劑補中益氣加煨薑，其功尤捷。

Whenever interrupting *nüè*-malaria, I normally use one *liǎng* (37.3 grams) each of *rén shēn* and *bái zhú*, and four *liǎng* (149.2 grams) of *shēng jiāng* that is roasted until cooked. The *nüè*-malaria stops when these are boiled and taken. Sometimes I use a large dose of *Bǔ Zhōng Yì Qì Tāng* F2-5 adding *wēi jiāng*; the results are especially quick.

**1-4-4** 一婦人頭暈唾痰，胸滿氣喘，得食稍緩，苦於白帶，二十餘年矣，諸藥不應。余曰：此氣虛而痰飲也，飲愈而帶始愈。遂用六味地黄丸，不月而驗。

A woman had dizziness and was spitting phlegm, with chest fullness and panting. When she ate, it moderated a little. She suffered from white discharge for more than twenty years. Various herbs had no response. I said: This is qì deficiency and phlegm-rheum.[31] The rheum recovered and the discharge began to recover. I then used *Liù Wèi Dì Huáng Wán* F2-16; it was effective in less than a month.

**1-4-5**一婦人耳鳴胸痞，內熱口乾，喉中若有一核，吞吐不利，月經不調，兼之帶下。余以為肝脾鬱結，用歸脾湯加半夏、山梔、升麻、柴胡，間以四七湯下白丸子而愈。

A woman had tinnitus, chest *pǐ*-glomus, internal heat, and dry mouth. She felt something like a pit in her throat that inhibited her ability to swallow or spit. Her menstruation was out of tune at the same time as her abnormal vaginal discharge. I took this as binding constraint of the liver and spleen. I used *Guī Pí Tāng* F2-3 adding *bàn xià, zhī zǐ, shēng má,* and *chái hú*. Between doses she used *Sì Qī Tāng* F1-16 to swallow *Bái Wán Zǐ* F1-15. She recovered.

**1-4-6** 一婦人吞酸胸滿，食少便泄，月經不調，服法制清氣化痰丸，兩膝漸腫，寒熱往來，帶下黄白，面黄體倦。余以為脾胃虛，濕熱下注，用補中益氣，倍用參、朮加茯苓、半夏、炮薑而愈。

A woman had sour swallowing, chest fullness, decreased food intake, diarrhea, and her menstruation was out of tune. She took *Fǎ Zhì Qīng Qì Huà Tán Wán* UFx-5. Both knees gradually swelled and she had alternating fever and chills, yellow and white vaginal

31. There seems to be a prescription missing here. However, looking in various editions, no missing words were found.

discharge, yellow face, and weariness of the body. I took this as spleen and stomach deficiency with damp heat pouring downward. I used *Bŭ Zhōng Yì Qì Tāng* F2-5, doubling the *rén shēn* and *bái zhú* and adding *fú líng, bàn xià,* and *pào jiāng*. She recovered.

若因怒，發熱少食，或兩腿赤腫，或指縫常濕，用六君加柴胡、升麻及補中益氣。

If it is due to anger, with fever and reduced food intake, and perhaps both legs are red and swollen or the crevices of the toes are constantly damp, use *Liù Jūn Zĭ Tāng* F2-6 adding *chái hú* and *shēng má* as well as *Bŭ Zhōng Yì Qì Tāng* F2-5.

**1-4-7**一婦人帶下，四肢無力，勞則倦怠。余曰：四肢者土也，此屬脾胃虛弱，濕痰下注，遂以補中益氣、《濟生》歸脾二藥治之，而愈。

A woman had abnormal vaginal discharge. Her four limbs were feeble. When taxed she was weary. I said: The four limbs are earth; this belongs to deficient weak spleen and stomach with phlegm damp pouring downward. I then used two medicines to treat her, *Bŭ Zhōng Yì Qì Tāng* F2-5 and *Jì Shēng Guī Pí Tāng* F2-3, and she recovered.

**1-4-8**一婦人年逾六十，帶下黃白，因怒胸膈不利，飲食少思。服消導利氣之藥，反痰喘胸滿，大便下血。余曰：此脾氣虧損，不能攝血歸源也。用補中益氣加茯苓、半夏、炮薑，四劑，諸症頓愈，又用八珍加柴胡、炒梔而安。

A woman who was more than sixty years of age had yellow and white vaginal discharge. Due to anger, her chest and diaphragm were inhibited with little thought of food and drink. She took herbs to disperse, lead out, and disinhibit qì, but contrary to expectations she developed phlegm panting, chest fullness, and blood in the stool. I said: This is enfeebled spleen qì with inability to contain the blood and return it to the source. I used four doses of *Bŭ Zhōng Yì Qì Tāng* F2-5 adding *fú líng, bàn xià,* and *pào jiāng,* and the various symptoms immediately recovered. Then I used *Bā Zhēn Tāng* F2-8 adding *chái hú* and stir-fried *zhī zĭ* and she was peaceful.

## 《女科撮要·卷上·血分水分》

## 1-5 Blood Division and Water Division (*xuè fēn shuǐ fèn*)[32]

二症或因飲食起居失養；或因六淫七情失宜，以致脾胃虧損，不能生發統攝，氣血乖違，行失常道。

These two conditions are due to loss of nourishment from food and drink or rising and dwelling [lifestyle]; or they are due to inappropriateness of the six excesses [external evils] and seven emotions. The result is enfeebled spleen and stomach with inability to engender and control [blood and fluids]; qì and blood separate and move in abnormal pathways.

若先因經水斷絕，後至四肢浮腫，小便不通，血化為水，名曰血分，宜用椒仁丸治之。若先小便不利，後至身面浮腫，經水不通，水化為血，名曰水分，宜用葶藶丸治之。

- If the menstrual flow is severed first and later she develops superficial swelling of the four limbs with obstruction of urine, blood has transformed into water; this is called *blood division*. It is appropriate to treat this with *Jiāo Rén Wán* F1-4.
- If urination is inhibited first and later she develops superficial swelling of body and face with obstruction of menstrual fluids, water has transformed into blood; this is called *water division*. It is appropriate to treat it with *Tíng Lì Wán* F1-5.

此屬形氣不足，邪淫隧道，必用此藥以宣導其邪，而佐以輔補元氣，庶使藥力有所仗而行，則邪自不能容，而真氣亦不至於復傷矣。

These conditions belong to insufficiency of the physical-body and qì with evil excesses tunneling through the pathways. You must use these herbs [mentioned above] to dredge out the evils and assist with herbs to support supplementation of original qì. When the supplementation gives the herbal power [of the formula] something to rely on, it can act; the evils automatically will not be tolerated and true qì will not sustain repeated damage.

32. These two conditions are not commonly discussed. They both involve edema and amenorrhea occurring together. In blood division, amenorrhea develops first; in water division, edema occurs first.

# 治驗
## Treatment Experience

**1-5-1**一婦人月經不調，晡熱內熱，飲食少思，肌體消瘦，小便頻數，服濟陰丸，月經不行，四肢浮腫，小便不通。余曰：此血分也。朝用椒仁丸，夕用歸脾湯漸愈，乃以人參丸代椒仁丸，兩月餘將愈。專用歸脾湯，五十餘劑而痊。

A woman whose menstruation was out of tune had late afternoon fever, internal heat, and little thought of food and drink. Her body became emaciated and she urinated frequently. She took *Jì Yīn Wán* UFx-6 but her menstruation did not move. She developed superficial swelling of the four limbs and urine did not pass. I said: This is the blood division. In the mornings I used *Jiāo Rén Wán* F1-4 and in the evenings I used *Guī Pí Tāng* F2-3. She gradually recovered. I then replaced *Jiāo Rén Wán* F1-4 with *Rén Shēn Wán* F1-6 for more than two months and she recovered. I next focused on *Guī Pí Tāng* F2-3 for more than fifty doses and she recuperated.

**1-5-2**一癧婦月經不調，小便短少；或用清熱分利之劑，小便不利，三月餘身面浮腫，月經不通。余曰：此水分也。遂朝用葶藶丸，夕用歸脾湯漸愈，乃用人參丸間服而愈。

The menstruation of a woman with scrofula was out of tune and she had short scant urination. Sometimes she used heat-clearing prescriptions to divide and disinhibit urination but it was still inhibited. After more than three months she developed superficial swelling of her body and face and her menstruation did not flow. I said: This is the water division. I then used *Tíng Lì Wán* F1-5 in the mornings and *Guī Pí Tāng* F2-3 in the evenings. She began to recover. I then used *Rén Shēn Wán* F1-6 between doses and she recovered.

已上二症，作脾虛水氣，用分利等藥而歿者多矣。惜哉!

For the above two conditions, take them as spleen deficiency with water qì. If you use herbs such as those to divide and disinhibit urination, many will die. What a pity!

# 《女科撮要·卷上·小便出血》
## 1-6 Blood in the Urine

婦人小便尿血；或因膏粱炙煿；或因醉飽入房；或因飲食勞役；或因六淫七情，以致元氣虧損，不能統攝歸源。

For women with blood in the urine, some cases are due to rich food that was roasted and broiled; or due to drunkenness, overeating, and entering the bedroom [sex]; or due to [inadequate] food and drink and taxation, or due to the six excesses [external evils] and seven emotions. These result in enfeebled original qì with inability to control [blood] and return it to its source.

若因怒動肝火者，用加味逍遙散調送髮灰；肝經風熱者，送子芩丸；久而血虛者，用八珍送髮灰。若膏粱積熱者，用清胃散加槐花、甘草；房勞所傷者，用六君加柴胡、升麻；風熱所傷者，用四君加防風、枳殼。凡久而虧損元氣者，用補中益氣為主；鬱結傷脾者，用《濟生》歸脾為主。

- If it is due to anger stirring up liver fire, mix *Jiā Wèi Xiāo Yáo Sǎn* F2-1 with *fà huī* [ash of head-hair] and swallow it.
- For wind heat of the liver channel, swallow *Zǐ qín Wán* UF-1.
- If it has lasted a long time and there is blood deficiency, use *Bā Zhēn Tāng* F2-8 to swallow *fà huī.*
- If rich food has accumulated heat, use *Qīng Wèi Sǎn* F2-10 adding *huái huā* and *gān cǎo.*
- If damaged by bedroom taxation, use *Liù Jūn Zǐ Tāng* F2-6 adding *chái hú* and *shēng má.*
- If damaged by wind heat, use *Sì Jūn Zǐ Tāng* F2-26 adding *fáng fēng* and *zhǐ qiào.*
- Whenever it has lasted a long time with enfeebled original qì, *Bǔ Zhōng Yì Qì Tāng* F2-5 is indicated.
- When binding constraint damages the spleen, *Jì Shēng Guī Pí Tāng* F2-3 is indicated.

## 治驗
## Treatment Experience

**1-6-1**一婦人尿血，因怒氣寒熱，或頭痛，或脅脹，用加味逍遙，諸症稍愈。惟頭痛，此陽氣虛，用補中益氣加蔓荊子而痊。後鬱怒，小腹內疞痛，次日尿血熱甚，仍用前散加龍膽草並歸脾湯，將愈，因飲食所傷，血仍作，徹夜不寐，心忡不寧，此脾血尚虛，用前湯而痊。

A woman had blood in her urine due to anger, with [sensations of] cold and heat and occasional headaches or rib-side distention. I used *Jiā Wèi Xiāo Yáo Sǎn* F2-1 and all the symptoms decreased somewhat. Only the headaches remained; this was yáng qì deficiency. I used *Bǔ Zhōng Yì Qì Tāng* F2-5 adding *màn jīng zǐ* and she recuperated. Later constrained anger led to colicky pain within the lower abdomen. The next day she had blood in the urine and a lot of heat. I still used the previous powder [*Jiā Wèi Xiāo Yáo Sǎn* F2-1] adding *lóng dǎn cǎo* and used *Guī Pí Tāng* F2-3 at the same time. She was on the verge of recovery. Then she started bleeding again due to damage from food and drink. She did not sleep for the whole night; her heart was fearful and not peaceful. Spleen blood was still deficient. I used the previous decoction [*Bǔ Zhōng Yì Qì Tāng* F2-5] and she recuperated.

**1-6-2**一婦人尿血，久用寒涼止血藥，面色痿黃，肢體倦怠，飲食不甘，晡熱作渴三年矣。此前藥復傷脾胃，元氣下陷而不能攝血也。蓋病久鬱結傷脾，用補中益氣以補元氣，用歸脾湯以解脾鬱，使血歸經。更用加味逍遙以調養肝血，不月諸症漸愈，三月而痊。

A woman had blood in her urine; for a long time she used cold and cool herbs to stop bleeding. For three years her face was withered yellow, her body weary, food and drink did not taste sweet, and late afternoon fever made her thirsty. This was due to the herbs she had taken repeatedly damaging the spleen and stomach, so original qì sank downward and was unable to contain blood. When disease lasts for a long time, it seems that binding constraint must damage the spleen. I used *Bǔ Zhōng Yì Qì Tāng* F2-5 to supplement original qì; I used *Guī Pí Tāng* F2-3 to resolve spleen constraint and make the blood return to its channel. I further used *Jiā Wèi Xiāo Yáo Sǎn* F2-1 to attune and nourish liver blood. All the symptoms gradually recovered in less than a month. She recuperated fully in three months.

# 《女科撮要·卷上·熱入血室》
# 1-7 Heat Entering the Blood Chamber

婦人傷寒；或勞役；或怒氣發熱，適遇經行，以致熱入血室；或血不行；或血不止，令人晝則明了安靜，夜則譫語如見鬼狀，用小柴胡加生地黃；血虛者，用四物加生地、柴胡。切不可犯胃氣。若病既愈而血未止；或熱未已，元氣素弱，用補中益氣；脾氣素鬱，用《濟生》歸脾；血氣素弱，用十全大補，庶無誤矣。

If women have fever from cold damage, or taxation, or anger during their menstrual period, the result is that heat can enter the blood chamber. Sometimes blood does not move and sometimes bleeding does not stop.

- If it lets her be clear and peaceful in the daytime but with delirious speech as if seeing ghosts at night, use *Xiǎo Chái Hú Tāng* F2-12 adding *shēng dì huáng*.
- For blood deficiency, use *Sì Wù Tāng* F2-51 adding *shēng dì huáng* and *chái hú*. Be sure not to offend stomach qì.
- If the disease has already recovered but bleeding does not stop, or fever does not cease and her original qì is usually weak, use *Bǔ Zhōng Yì Qì Tāng* F2-5.
- If spleen qì is usually constrained, use *Jì Shēng Guī Pí Tāng* F2-3.
- If blood and qì are usually weak, use *Shí Quán Dà Bǔ Tāng* F2-7.

[If one follows the above guidelines,] in many cases there will be no mistake.

## 治驗
## Treatment Experience

**1-7-1**一婦人經行，感冒風寒，日間安靜，至夜譫語，用小柴胡加生地治之，頓安。但內熱頭暈，用補中益氣加蔓荊子而愈。後因怒惱，寒熱譫語，胸脅脹痛，小便頻數，月經先期，此是肝火血熱妄行，用加味逍遙加生地而愈。

A woman had external contraction of wind and cold while menstruating. She was peaceful in the daytime but spoke deliriously when night arrived. I treated her with *Xiǎo Chái*

*Hú Tāng* F2-12 adding *shēng dì huáng* and she was immediately peaceful. Only internal heat and dizziness remained. I used *Bǔ Zhōng Yì Qì Tāng* F2-5 adding *màn jīng zǐ* and she recovered. Later due to anger, she had [sensations of] cold and heat, delirious speech, distention and pain of the chest and rib-sides, frequent urination, and early menstruation. This was liver fire with reckless movement of hot blood. I used *Jiā Wèi Xiāo Yáo Sǎn* F2-1 adding *shēng dì huáng* and she recovered.

**1-7-2**一婦人因怒，寒熱頭痛，譫言妄語，日晡至夜益甚，而經暴至。蓋肝藏血，此怒動火，而血妄行。用加味逍遙散加生地治之，神思頓清，但食少體倦，月經未已。蓋脾統血，此脾氣虛不能攝，用補中益氣治之，月經漸止。

Due to anger, a woman had [sensations of] cold and heat, headache, and raving delirious speech that increased greatly from sundown until nighttime. Her menstrual period suddenly arrived. Now, the liver stores blood, but here anger stirred up fire so blood moved recklessly. I treated it with *Jiā Wèi Xiāo Yáo Sǎn* F2-1 adding *shēng dì huáng*. Her mental state immediately cleared, but she ate little, her body was weary, and her menstrual period did not cease. Now, the spleen controls blood; this was inability of the deficient spleen qì to contain it. I treated her with *Bǔ Zhōng Yì Qì Tāng* F2-5, and her menstruation gradually stopped.

**1-7-3**一婦人懷抱素鬱，感冒經行譫語，服發散之劑，不應；用寒涼降火，前症益甚，更加月經不止，肚腹作痛，嘔吐不食，痰涎自出，此脾胃虛寒，用香砂六君，脾胃漸健，諸症漸退，又用歸脾湯而痊愈。

A woman held on to her usual constraint. She suffered external contraction during menstruation and had delirious speech. She took a prescription to disperse it but did not respond. She used cold and cooling herbs to descend fire, but her previous symptoms increased a lot. Furthermore her menstruation did not stop, and she had belly ache and vomiting. She did not eat and spontaneously drooled phlegm. This was deficient cold spleen and stomach. I used *Xiāng Shā Liù Jūn Zǐ Tāng* UF-2. Her spleen and stomach gradually strengthened and all the symptoms gradually receded. Later I used *Guī Pí Tāng* F2-3 and she was completely cured.

# 《女科撮要·卷上·師尼寡婦寒熱》
## 1-8 Cold and Heat in Nuns and Widows[33]

宋褚氏療師尼寡婦，別制方藥，謂獨陰無陽，致血氣交爭，乍寒乍熱如瘧；或腰背作痛而寒熱，其肝脈弦出寸口，是其症也。若室女出嫁，愆期而寒熱亦然。蓋男子精盛，則思室，女子血盛以懷胎，此天地自然之理也。

Master Chǔ of the *Sòng* dynasty[34] treated nuns and widows by preparing different formulas and herbs [than for married women]. He said solitary yīn [an unmarried woman] without yáng [a man] results in contentious interaction of blood and qì, with alternating chills and fever like *nüè*-malaria; perhaps there is back pain with [sensations of] cold and heat. The liver pulse is bowstring and goes beyond the *cùn kǒu;*[35] this is the disease. When there are [sensations of] cold and heat in an unmarried girl whose wedding has fallen behind schedule, it is also like this. Now, when a male's *jīng*-essence fills up, he thinks of the bedroom; when a female's blood fills up, she cherishes pregnancy. This is the natural principle of heaven and earth.

治以小柴胡加生地；久而血虚，佐以四物。若兼怒動肝火而寒熱者，佐以加味逍遙散；若兼虧損肝經而寒熱者，佐以八珍湯；若兼虧損元氣而寒熱者，佐以補中益氣湯；若兼鬱傷脾氣而寒熱者，佐以《濟生》歸脾湯。此症多兼經候不調，當詳孰為緩急而治之。

Treat it using *Xiǎo Chái Hú Tāng* F2-12 adding *shēng dì huáng.*

- If it has lasted a long time and blood is deficient, assist with *Sì Wù Tāng* F2-51.
- If if there is anger stirring up liver fire at the same time as [sensations of] cold and

33. This chapter is about the negative heath effects for women of reproductive age who do not have heterosexual sex with a goal of reproduction: nuns, widows, unmarried girls, women whose husbands are away for long periods of time, and so forth..
34. This refers to *Chǔ Shì Yí Shū* 褚澄《褚氏遺書》南齊 (The Lost Book of Master Chǔ) by Chǔ Chéng, Southern *Qí* dynasty (420—589 CE). Later, Xǔ Shūwēi 許叔微 who lived from about 1075 to 1156 (Southern *Sòng*) misattributed statements to Chǔ Chéng and also gave the wrong dynasty. Here, Xuē Jǐ must have used Xǔ Shūwēi as a source as these statements are not all found in *Chǔ Shì Yí Shū*.
35. This means the pulse is long. In other books it is described as going up the base of the thumb to the region of Yú Jì (LU 10).

heat, assist with *Jiā Wèi Xiāo Yáo Sǎn* F2-1.

- If the liver channel is enfeebled at the same time as [sensations of] cold and heat, assist with *Bā Zhēn Tāng* F2-8.
- If original qì is enfeebled at the same time as [sensations of] cold and heat, assist with *Bǔ Zhōng Yì Qì Tāng* F2-5.
- If constraint damages spleen qì at the same time as [sensations of] cold and heat, assist with *Jì Shēng Guī Pí Tāng* F2-3.

This pattern is often found when the timing of menstruation out of tune; treat it according to the specifics and whether it is chronic or acute.

## 治驗
## Treatment Experience

**1-8-1**一寡婦因怒，致不時寒熱，久而不已，肝脈弦緊，用小柴胡加生地治之而愈。但見風寒熱仍作，此是脾胃氣虛，用加味歸脾、補中益氣二湯，兼服而止。

Due to anger, a widow ended up with [sensations of] cold and heat at no particular time. This went on for a long while without stopping. Her liver pulse was bowstring and tight. I treated her with *Xiǎo Chái Hú Tāng* F2-12 adding *shēng dì huáng* and she recovered. However she met with wind and suffered [sensations of] cold and heat again. This was spleen and stomach qì deficiency. I used two decoctions, *Jiā Wèi Guī Pí Tāng* F2-4 and *Bǔ Zhōng Yì Qì Tāng* F2-5. She took them together and it stopped.

**1-8-2**一婦人因夫經商久不歸，發寒熱，月經旬日方止。服降火涼血，反潮熱內熱，自汗盜汗，月經頻數。余曰：熱汗，氣血虛也；經頻，肝脾虛也。用歸脾湯、六味丸而愈。常治兼症，既愈而寒熱，當仍用本症葯。

Because the husband of a woman was away on business for a long time and did not return, she suffered fever and chills and her menstrual period went on for ten days before it stopped. She took herbs to descend fire and cool the blood, but contrary to expectations she ended up with tidal fevers, internal heat, spontaneous sweating, night sweating, and her menstrual period occurred frequently. I said: Her hot sweating means qì and blood are deficient; her frequent menstruation means the liver and spleen are deficient. I used *Guī Pí Tāng* F2-3 and *Liù Wèi Wán* F2-16 and she recovered. Normally when treating all these symptoms, if the patient has already recovered and then suffers [sensations of] cold and heat, one should still use herbs for the root condition.

**1-8-3**一室女寒熱，左手脈弦長而出寸口，用小柴胡加生地、烏梅治之，而愈，既嫁而諸症悉痊。

An unmarried girl had [sensations of] cold and heat. Her left pulse was bowstring and long, going beyond *cùn kǒu*. I treated her with *Xiǎo Chái Hú Tāng* F2-12 adding *shēng dì huáng* and wū méi and she recovered. After she married, all symptoms completely cleared up.

**1-8-4**一室女久患寒熱，月經不調，先以小柴胡加生地，治之少愈，更以生地黃丸而痊。

An unmarried girl suffered [sensations of] cold and heat for a long time with out of tune menstruation. I first treated her with *Xiǎo Chái Hú Tāng* F2-12 adding *shēng dì huáng*, and there was a little improvement. I further used *Shēng Dì Huáng Wán* F1-32 and it cleared up.

**1-8-5**一放出宮女，年逾三十，兩胯作痛，肉色不變，大小便中作痛如淋，登廁尤痛。此瘀血漬入隧道為患，乃男女失合之症也，難治。後潰不斂，又患瘰癧而歿。此婦為吾鄉湯氏妾，湯為商常在外，可見此婦在內久懷憂鬱，及出外又不能如願，是以致生此疾。

A released palace maiden[36] was more than thirty years old. Both hips were painful but there was no change in the color of the flesh. Her urination and bowel movements were painful as if she had lín-dribbling, and getting up from the latrine was especially painful.

36. A released palace maiden: A woman who has worked in the imperial palace but was allowed to retire. During her service she was not allowed to marry.

She suffered from blood stasis soaking into the tunnel pathways;[37] it was a condition due to loss of joining of male and female and is difficult to treat. Later the blood stasis burst open and would not close up. She then suffered scrofula and died. This woman was the concubine of Mr. Tāng from my hometown. Tāng was frequently away from home on business. It is apparent that when this woman was on the inside [of the palace] she held onto worry and constraint for a long time, and when she was let out [of the palace] she was still unable to do as she wished, so it resulted in engendering this disease.

愈見瘰癧流注，乃七情氣血損傷，不可用攻伐皎然矣 。按《 精血篇 》云：女人天癸既至，逾十年無男子合，則不調 。未逾十年，思男子合，亦不調 。不調則舊血不出，新血誤行；或漬而入骨；或變而為腫；或雖合而難子，合多則瀝枯虛人，產乳眾則血枯殺人 。觀其精血，思過半矣 。

Even more, when scrofula or streaming sores appear, it is due to the seven emotions damaging qì and blood; one clearly cannot use attacking methods. Note that *Jīng Xuè Piān* says[38]: "Once a girl's *tiān guǐ* has arrived, if she goes for more than ten years without joining with a male, she becomes out of tune.[39] If less than ten years have passed but she longs to join with a male, she is also out of tune. When she is out of tune, old blood does not leave and new blood moves erroneously. Perhaps it soaks into the bones, or it mutates and becomes swellings.[40] Perhaps even if she joins [with a male at that late point], it is difficult to become pregnant. When someone frequently joins with a male, [blood] trickles and she becomes withered and deficient; when someone gives birth and lactates a lot, blood withers and it kills her. If you observe one's *jīng*-essence and blood, you have already understood more than half."

37. Tunnel pathways (*suì dào* 隧道): This odd phrase may refer to the blood vessels, or perhaps the regions where blood collects in the female reproductive system. Based on her symptoms related to the hips, urination, and bowel movement, it may refer to any place that blood flows in the lower burner. In any case, because she had infrequent sexual relations and never achieved pregnancy and because of emotional constraint, her reproductive blood became static and caused the development of symptoms.
38. From the *Chǔ Shì Yí Shū* 《 褚氏遺書 》(Lost Book of Master Chǔ) by Chǔ Chéng 褚澄, Southern *Qí* dynasty 南齊 (420—589 CE).
39. This could refer to out of tune menstruation, but could mean a broader range of disharmonies or maladjustments.
40. *Swellings* probably means *lumps* here, including scrofula or abdominal masses.

**1-8-6**一室女年十七，瘰久不愈，天癸未通，發熱咳嗽，飲食少思；或欲用通經丸。余曰：此症潮熱，經候不調者，不治，所喜脈不澀，且不潮熱，尚可治。但養氣血，益津液，其經自行。惑於速效，仍用之。余曰：非其治也，此乃慓悍之劑，大助陽火，陰血得之則妄行，脾胃得之則愈虛。經果通而不止，飲食愈少，更加潮熱，遂致不救。

A seventeen year old unmarried girl had scrofula for a long time without recovering. Her *tiān guǐ* had never flowed. She had fever, cough, and little thought of food or drink. Someone wanted her to use *Tōng Jīng Wán* UFx-2. I said: "This disease of tidal fever and out of tune menstrual timing cannot be treated [that way]. I am pleased that the pulse is not rough and there are no tidal fevers at this time, so it is still treatable. We must only nourish qì and blood and boost *jīnyè*-fluids. Then menstruation will move on its own." She was mislead by [the promise of] quick results and used *Tōng Jīng Wán* UFx-2 anyway. I said: "This is not the [proper] treatment. This prescription is swift and fierce and will strongly aid yáng fire. When yīn blood receives it, it will move recklessly. When the spleen and stomach receive it, they will become more deficient." As a result [of her taking *Tōng Jīng Wán*], her menstruation flowed and did not stop, eating and drinking decreased even more, it further increased her tidal fevers, and subsequently she could not be saved.

# 《女科撮要·卷上·歷節痛風》
# (即白虎歷節風)
## 1-9 Joint-Running Painful Wind
## (means white tiger joint-running wind)[41]

歷節痛，或因飲食起居失節；或因七情六淫失宜，以致脾胃虧損，腠理不密，外邪所侵；或為肝火內動，肝血耗損；或為肢體疼痛；或為肢節難伸；或為卒然掣痛；或為走痛無常；或內熱晡熱，自汗盜汗；或經候不調，飲食不甘。

Sometimes joint-running pain is due to loss of regularity of food and drink or rising and dwelling [lifestyle], or due to inappropriateness of the seven emotions and the six excesses [external evils]. This results in debility of the spleen and stomach, the *còu lǐ*[42] do not close, and one is invaded by external evils. Perhaps it becomes liver fire stirring internally and consuming liver blood. Sometimes it becomes painful limbs and body; or it becomes difficulty stretching out the joints of the limbs; or it becomes sudden pulling pain; or it becomes wandering changeable pain. At times there is internal heat, late afternoon fever, spontaneous sweating, and night sweating; or the timing of menstruation is out of tune and food and drink do not taste sweet.

其治法：屬風邪者，小續命湯；走注疼痛者，漏蘆散；骨節疼痛者，四生丸；濕熱痛者，清燥湯，兼痰佐以二陳；肝火者，加味逍遙散加羌活、川芎；脾鬱者，加味歸脾加羌活、川芎；血虛者，四物加羌活、川芎；氣虛者，四君加羌活、川芎；氣血俱虛者，八珍加羌活、川芎；月經先期而痛者，加味逍遙散為主；月經過期而痛者，補中益氣為主。

The treatment method:

- If it belongs to wind evils, use *Xiǎo Xù Mìng Tāng* F1-20.

41. Joint-running painful wind (*lì jié tong fēng* 歷節痛風) is a painful wind condition with spontaneous sweating, shortness of breath, aching joints, and inability to bend and stretch. White tiger joint-running wind (*bái hǔ lì jié fēng* 白虎歷節風) is a synonym.
42. *Còu lǐ* 腠理 is often translated as pores. Wiseman glosses it as *interstices*. This is the anatomical entity within the skin that opens to allow sweating but is held closed by *wèi* qì most of the time to prevent invasion by exterior evils.

- For traveling influx [moving *bì*-obstruction] pain, use *Lòu Lú Săn* F2-80.
- For painful bones and joints, use *Sì Shēng Wán* UF-18.
- For damp heat pain, use *Qīng Zào Tāng* F2-72.
    - With phegm at the same time, use *Èr Chén Tāng* F2-42.
- For liver fire, use *Jiā Wèi Xiāo Yáo Săn* F2-1 adding *qiāng huó* and *chuān xiōng*.
- For spleen constraint, use *Jiā Wèi Guī Pí Tāng* F2-4 adding *qiāng huó* and *chuān xiōng*.
- For blood deficiency, use *Sì Wù Tāng* F2-51 adding *qiāng huó* and *chuān xiōng*.
- For qì deficiency, use *Sì Jūn Zĭ Tāng* F2-26 adding *qiāng huó* and *chuān xiōng*.
- For deficiency of both qì and blood, use *Bā Zhēn Tāng* F2-8 adding *qiāng huó* and *chuān xiōng*.
- For pain that comes before menstruation, *Jiā Wèi Xiāo Yáo Săn* F2-1 is indicated.
- For pain that comes after menstruation, *Bŭ Zhōng Yì Qì* F2-5 is indicated.

大抵痛而不敢按者，屬病氣元氣俱實也；手按而痛緩者，病氣元氣俱虛也。若勞役而作痛者，元氣虛也；飲食失宜而作痛者，脾胃虛也；怒惱而作痛者，肝火也；經行而作痛，血虛也。凡此皆固元氣為主，而佐以治病之藥。

Generally speaking:

- Pain that one does not dare to press belongs to excess of both disease qì and original qì.
- If pain moderates when pressed, disease qì and original qì are both deficient.
- If there is pain after taxation, original qì is deficient.
- When inappropriate diet causes pain, the spleen and stomach are deficient.
- If anger makes pain, it is liver fire.
- If menstruation causes pain, it is blood deficiency.

Whenever joint-running pain occurs, securing original qì is always indicated and then assist with herbs to treat the disease.

## 治驗
## Treatment Experience

**1-9-1**一婦人自汗盜汗，發熱晡熱，體倦少食，月經不調，吐痰甚多，二年矣。遍身作痛，天陰風雨益甚。用小續命湯而痛止，用補中益氣、加味歸脾二湯，三十餘劑而愈。自汗等症，皆鬱結傷損脾氣，不能輸養諸臟所致。故用前二湯，專主脾胃。若用寒涼降火，理氣化痰，復傷生氣，多致不起。

For two years, a woman had spontaneous sweating, night sweating, fever, late afternoon fever, weariness of the body, reduced food intake, and out of tune menstruation. She spit quite a lot of phlegm. Her entire body was painful; it increased a lot when the weather was cloudy, windy, or rainy. I used *Xiǎo Xù Mìng Tāng* F1-20 and the pain stopped; I used more than thirty doses of two decoctions, *Bǔ Zhōng Yì Qì Tāng* F2-5 and *Jiā Wèi Guī Pí Tāng* F2-4 and she recovered. The spontaneous sweating and similar symptoms were all caused by binding constraint damaging spleen qì with inability to transport and nourish all the *zàng*-organs. Thus I used the above two decoctions and focused on governing the spleen and stomach. If I had used cold and cool herbs to descend fire, or rectified qì and transformed phlegm, I would have repeatedly damaged her life qì, which often incurs death.

**1-9-2**一婦人因怒，月經去多，發熱作渴，左目緊小，頭項動掉，四肢抽搐，遍身疼痛，此怒動肝火，肝血虛而內生風，用加味逍遙加鉤藤數劑，諸症漸愈；又用八珍湯，調理而痊。

Due to anger, a woman's menstrual period bled a lot with fever that led to thirst. Her left eye was tight and small, her head and neck moved and drooped, her four limbs twitched, and her entire body was painful. This was anger stirring up liver fire with liver blood deficiency and internally generated wind. I used several doses of *Jiā Wèi Xiāo Yáo Sǎn* F2-1 adding *gōu téng* and all the symptoms gradually recovered. I then used *Bā Zhēn Tāng* F2-8 to attune and rectify her and she recuperated.

**1-9-3**一婦人月經先期，素有痛症，每勞必作，用眾手重按，痛稍止。此氣血虛而有火，用十全大補加獨活治之而痛痊，用六味丸、逍遙散而經調。

A woman with early menstruation usually had painful symptoms that would occur when she taxed herself. Pressing heavily with many hands stopped the pain a little. This was qì and blood deficiency with fire. I treated it using *Shí Quán Dà Bǔ Tāng* F2-7 adding dú huó and the pain recuperated. I used *Liù Wèi Wán* F2-16 and *Xiāo Yáo Sǎn* F2-2 and her menstruation attuned itself.

**1-9-4**一婦人歷節作痛，發熱作渴，飲食少思，月經過期，諸藥不應，脈洪大，按之微細，用附子八物四劑而痛止，用加味逍遙而元氣復，六味丸而月經調。

A woman had joint-running pain with fever that made thirst, little thought of food and drink, and late menstruation. It did not respond to any herbs. Her pulse was surging and large but faint and fine when pressed. I used four doses of *Fù zǐ Bā Wù Tāng* F2-77 and the pain stopped. I used *Jiā Wèi Xiāo Yáo Sǎn* F2-1 and original qì returned. I used *Liù Wèi Wán* F2-16 and her menstruation attuned itself.

**1-9-5**一婦人體肥胖，素內熱，月經先期，患痛風，下體微腫痛甚，小便頻數，身重脈緩，症屬風濕，而血虛有熱。先用羌活勝濕湯四劑，腫痛漸愈；用清燥湯數劑，小便漸清；用加味逍遙十餘劑，內熱漸愈。為飲食停滯，發熱仍痛，面目浮腫，用六君加柴胡、升麻而愈。又因怒氣，小腹痞悶，寒熱嘔吐，此木侮脾土。用前藥加山梔、木香而安。惟小腹下墜，似欲去後，此脾氣下陷，用補中益氣而愈。後因勞役、怒氣，作嘔吐痰，遍身腫痛，月經忽來寒熱。用六君加柴胡、山梔以扶元氣清肝火，腫痛嘔吐悉退，用補中益氣以升陽氣健營氣，月經寒熱悉瘥。

A woman who was plump usually had internal heat and early menstruation. She suffered painful wind; her lower body was slightly swollen and was extremely painful. She also had frequent urination, heaviness of the body, and a moderate pulse. Her symptoms belonged to wind damp and blood deficiency with heat. I first used four doses of *Qiāng Huó Shèng Shī Tāng* F2-76 and the swelling and pain gradually recovered. I used several doses of *Qīng Zào Tāng* F2-72 and her urination gradually cleared. I used more than ten doses of *Jiā Wèi Xiāo Yáo Sǎn* F2-1 and the internal heat gradually recovered. For food retention, fever, the remaining pain, and superficial swelling of the face and eyes, I used *Liù Jūn Zǐ Tāng* F2-6 adding *chái hú* and *shēng má* and she recovered. Later, due to anger, she developed *pǐ*-glomus with oppression in her lower abdomen, [sensations of] cold and heat, and vomiting. This was wood insulting spleen earth. I used the previous herbs adding *zhī zǐ* and *mù xiāng* and she was peaceful. Only her lower abdomen felt downward pressure [a term for tenesmus] as if she was about to have a bowel movement. This was spleen qì sinking downward. I used *Bǔ Zhōng Yì Qì* F2-5 and she recovered. Later, due to taxation and anger, she began vomiting phlegm. Her entire body became swollen and painful and her menstruation suddenly came with [sensations of] cold and heat. I used *Liù Jūn Zǐ Tāng* F2-6 adding *chái hú* and *zhī zǐ* to support original qì and clear liver fire. The swelling, pain, and vomiting receded completely. I used *Bǔ Zhōng Yì Qì* F2-5 to raise up yáng qì and strengthen *yíng* qì, and her menstruation and [sensations of] cold and heat completely recovered.

**1-9-6**一婦人飲食少思，畏見風寒，患痛風，嘔吐寒熱，脈弦緊。用附子八物，四肢痛愈。用獨活寄生，腰痛亦痊，惟兩膝腫痛，用大防風而消，用加味歸脾、逍遙而元氣復。

A woman had little thought of food and drink, feared seeing wind and cold, and suffered painful wind. She also had vomiting and [sensations of] cold and heat. Her pulse was bowstring and tight. I used *Fù zǐ Bā Wù Tāng* F2-77 and the pain of the four limbs recovered. I used *Dú Huó Jì Shēng Tāng* F2-75 and the low back pain also recuperated. Only both knees were still swollen and painful. I used *Dà Fáng Fēng Tāng* F2-74 and it dispersed. I used *Jiā Wèi Guī Pí Tāng* F2-4 and *Xiāo Yáo Sǎn* F2-2 and her original qì returned.

# 《女科撮要·卷上·流注》
## 1-10 Streaming Sores (*liú zhù*)[43]

婦人流注；或因憂思鬱怒，虧損肝脾；或因產後勞役，復傷氣血，以致營氣不從，逆於肉理；或因腠理不密，外邪客之；或濕痰流注；或跌撲血滯；或產後惡露。蓋氣流而注，血注而凝。或生於四肢關節；或流於胸腹腰臀；或結塊；或漫腫，皆屬虛損。

Streaming sores in women are due to worry, thought, and constrained anger which enfeeble the liver and spleen. Perhaps this is due to postpartum taxation repeatedly damaging qì and blood with the result that *yíng* qì is not compliant and counterflows into the textured layers of the flesh (*ròu lǐ*); or due to unclosed *còu lǐ* allowing external evils to settle into them; or damp phlegm flows (*liú*) and pools (*zhù*); or falls and knocks make blood stagnation; or postpartum lochia. Now, qì flows (*liú*) and then pools (*zhù*); blood pools and then congeals. Perhaps [these sores] are engendered in the joints of the four limbs; or flow into the chest, abdomen, low back, and buttocks; or bind into lumps; or overflow and swell. All these belong to [the category of] deficiency harm.

急用蔥熨及益氣養榮湯，則未成自消，已成自潰。若久而腫起作痛，肢體倦怠，病氣有餘，形氣不足，尚可治。若漫腫微痛，屬形氣病氣俱不足，最難治。

Quickly iron the sores with scallions [see *Shén Xiào Cōng Yùn Fǎ* F1-25] and use *Yì Qì Yǎng Róng Tāng* F1-27; sores that are undeveloped will automatically disperse and those that have already developed will automatically burst open.

- If they have lasted a long time, so painful swelling arises and the body is weary, there is surplus disease qì and insufficient body qì; it still can be treated.
- If they overflow and swell with mild pain, it belongs to insufficiency of both body qì and disease qì, and is most difficult to treat.

不作膿；或膿成不潰，氣血虛也，用八珍湯。憎寒畏寒，陽氣虛也，十全大補湯。晡熱內熱，陰血虛也，四物加參、朮。作嘔欲

43. Streaming sores (*liú zhù* 流注) are sores that discharge pus. The term literally means flowing (*liú*) and pooling (*zhù*).

嘔，胃氣虛也，六君加炮薑。食少體倦，脾氣虛也，補中益氣加茯苓、半夏。四肢逆冷，小便頻數，命門火衰也，八味丸。小便頻數，痰盛作渴，腎水虧損也，六味丸。月經過期，多日不止，肝脾虛也，八珍湯加柴胡、丹皮。凡潰而氣血虛弱不斂者，更用十全大補湯，煎膏外補之。久潰而寒邪凝滯不斂者，用豆豉餅祛散之。其潰而內有膿管不斂者，用針頭散腐化之，自愈。若不補氣血，不節飲食，不慎起居，不戒七情；或用寒涼剋伐，俱不治。

- If they do not make pus, or they make pus but do not burst open, qì and blood are deficient; use *Bā Zhēn Tāng* F2-8.
- If the patient hates and fears cold, yáng qì is deficient; use *Shí Quán Dà Bǔ Tāng* F2-7.
- If there is late afternoon fever and internal heat, yīn blood is deficient; use *Sì Wù Tāng* F2-51 adding *rén shēn* and *bái zhú*.
- Nausea with desire to vomit means stomach qì is deficient; use *Liù Jūn Zǐ Tāng* F2-6 adding *pào jiāng*.
- Decreased food intake with a tired body means spleen qì deficiency; use *Bǔ Zhōng Yì Qì Tāng* F2-5 adding *fú líng* and *bàn xià*.
- Counterflow cold of the four limbs and frequent urination means debility of *mìng mén* fire; use *Bā Wèi Wán* F2-17.
- Frequent urination, flourishing phlegm, and thirst means enfeebled kidney water; use *Liù Wèi Wán* F2-16.
- Late menstruation that lasts many days without stopping means liver and spleen deficiency; use *Bā Zhēn Tāng* F2-8 adding *chái hú* and *mǔ dān pí*.
- Whenever the sores burst open, if qì and blood are deficient they won't close up; in addition [to the internal prescriptions given above] supplement by boiling *Shí Quán Dà Bǔ Tāng* F2-7 into a paste and applying it externally.
- If the sores have been open for a long time but cold evils congeal and stagnate so they don't close up, use *Dòu Chǐ Bǐng* F1-26 to drive out and scatter the evils.
- If the sores burst open but internally there is a pus tube [fistula] that doesn't close up, use *Zhēn Tóu Sǎn* UF-17 to dissolve it, and the patient will spontaneously recover.

If one fails to supplement qì and blood, fails to regulate food and drink, is not careful with rising and dwelling [lifestyle], does not avoid the seven emotions, or uses cold and cooling formulas to control and attack - all these things make the condition untreatable.

## 治驗
## Treatment Experience

**1-10-1**一婦人左臂患之，年許不潰，堅硬不痛，肉色不變，脈弱少食，月經過期，日晡發熱，勞役則痛，遂與參、耆、歸、朮、川芎、芍藥、熟地、貝母、遠志、香附、桔梗、丹皮、甘草，百餘貼而消。

A woman suffered this condition on her left arm; it did not burst open for about a year. It was hard but not painful. The color of the flesh did not change and her pulse was weak. She had reduced food intake, late menstruation, and fevers at sunset. When taxed, it was painful. I then gave her more than a hundred doses of *rén shēn, huáng qí, dāng guī, bái zhú, chuān xiōng, sháo yào, shú dì huáng, bèi mǔ, yuǎn zhì, xiāng fù, jié gěng, mǔ dān pí,* and *gān cǎo* to be applied topically and it dispersed.

**1-10-2**一婦人暴怒，腰腫一塊，胸膈不利，時或氣走作痛，與方脈流氣飲，數劑而止，更以小柴胡對四物，加香附、貝母，月餘而愈。

A woman had explosive anger. A lump swelled on her lower back. Her chest and diaphragm were inhibited with occasional radiating qì that made pain. I gave several doses of *Fāng Mài Liú Qì Yǐn Zǐ* F1-29 and it stopped. Further, for more than a month I used *Xiǎo Chái Hú Tāng* F2-12 paired with *Sì Wù Tāng* F2-51 adding *xiāng fù* and *bèi mǔ,* and she recovered.

**1-10-3**一婦人因怒，脅下腫痛，胸膈不利，脈沉滯，以方脈流氣飲，數劑少愈；以小柴胡對二陳，加青皮、桔梗、貝母，數劑頓退；更以小柴胡湯對四物，二十餘劑而痊。

Due to anger, a woman had swelling and pain below her rib-sides. Her chest and diaphragm were inhibited and her pulse was sunken and stagnant. I used several doses of *Fāng Mài Liú Qì Yǐn Zǐ* F1-29 and she recovered a little. I used several doses of *Xiǎo Chái Hú Tāng* F2-12 paired with *Èr Chén Tāng* F2-42, adding *qīng pí, jié gěng,* and *bèi mǔ,* and it instantly receded. I further used more than twenty doses of *Xiǎo Chái Hú Tāng* F2-12 paired with *Sì Wù Tāng* F2-51 and she recuperated.

**1-10-4**一婦人因閃胸肩患腫，遍身痛，遂以黑丸子二服而痛止，以方脈流氣飲二劑而腫消，更以二陳對四物，加香附、枳殼、桔梗而全愈。

A woman suffered swelling due to a sprained chest and shoulder; her entire body was painful. I then used two doses of *Hēi Wán Zǐ* UF-3 and the pain stopped. I used two doses of *Fāng Mài Liú Qì Yǐn Zǐ* F1-29 and the swelling dispersed. I further used *Èr Chén Tāng* F2-42 paired with *Sì Wù Tāng* F2-51 adding *xiāng fù, zhǐ qiào,* and *jié gěng* and she completely recovered.

**1-10-5**一婦人腿患筋攣骨痛，諸藥不應，脈遲緊，用大防風湯，二劑頓退，又二劑而安。又一婦患之亦然，先用前湯二劑，更服黑丸子而痊。此二患若失治，潰成敗證。

A woman suffered sinew spasms and bone pain in her legs. It did not respond to various herbs. Her pulse was slow and tight. I used two doses of *Dà Fáng Fēng Tāng* F2-74 and it immediately receded. She was peaceful after two more doses. A different woman suffered the same thing. I first used two doses of the above decoction. She further took *Hēi Wán Zǐ* UF-3 and completely recuperated. If these two patients were not treated properly, it would burst open and become a conquering pattern.

**1-10-6**一婦人潰後發熱，予以為虛，彼不信，乃服敗毒藥，果發大熱，竟至不救。

A woman had fever after [her sores] burst open. I took it as deficiency, but she did not believe me so she took herbs to conquer toxins. This resulted in high fever and in the end she could not be saved.

夫潰瘍雖有表證，發熱宜以托裏為主，佐以表散之劑，何況瘰癧流注乎?若氣血充實，經絡通暢，決無患者。此證之因，皆由氣血素虧；或七情所傷，經絡鬱結；或腠理不密，六淫外侵，隧道壅塞。若不審其所因，辨其虛實，鮮不誤人。

Although there are exterior patterns for open sores, in fever it is appropriate to take drawing out the interior[44] as governing and assist with prescriptions to scatter the exterior. What are the circumstances of scrofula and streaming sores? If qì and blood are filled up and the channels and *luò*-networks are unobstructed, this suffering will not develop. All causes of these symptoms are usually from lack of qì and blood; or damage by the seven emotions with binding constraint of the channels and *luò*-networks; or the *còu lǐ* do not close so the six excesses invade externally and the tunnels are obstructed. If one fails to examine what caused it, differentiating the patient's deficiency or excess, few will not be led astray.

## 《女科撮要·卷上·瘰癧》
## 1-11 Scrofula

婦人瘰癧；或因胎產血崩，虧損腎肝；或因憂思鬱怒，傷損肝脾；或因恚怒風熱，肝膽血燥；或因水涸血虛，筋攣則累累然如貫珠，故多生於耳前後、項側、胸脅間。

Sometimes scrofula in a woman is due to bēng-flooding during childbirth which enfeebles the kidneys and liver; or due to worry, thought, and constrained anger which damage the liver and spleen; or due to rage becoming wind heat which dry out liver-gallbladder blood; or due to water drying up and blood deficiency. When the sinews contact, the [scrofula nodes] are countless like a string of pearls. Thus many are engendered behind the ears, on the side of the neck, and between the chest and rib-sides.

若寒熱腫痛，乃肝經氣動而為病；用柴胡梔子散以清肝火為主，而佐以逍遙散以養肝血。若寒熱既止，而核不消，乃肝經之血亦病；用加味四物湯以養肝血為主，而佐以柴胡梔子散以清肝火。若初生如豆粒，附著於筋，肉色不變，內熱口乾，精神倦怠，久不消潰，乃肝脾虧損；用逍遙散、歸脾湯、六味丸健脾土，培肝木；切不可輕用散堅追毒之劑。

44. Drawing out the interior (*tuō lǐ* 托裹): Also translated as internal expression. This is a treatment method of pushing toxins (including their manifestation as pus) outward from the inside of the body by supplementing right qì.

- If there are [sensations of] cold and heat with swelling and pain, the illness is from qì stirring in the liver channel; govern the treatment with *Chái Hú Zhī Zǐ Sǎn* UF-4 to clear liver fire and assist with *Xiāo Yáo Sǎn* F2-2 to nourish liver blood.
- If [sensations of] cold and heat have already stopped but the nodes do not disperse, there is also blood disease of the liver channel; govern the treatment with *Jiā Wèi Sì Wù Tāng* F2-52 to nourish liver blood and assist with *Chái Hú Zhī Zǐ Sǎn* [not given] to clear liver fire.
- If the nodes are initially like beans adhering to the sinews and the color of the flesh is unchanged, with internal heat, dry mouth, and weary *jīng-shén*, and if it lasts a long time without dispersing or bursting open, it is enfeebled liver and spleen; use *Xiāo Yáo Sǎn* F2-2, *Guī Pí Tāng* F2-3, and *Liù Wèi Wán* F2-16 to strengthen spleen earth and bank up liver wood.

Be sure not to carelessly use prescriptions to scatter hardness and chase toxins.

《外臺秘要》云：肝腎虛熱，則生瘰矣。《病機》云：瘰癧不系膏粱丹毒；因虛勞氣鬱所致。補形氣，調經脈，其瘡當自消散。誤下之，先犯病禁經禁。若久潰脈浮大，邪火盛也；而色㿠白，金剋木也，皆不治。若赤脈貫瞳子，有幾條則幾年死。

*Wài Tái Mì Yào*[45] says: "When there is deficiency heat of the liver and kidneys, it engenders scrofula." *Bìng Jī*[46] says: Scrofula is not related to rich food or cinnabar toxins; it is due to deficiency taxation and qì constraint. If you supplement the body's qì and attune the channel-vessels, the sores should automatically disperse and scatter. If you mistakenly descend [promote a bowel movement], you first violate the disease and channel prohibitions. If they have been open for a long time with a floating large pulse, evil fire flourishes. If the complexion is somber white, metal controls wood. All these are untreatable. When a few red vessels thread through the pupils of the eye, she will die in a few years.

45. *Wài Tái Mì Yào*《外臺秘要》was published in 752 (*Táng*) and written by Wáng Tāo 王燾.
46. Disease Mechanisms (*Bìng Jī*《病機》) or Essentials of Disease Mechanisms (*Bìng Jī Yào*《病機要》) is also mentioned in Section 2-7. This seems to refer to a lost book written by Zhāng Jiégǔ 張潔古 (*Jīn* dynasty).

## 治驗
## Treatment Experience

**1-11-1**一婦人久而不愈；或以為木旺之症，用散腫潰堅湯伐之，腫硬益甚。余以為肝經氣血虧損，當滋化源，用六味地黃丸、補中益氣湯，至春而愈。

A woman had this for a long time without recovering. Perhaps it was taken as a symptom of wood at peak strength so they used *Sàn Zhǒng Kuì Jiān Tāng* UFx-7 to cut it down. The swelling and hardness increased a lot. I took it as enfeebled qì and blood of the liver channel so the source should be enriched and transformed. I used *Liù Wèi Dì Huáng Wán* F2-16 and *Bǔ Zhōng Yì Qì Tāng* F2-5 until spring when she recovered.

此症若肝經風火暴病，元氣無虧，宜用前湯。若風不旺而自病，宜用瀉青丸；虛者，用地黃丸。若水不能生木，亦用此丸。若金來剋木，宜補脾土生腎水。大凡風木之病，但壯脾土，則木自不能剋矣。若行伐肝，則脾胃先傷，而木反來剋土矣。

- If this disease is sudden intense wind fire in the liver channel and original qì is not lacking, it is appropriate to use the above decoction [*Sàn Zhǒng Kuì Jiān Tāng* UFx-7].
- If wind is not at peak strength but [wood] alone is ill, it is appropriate to use *Xiè Qīng Wán* F1-30.
- In deficiency, use *Dì Huáng Wán* F2-16. If water is unable to engender wood, also use this pill.
- If metal comes to control wood, it is appropriate to supplement spleen earth and engender kidney water.

In most cases of wind-wood disease, if spleen earth alone is invigorated, wood is automatically unable to control it. If you act to cut down the liver, the spleen and stomach are damaged first and then, contrary to expectations, wood comes to control earth.

**1-11-2**一婦人患之，恐不起，致少寐，年餘癧破，膿水淋漓，經水或五十日或兩月餘一至，誤服通經丸，展轉無寐，午前惡寒，午後發熱。余以為思慮虧損脾血，用歸脾湯作丸，午前以六君子送下，午後以逍遙散送下，兩月餘得寐，半載後經行如期，年餘而瘡愈。

A woman suffered this [scrofula]. She was afraid she would die and this resulted in insomnia. After more than a year, the scrofula broke open and pus-water trickled out. Sometimes her menstrual flow arrived after fifty days and sometimes it was more than two months. She mistakenly used *Tōng Jīng Wán* UFx-2, and then she tossed and turned without sleeping. Before noon she had aversion to cold; after noon she had fever. I took this as thought and contemplation enfeebling spleen blood. I used *Guī Pí Tāng* F2-3 made into pills. Before noon she swallowed them with *Liù Jūn Zǐ Tāng* F2-6; after noon she swallowed them with *Xiāo Yáo Sǎn* F2-2. After more than two months she was able to sleep, after half a year her menstruation moved on schedule. The sores recovered after more than a year.

**1-11-3**一瘰婦潰後，發熱煩躁作渴，脈大而虛，以當歸補血湯，六劑而寒熱退；又以聖愈湯，數劑而痊愈。更以八珍加貝母、遠志，三十餘劑而斂。

After her scrofula burst open, a woman had fever, vexation, and agitation which made her thirsty. Her pulse was large but deficient. I used six doses of *Dāng Guī Bǔ Xuè Tāng* F2-9 and the [sensations of] cold and heat receded. Then I used several doses of *Shèng Yù Tāng* F1-11 and she completely recovered. I further used more than thirty doses of *Bā Zhēn Tāng* F2-8 adding *bèi mǔ* and *yuǎn zhì* and the sores closed up.

**1-11-4**一婦人項結核，寒熱頭痛，脅乳脹痛，內熱口苦，小便頻數。症屬肝火血虛，用四物加柴胡、山梔、膽草而愈，又用加味逍遙散而安。

A woman had nodules on her nape, [sensations of] cold and heat, headache, distended painful rib-sides and breasts, internal heat, bitter mouth, and frequent urination. The symptoms belonged to liver fire with blood deficiency. I used *Sì Wù Tāng* F2-51 adding *chái hú, zhī zǐ,* and *lóng dǎn cǎo* and she recovered. Then I used *Jiā Wèi Xiāo Yáo Sǎn* F2-1 and she was peaceful.

**1-11-5**一婦人瘰癧後，遍身作癢，脈大按而虛，以十全大補加香附治之而愈。

After a woman suffered scrofula, her entire body began itching and her pulse was large but it was deficient when pressed. I treated her using *Shí Quán Dà Bǔ Tāng* F2-7 adding *xiāng fù* and she recovered.

大凡潰後，午前癢作氣虛，午後癢作血虛。若作風症治之，必死。

Generally after [scrofula sores] burst open, itching before noon is from qì deficiency; itching after noon is from blood deficiency. If it is treated as a wind pattern she will die.

**1-11-6**一婦人項核腫痛，察其氣血俱實，先以必效散一服下之，更以益氣養榮湯補之，三十餘劑而消。

A woman had swollen painful nodes on her nape. I observed that her qì and blood were both in excess. I first descended her [promoted a bowel movement] with one dose of *Bì Xiào Sǎn* F1-34. I further supplemented her with more than thirty doses of *Yì Qì Yǎng Róng Tāng* F1-27, and the nodes dispersed.

常治此症，若必欲出膿，但虛弱者，先用前湯，待其氣血稍充，乃用必效散，去其毒，仍用補藥，無不效。未成膿者，灸肘尖調經解鬱，及隔蒜灸，多自消。有膿即針之。若氣血復而核不消，卻服散堅之劑。月許不應，氣血不損，須用必效散。其毒一下，即多服益氣養榮湯。如不應，亦灸肘尖。如瘡口不斂者，更用豆豉餅、琥珀膏。若氣血俱虛，或不慎飲食七情者，不治。然此症以氣血為主，氣血壯實，不用追蝕之劑，亦能自腐。但取去使易於收斂耳。血虛而用追蝕，不惟徒治，適足以敗矣。

I often treat this disease.

- If it is about to exude pus but the patient is deficient and weak, I first use the previous decoction [*Yì Qì Yǎng Róng Tāng* F1-27] and wait for qì and blood to fill up a little. Then I use *Bì Xiào Sǎn* F1-34 to remove the toxins. I still use supplementing herbs and it never fails to be effective.

- If pus has not developed, I apply moxbustion to Zhǒu Jiān [non-channel][47] to attune the channels and resolve constraint, as well as garlic-isolated moxibustion [on the nodes], and many spontaneously disperse.
- When there is pus, needle it.
- If qì and blood return but the nodes do not disperse, then the patient can take a prescription to scatter hardness.
    - If there is no response in about a month and qì and blood are not harmed, one must use *Bì Xiào Sǎn* F1-34. Once the toxins have descended [with a bowel movement], take a lot of *Yì Qì Yǎng Róng Tāng* F1-27.
    - If she does not respond, again apply moxibustion to Zhǒu Jiān [non-channel].
- If an open sore does not close up, further use *Dòu Chǐ Bǐng* F1-26 and *Hǔ Pò Gāo* F1-35.
- If both qì and blood are deficient, or the patient is incautious with food and drink and the seven emotions, it is untreatable.
- Like this, qì and blood are governing for this condition. Do not use prescriptions to expel and erode [the scrofula nodes] even if qì and blood are robust, as they will be able to break down on their own. However, removing [the decayed flesh] makes it easier [for the sores] to close up. If there is blood deficiency but you use herbs to expel and erode, it is not simply a wasted treatment; it is enough to conquer [the patient].

47. *Zhǒu Jiān* 肘尖 means *tip of the elbow*, and that is exactly where it is located. It treats scrofula and is a moxibustion-only point.

## 《女科撮要·卷上·乳癰乳岩》
## 1-12 Breast Abscess and Breast Rock[48]

婦人乳癰，屬膽胃二腑熱毒，氣血壅滯。故初起腫痛，發於肌表，肉色焮赤，其人表熱發熱；或發寒熱；或憎寒頭痛，煩渴引冷，用人參敗毒散、神效瓜蔞散、加味逍遙散治之，其自消散。若至數日之間，膿成潰竅，稠膿湧出，膿盡自愈。若氣血虛弱；或誤用敗毒，久不收斂，膿清脈大，則難治。

*Breast abscesses* in women belong to heat and toxins of two *fǔ*-organs: the gallbladder and the stomach. Qì and blood become obstructed and stagnant. Therefore it initially arises with swelling and pain that develops on the surface of the muscles. The color of the flesh is scorching red, the person has exterior heat and fever; or fever and chills; or aversion to cold with headache, vexation, and thirst for cold drinks.

- Treat it with *Rén Shēn Bài Dú Sǎn* F1-31, *Shén Xiào Guā Lóu Sǎn* F1-36, and *Jiā Wèi Xiāo Yáo Sǎn* F2-1. It will spontaneously scatter and disperse.
- If after the space of several days, pus develops, breaks through an opening, and thick pus gushes out, it will spontaneously recover when it finishes discharging pus.
- If qì and blood are deficient and weak or someone has mistakenly used herbs to conquer toxins, and it does not close up for a long time, with clear pus and a large pulse, it is difficult to treat.

乳岩屬肝脾二臟鬱怒，氣血虧損，故初起小核，結於乳內，肉色如故，其人內熱夜熱，五心發熱，肢體倦瘦，月經不調，用加味歸脾湯、加味逍遙散、神效瓜蔞散，多自消散。若荏苒日月漸大，壘岩色赤，出水腐潰深洞，用前歸脾湯等藥，可延歲月。若誤用攻伐，危殆迫矣。

*Breast rocks* belong to constrained anger of two *zàng*-organs: the liver and the spleen. Qì and blood are enfeebled, so initially a small node is bound up within the breast but the color of the flesh is unchanged. The person has internal heat, nighttime heat, and five heart fever. Her body is weary and thin, and her menstruation is out of tune. Use *Jiā Wèi Guī Pí Tāng* F2-4, *Jiā Wèi Xiāo Yáo Sǎn* F2-1, and *Shén Xiào Guā Lóu Sǎn* F1-36; many breast

48. In some cases, breast rocks may be equivalent to breast cancer. For a description, see below.

rocks will spontaneously scatter and disperse.

- If it goes unnoticed for days or months, it gradually enlarges and red colored rocks pile up. They discharge water, break down, and burst open into deep caves. Use *Guī Pí Tāng* F2-3 and the other herbs mentioned above. This can prolong the person's years [of life].
- If one mistakenly uses attacking herbs, great danger approaches.

大凡乳症，若因恚怒，宜疏肝清熱。焮痛寒熱，宜發表散邪。腫焮痛甚，宜清肝消毒，並隔蒜灸。不作膿，或膿不潰，補氣血為主。不收斂，或膿稀，補脾胃為主。膿出反痛，或發寒熱，補氣血為主。或晡熱內熱，補血為主。若飲食少思；或作嘔吐，補胃為主。飲食難化，或作泄瀉，補脾為主。勞碌腫痛，補氣血為主。怒氣腫痛，養肝血為主。兒口所吹，須吮通揉散。成癰，治以前法。潮熱暮熱，亦主前藥。

In breast conditions:

- If it is due to rage and anger, it is appropriate to course the liver and clear heat.
- For scorching pain with [sensations of] cold and heat, it is appropriate to express the exterior [promote sweating] and scatter evils.
- When swelling and scorching pain are severe, it is appropriate to clear the liver and disperse toxins; at the same time perform garlic-isolated moxibustion (F1-24).
- If it doesn't form pus or the pus does not exude, supplementing qì and blood governs the treatment.
- If it does not close up or the pus is thin, supplementing the spleen and stomach is governing.
- If it exudes pus but, contrary to expectations, there is pain or fever and chills, supplementing qì and blood is governing.
- If there is occasional late afternoon fever and internal heat, supplementing blood is governing.
- If there is little thought of food and drink or vomiting, supplementing the stomach is governing.
- If food and drink are difficult to transform [leading to undigested food in the stool] or if it becomes diarrhea, supplementing the spleen is governing.
- In taxation with swelling and pain, supplementing qì and blood is governing.
- If there is anger with swelling and pain, nourishing liver blood is governing.
- If it is blown on by the child's mouth, [the stagnant milk] must be sucked out and the breast kneaded to scatter it.

- If it develops into an abscess, treat using the above formulas.
- Tidal fevers with heat at dusk are also governed by the above herbs.

大抵男子多由房勞，耗傷肝腎。婦人鬱怒，虧損肝脾。治者審之。

Generally speaking, males often damage their liver and kidneys from bedroom taxation. Females harm their liver and spleen from constrained anger. Someone treating patients should know this.

（世以孕婦患此，名曰內吹。然其所致之因則一，惟用藥不可犯其胎耳。）

(For generations, when pregnant woman suffered this, they called it internal *blowing*.[49] Even though the cause is the same [as in women who are not pregnant], one should only use herbs that cannot assail the fetus.)

## 治驗
## Treatment Experience

**1-12-1**一婦人內熱脅脹，兩乳不時作痛，口內不時辛辣，若臥而起急，則臍下牽痛。此帶脈為患，用小柴胡加青皮、黃連、山梔二劑而瘥。

A woman had internal heat, rib-side distention, pain in both breasts at no particular time, and a hot spicy taste in her mouth at no particular time. If she got up quickly from lying down, she felt pain radiating downward from her umbilicus. This was an illness of the dài vessel. I used two doses of *Xiǎo Chái Hú Tāng* [F2-12] adding *qīng pí, huáng lián,* and *zhī zǐ* and she got better.

49. One of the causes of breast abscess was said to be the baby blowing wind on the breast [mentioned above]. It is called *internal blowing* in a pregnant woman because the fetus is still inside the mother.

**1-12-2**一婦人因怒兩乳腫，兼頭痛寒熱，用人參敗毒散二劑，表症已退；用小柴胡加芎、歸、枳殼、桔梗，四劑而消。

Due to anger, both of a woman's breasts were swollen. At the same time she had headaches and [sensations of] cold and heat. I used two doses of *Rén Shēn Bài Dú Sǎn* F1-31 and the exterior pattern ceased; I used four doses of *Xiǎo Chái Hú Tāng* F2-12 adding *chuān xiōng, dāng guī, zhǐ qiào,* and *jié gěng* and the swelling dispersed.

**1-12-3**一婦人久鬱，右乳內腫硬，用八珍湯加遠志、貝母、柴胡、青皮及隔蒜灸，兼服神效栝蔞散，兩月餘而消。

A woman had constraint for a long time. There was swelling and hardness inside her right breast. I used *Bā Zhēn Tāng* F2-8 adding *yuǎn zhì, bèi mǔ, chái hú,* and *qīng pí* as well as garlic-isolated moxibustion [on the lump]. At the same time she took *Shén Xiào Guā Lóu Sǎn* F1-36 and it dispersed after more than two months.

**1-12-4**一婦人左乳內腫如桃，不痛不赤，發熱漸瘦，用八珍加香附、遠志、青皮、柴胡百餘劑，又兼服神效瓜蔞散三十餘劑，膿潰而愈。

There was a swelling the size of a peach[50] inside a woman's left breast. It was not red or painful. She had fever and gradually lost weight. I used more than a hundred doses of *Bā Zhēn Tāng* F2-8 adding *xiāng fù, yuǎn zhì, qīng pí,* and *chái hú*. Later she took more than thirty doses of *Shén Xiào Guā Lóu Sǎn* F1-36 at the same time [as the other formula]. Pus exuded and she recovered.

**1-12-5**一婦人鬱久，左乳內結核如杏許，三月不消，心脈澀而脾脈大，按之無力，以八珍加貝母、遠志、香附、柴胡、青皮、桔梗，五十餘劑而潰，又三十餘劑而愈。

A woman who had constraint for a long time developed a nodule about the size of an almond in her left breast. It did not diserse for three months. Her heart pulse was rough and the spleen pulse was large but forceless when pressed. She took more than fifty doses of *Bā Zhēn Tāng* F2-8 adding *bèi mǔ, yuǎn zhì, xiāng fù, chái hú, qīng pí,* and *jié gěng* and it burst open. She recovered after more than thirty additional doses.

50. Peaches were probably smaller in ancient times.

**1-12-6**一婦人稟實性躁，懷抱久鬱，左乳內結一核，按之微痛，以連翹飲子二十餘劑少退，更以八珍加青皮、香附、桔梗、貝母，二十餘劑而消。

A woman had constitutional excess and a restless temperament; she held onto constraint for a long time. A node was bound up inside her left breast; it was slightly painful when pressed. I used more than twenty doses of *Lián Qiáo Yǐn Zǐ* F1-33 and it decreased in size. I further used more than twenty doses of *Bā Zhēn Tāng* F2-8 adding *qīng pí, xiāng fù, jié gěng,* and *bèi mǔ* and it dispersed.

**1-12-7**一婦人發熱作渴，至夜尤甚，兩乳忽腫，肝脈洪數，乃熱入血室也，用加味小柴胡湯，熱止腫消。

A woman had fever that made her thirsty; when night arrived it was especially severe. Both breasts suddenly swelled up. Her liver pulse was surging and rapid so heat had entered the blood chamber. I used *Jiā Wèi Xiǎo Chái Hú Tāng* F2-13. The fever stopped and the swelling dispersed.

**1-12-8**一婦人因怒，左乳作痛發熱，表散太過，腫熱益甚，用益氣養榮湯，數劑熱止膿成，不從用針，腫脹熱渴，針膿大泄，仍以前湯，月餘始愈。

Due to anger, the left breast of a woman became painful and she had fever. She used exterior scattering herbs excessively and then the swelling and fever increased a lot. I used several doses of *Yì Qì Yǎng Róng Tāng* F1-27; the fever stopped and pus developed. She did not comply with the use of a needle,[51] and had swelling, distention, fever, and thirst. It was needled but the pus did not drain out. I continued to use the previous formula, and she began to recover after more than a month.

此症若膿成未破，有薄皮剝起者，用代針之劑，其膿自出。不若及時用針，不致大潰。若膿血未盡，輒用生肌，反助其邪。慎之！

In this condition, if pus develops but the abscess has not broken open and there is thin skin starting to peel off, use prescriptions to take the place of the needle; the pus will

51. This probably means she refused to have it lanced.

spontaneously discharge. If not, prompt use of the needle will not result in a large open sore. If pus and blood are not fully discharged, using herbs to engender flesh assists the evil, contrary to expectations. Be careful of this!

**1-12-9**一婦人因怒，左乳作痛，胸膈不利，以方脈流氣飲加木香、青皮，四劑而安。

Due to anger, a woman's left breast was painful, with inhibited chest and diaphragm. I used four doses of *Fāng Mài Liú Qì Yǐn Zǐ* F1-29 adding *mù xiāng* and *qīng pí* and she was peaceful.

**1-12-10**一婦人膿清腫硬，面黃食少，內熱晡熱，自汗盜汗，月經不行，此肝脾氣血俱虛，用十全大補加遠志、貝母及補中益氣，各三十餘劑，外用蔥熨患處，諸症尋愈。

A woman had clear pus in a hard swelling, yellow face, reduced food intake, internal heat, late afternoon fever, spontaneous sweating, night sweating, and her menstruation did not move. This was qì and blood deficiency of the liver and spleen. I used more than thirty doses each of *Shí Quán Dà Bǔ Tāng* F2-7 adding *yuǎn zhì* and *bèi mǔ* as well as *Bǔ Zhōng Yì Qì Tāng* F2-5. Externally I ironed the affected site with scallions [see *Shén Xiào Cōng Yùn Fǎ* F1-25], and the various symptoms recovered soon after.

**1-12-11**一婦人膿成脹痛，余欲針之，不從，數日始針，出敗膿三四碗許，虛症蜂起，幾至危殆，用大補兩月餘而安。

A woman developed pus with distention and pain. I wanted to needle it but she would not comply. It was several days before she let me needle it and about three or four bowlfuls of conquered pus were discharged. Deficiency symptoms arose in swarms and several reached a dangerous state. I used *Shí Quán Dà Bǔ Tāng* F2-7 for more than two months and she was peaceful.

若元氣虛弱，不作膿者，用益氣養榮湯補之，膿成即針。若腫痛寒熱，怠惰食少，或至夜熱甚，用補中益氣湯兼逍遙散，補之為善。

- If original qì is deficient and weak, and it does not develop pus, supplement with *Yì Qì Yǎng Róng Tāng* F1-27; when it develops pus, needle it.
- If there is swelling, pain, [sensations of] cold and heat, laziness, and reduced food intake, or if the nighttime fevers become severe, it is good to supplement with *Bǔ Zhōng Yì Qì Tāng* F2-5 and *Xiāo Yáo Sǎn* F2-2 at the same time.

**1-12-12**一產婦因乳少，服藥通之，致乳房腫脹，發熱作渴，以玉露散補之而愈。

A woman who had given birth took herbs to free the flow for scant milk. This resulted in breast swelling and distention with fever that led to thirst. I supplemented her with *Yù Lù Sǎn* F1-10 and she recovered.

夫乳汁乃氣血所化，在上為乳，在下為經。若沖任之脈盛，脾胃之氣壯，則乳汁多而濃，衰則淡而少，所乳之子，亦弱而多病。又有屢產無乳，或大便澀滯，乃亡津液也，當滋化源。

Now, breast milk is transformed from qì and blood; when [qì and blood] are above they becomes milk and when below they becomes menstruation. If the chōng and rèn vessels fill up and spleen-stomach qì is vigorous, there is plenty of milk and it is thick; if they are debilitated, it is thin and scant. A child who is nursed with it will also become weak and frequently ill. Women who repeatedly give birth may have no milk and sometimes their bowel movement is rough and stagnant; this is collapse of *jīnyè*-fluids. One should nourish and transform the source.

**1-12-13**一婦人右乳內結三核，年餘不消，朝寒暮熱，飲食不甘。此乳岩，以益氣養榮湯，百餘劑，血氣漸復，更以木香餅熨之，喜其謹疾，年餘而消。

A woman had three nodes bound up inside her right breast. They did not disperse for more than a year. She was cold in the mornings and hot in the evenings. Food and drink did not taste sweet. This was breast rocks. I used more than a hundred doses of *Yì Qì Yǎng Róng Tāng* F1-27 and her blood and qì gradually returned. I further ironed it with *Mù Xiāng Bǐng* F1-23. Happily this took care of her disease and it dispersed after more than a year.

**1-12-14**至英内年二十有五，素虛弱，多鬱怒。時疫後，脾胃愈虛，飲食愈少，又值氣忿，右乳脅下紅腫，膺內作痛。用炒麩皮熨之，腫雖少散，內痛益甚，轉側胸中，如物懸墜，遂與加減四物湯，內腫如鵝卵，外大如盤，胸脅背心相引而痛，夜熱勢甚。

I am Yóu Zhìyīng; my wife was twenty-five years old at the time this happened. She was usually deficient and weak and she had a lot of constrained anger. After a seasonal epidemic, her spleen and stomach were even more deficient. She ate and drank little and then she happened to get angry again. Her right breast and the region below her rib-side became red and swollen with pain inside her bosom. It was ironed with stir-fried wheat bran (*fū pí*). Although the swelling scattered a little, the pain inside increased a lot, moving about inside her chest like something was suspended and sagging. Someone then gave her *Jiā Jiǎn Sì Wù Tāng* [*Jiā Wèi Sì Wù Tāng* F2-52 or a different modification of *Sì Wù Tāng* F2-51]. Inside, the swelling grew to the size of a goose egg; outside the affected site was the size of a plate. Pain radiated through her chest, rib-sides, upper back, and heart; at night the heat was extreme.

時治者皆以攻毒為言。叩諸先生，乃云：此病後脾弱，而復怒傷肝，治法惟主於健脾氣，平肝火，則腫自消，而病自愈矣。《聖惠方》以八物加陳皮、黃耆、柴胡、山梔、白芷，服八劑，病減六七；去白芷加青皮、木香、桔梗，又六劑而痊愈。奏功之奇，獲效之速，蓋出於尋常萬萬也。感激濃恩，昕夕不忘，錄此乞附醫案，以詔後之患者，毋為攻毒者之所惑也。

At the time, the people treating her all talked about attacking toxins. I invited various doctors. [Xuē Jǐ] then said: The spleen was weak after this [seasonal epidemic] disease and on top of that, anger damaged the liver. When the treatment method is governed soley by strengthening spleen qì and leveling liver fire, the swelling will automatically disperse and the disease will automatically recover. We used *Bā Wù Tāng* from *Shèng Huì Fāng*[52] adding *chén pí, huáng qí, chái hú, zhī zǐ,* and *bái zhǐ*. She took eight doses and the disease decreased to six or seven [out of ten]; we removed *bái zhǐ* and added *qīng pí, mù xiāng,* and *jié gěng*. She completely recovered after another six doses. The extraordinary effectivenss and the speed of efficacy surpassed the usual [results from other doctors] by

52. This formula is not found in *Shèng Huì Fāng*. *Bā Wù Tāng* is an alternate name for *Bā Zhēn Tāng* F2-8 or it could refer to *Fù Zǐ Bā Wù Tāng* F2-77 but neither formula is from from *Shèng Huì Fāng*. *Shèng Huì Fāng* refers to *Tài Píng Shèng Huì Fāng*《太平聖惠方》(Sagely Formulas for Universal Relief from the Era of Great Peace), written for the *Sòng* dynasty government.

ten-thousand times ten-thousand. I am grateful for your deep kindness which will not be forgotton from dawn to sunset. I record this appended medical case to instruct later people who suffer: Do not be mislead by people who want to attack toxins.

晚生尤至英頓首再拜書

I, Yóu Zhìyīng, respectfully wrote this bowing twice

**1-12-15**一婦人乳内結核年餘，晡熱少食，余欲用益氣養榮湯治之；彼以為緩，乃服行氣之劑，其勢愈甚，潰而日出清膿而歿 。

A woman had a nodule inside her breast for more than a year, with late afternoon fever and reduced food intake. I wanted to treat it with *Yì Qì Yǎng Róng Tāng* [F1-27]. She thought this was [too] slow-acting so she took a prescription to move qì. The situation became more severe. It burst open and every day it discharged clear pus until she died.

**1-12-16**郭氏妾，乃放出宮女，乳内結一核如栗，亦服流氣等藥，大如覆碗，堅硬如石，出水而歿 。

Mister Guō's concubine was a released palace maiden. She had a node the size of a chestnut bound up inside her breast. She also took herbs of the type that makes qì flow and then the node enlarged to the size of an overturned bowl and became hard as a rock. It discharged water and she died.

# 《女科撮要·卷上·血風瘡》
## 1-13 Blood Wind Sores

婦人血風瘡，因肝脾二經風熱鬱火血燥所致。其外症身發疙瘩；或如丹毒，癢痛不常，搔破成瘡，膿水淋漓。其內症月經無定，小便不調，夜熱內熱，自汗盜汗，惡寒憎寒，肢體倦怠，飲食不甘，寒熱往來。

Blood wind sores in women are due to wind heat in both the liver and spleen channels with constrained fire and blood dryness. The external symptoms include eruptions of swellings on the body. Some are similar to cinnabar toxins with itching and pain at times; they break open when scratched and become sores with pus trickling out. The internal symptoms include menstruation that does not occur at fixed times, out of tune urination, nighttime fevers, internal heat, spontaneous sweating, night sweating, aversion to cold, hating coldness, weariness of the body, food and drink do not taste sweet, and alternating fever and chills.

若發熱作痛，乃肝經風熱血燥，用當歸飲加柴胡、山梔。若體倦食少，口乾潮熱，乃肝脾鬱火傷血，用加味逍遙散。若疙瘩痛癢，寒熱往來，乃肝經風熱傷血，用小柴胡加山梔、黃連。若夜間發熱，作渴譫語，乃熱入血室，用小柴胡加生地黃；血虛，四物合小柴胡湯。若無寐盜汗，內熱晡熱，乃脾經血虛，用歸脾湯；兼寒熱，加山梔、熟地。若用風藥，復傷陰血，反致他症。

- If feverish and painful, it is wind heat of the liver channel with blood dryness; use *Dān Guī Yǐn* F1-12 adding *chái hú* and *zhī zǐ*.
- If the body is weary, eating little, dry mouth, and tidal fevers, it is constrained fire of the liver and spleen damaging blood; use *Jiā Wèi Xiāo Yáo Sǎn* F2-1.
- If there are swellings that are painful and itch with alternating fever and chills, it is wind heat of the liver channel damaging blood; use *Xiǎo Chái Hú Tāng* F2-12 adding *zhī zǐ* and *huáng lián*.
- If there are fevers at night with thirst and delirious speech, it is heat entering the blood chamber; use *Xiǎo Chái Hú Tāng* F2-12 adding *shēng dì huáng*;
    - With blood deficiency, use *Sì Wù Tāng* F2-51 combined with *Xiǎo Chái Hú Tāng* F2-12.

- If there is insomnia, night sweating, internal heat, and late afternoon fever, it is blood deficiency of the spleen channel; use *Guī Pí Tāng* F2-3;
    - With [sensations of] cold and heat at the same time, add *zhī zǐ* and *shú dì huáng*.

If you use herbs for wind, it will repeatedly damage yīn blood, and contrary to expectations, it will result in other symptoms.

## 治驗
## Treatment Experience

**1-13-1**一婦人素清苦，四肢患此，誤用敗毒寒涼，晡熱內熱，自汗盜汗，月經不行，口乾咽燥，此鬱結傷脾，四肢者脾主之，用歸脾湯數劑，後兼逍遙散，五十餘劑而愈。

A woman was poor but clean and honest. She suffered this on all four limbs and mistakenly used cold and cool herbs to conquer toxins. She had late afternoon fever, internal heat, spontaneous sweating, and night sweating. Her menstruation did not move and her mouth and throat were dry. This was binding constraint damaging the spleen. The spleen governs the four limbs. I used several doses of *Guī Pí Tāng* F2-3. Later I used *Guī Pí Tāng* F2-3 along with *Xiāo Yáo Sǎn* F2-2 for more than fifty doses and she recovered.

**1-13-2**一婦人性躁，寒熱口苦，脅痛耳鳴，腹脹溺澀年餘矣，症屬肝火，用四君加柴胡、炒山梔、炒龍膽數劑，乃與逍遙散兼服而瘡愈，又與六味丸及逍遙散，七十餘劑，諸症悉退。

A woman was impetuous by temperament. For more than a year, she had [sensations of] cold and heat, bitter mouth, rib-side pain, tinnitus, abdominal distention, and rough urination. These symptoms belong to liver fire. I used several doses of *Sì Jūn Zǐ Tāng* F2-26 adding *chái hú*, stir-fried *zhī zǐ*, and stir-fried *lóng dǎn cǎo*. I then gave her *Xiāo Yáo Sǎn* F2-2 to take at the same time and the sores recovered. I then gave her more than seventy doses of *Liù Wèi Wán* F2-16 and *Xiāo Yáo Sǎn* F2-2. All her symptoms receded.

若有愈後身起白屑，搔則肌膚如帛所隔，此氣血虛不能營於腠理，用大補之劑。若有愈後發熱，身起疙瘩癢痛，搔破膿水淋漓，經候不調，此肝火血熱，用四物加柴胡、山梔、白朮、茯苓、丹皮、甘草。

- After recovery, if white flakes arise on the body and it feels like the muscles and skin are covered with silk cloth when scratching, this is qì and blood deficiency with inability to nourish the *còu lǐ*; use strongly supplementing prescriptions.
- After recovery, it is liver fire with blood heat if there is fever with bumps arising on the body that itch and are painful; they break open when scratched and pus-water trickles out. The timing of menstruation is also out of tune; use *Sì Wù Tāng* F2-51 adding *chái hú, zhī zǐ, bái zhú, fú líng, mǔ dān pí,* and *gān cǎo.*

**1-13-3**一婦人日晡身癢，月餘口乾，又月餘成瘡，服袪風之劑，膿水淋漓，午前畏寒，午後發熱，殊類風症。余謂此肝經鬱火，外邪所搏，用補中益氣加山梔、鉤藤，又以逍遙散加川芎、貝母而愈。

A woman's body itched at sundown. For more than a month she had dry mouth. Sores had also developed for more than a month. She took prescriptions to dispel wind and then pus-water trickled. Before noon she feared cold and after noon she had fever. This is a specific type of wind pattern I call *constrained fire of the liver channel wrestling with external evils.* I used *Bǔ Zhōng Yì Qì Tāng* F2-5 adding *zhī zǐ* and *gōu téng.* I then used *Xiāo Yáo Sǎn* F2-2 adding *chuān xiōng* and *bèi mǔ* and she recovered.

**1-13-4**一婦人瘙癢，發熱，日晡益甚，膚見赤痕，月經過期。此血虛有熱，以逍遙散倍加熟地，熱止癢退，更以四物加柴胡、參、耆、炙草、茯苓，調理遂愈。

A woman had itching and fever that increased a lot at sunset. Red marks appeared on her skin and her menstrual period was late. This was blood deficiency with heat. I used *Xiāo Yáo Sǎn* F2-2 adding a double dose of *shú dì huáng.* The heat stopped and the itching receded. I further used *Sì Wù Tāng* F2-51 adding *chái hú, rén shēn, huáng qí, zhì gān cǎo,* and *fú líng* to attune and rectify and then recovered.

**1-13-5**一女子十二歲，善怒，遍身作癢，用柴胡、川芎、山梔、芍藥以清肝火，以生地、當歸、黃芩涼肝血，以白朮、茯苓、甘草健脾土而愈。半載後，遍身起赤痕，或時眩暈，此肝火熾甚，血得熱而妄行，是夜果經至。

A twelve year old girl tended to get angry. She itched all over her entire body. I used *chái hú, chuān xiōng, zhī zǐ,* and *sháo yào* to clear liver fire. I used *shēng dì huáng, dāng guī,* and *huáng qín* to cool liver blood. I used *bái zhú, fú líng,* and *gān cǎo* to strengthen spleen earth and she recovered. Half a year later, red marks arose over her entire body and sometimes she was dizzy. This was intense blazing of liver fire. The blood became hot and moved recklessly. That night it resulted in the arrival of her [first] menstrual period.

## 《女科撮要·卷上·臁瘡》
## 1-14 Shank Sores (*lián chuāng*)

婦人兩臁生瘡；或因胎產，飲食失宜，傷損脾胃；或因憂思鬱怒，虧損肝脾，以致濕熱下注；或外邪所侵。外臁屬足三陽可治，內臁屬足三陰難治。

Sometimes sores engendered on the shanks of women are due to pregnancy and childbirth when food and drink are inappropriate, damaging the spleen and stomach; or they are due to worry, thought, and constrained anger which enfeeble the liver and spleen and result in damp heat pouring downward; or attack by external evils. Lateral shank sores belong to the three yáng channels and are treatable; medial shank sores belong to the three yīn channels and are difficult to treat.

若初起發腫赤痛，屬濕毒所乘，用人參敗毒或檳蘇敗毒散。若漫腫作痛；或不腫不痛，屬脾虛濕熱下注，用補中益氣或八珍湯。若膿水淋漓，體倦少食，內熱口乾，屬脾氣虛弱，用補中益氣加茯苓、酒炒芍藥。若午後頭目不清，屬陰火，用前湯加酒炒黑黃柏。若午後發熱體倦，屬血虛，用前湯加川芎、熟地。若懷抱不樂而甚，用歸脾湯加山梔、柴胡。若恚怒氣逆而甚，用補中益氣加川芎、山梔。若內熱體倦，痰涎口瘡，屬脾腎虛熱，用六味丸。若肢體畏寒，飲食少思，屬脾腎虛寒，用八味丸。

- If there is swelling, redness, and pain during the initial eruption, it corresponds to damp toxins taking advantage; use *Rén Shēn Bài Dú Sǎn* F1-31 or *Bīng Sū Bài Dú Sǎn* UF-5.
- If there is fullness with or without swelling and pain, it belongs to spleen deficiency with damp heat pouring downward; use *Bǔ Zhōng Yì Qì Tāng* F2-5 or *Bā Zhēn Tāng* F2-8.
- If pus-water trickles out and the body is weary with reduced food intake, internal heat, and dry mouth, it belongs to deficient spleen and weak qì; use *Bǔ Zhōng Yì Qì Tāng* F2-5 adding *fú líng* and *sháo yào* stir-fried with liquor.
- If the head and eyes are not clear after noon, it belongs to yīn fire; use the previous decoction adding *huáng bǎi* stir-fried with liquor until black.
- If there is after noon fever and weariness of the body, it belongs to blood deficiency; use the previous decoction adding *chuān xiōng* and *shú dì huáng*.
- If she is holding onto unhappiness and the condition is severe; use *Guī Pí Tāng* F2-3 adding *zhī zǐ* and *chái hú*.
- If rage and anger make qì counterflow and the condition is severe; use *Bǔ Zhōng Yì Qì Tāng* F2-5 adding *chuān xiōng* and *zhī zǐ*.
- If there is internal heat, weariness of the body, phlegm drool, and mouth sores, it belongs to deficient hot spleen and kidneys; use *Liù Wèi Wán* F2-16.
- If her body fears cold with little thought of food and drink, it belongs to deficient cold spleen and kidneys; use *Bā Wèi Wán* F2-17.

大抵色赤屬熱毒易治，色黯屬脾腎虛寒難治，設誤用攻伐，復傷胃氣，難保其生。

Generally speaking, red color belongs to heat toxins and is easy to treat; a dull color belongs to deficient cold spleen and kidneys and is difficult to treat. If you mistakenly use attacking herbs, you repeatedly damage stomach qì and it is difficult to protect her life.

## 治驗
## Treatment Experience

**1-14-1**一婦人患之，四畔微赤，作痛重墜，膿水淋漓，胸膈不利，飲食少思，內熱口苦，夜間少寐，此屬脾虛鬱傷。用歸脾湯解鬱結而生脾血，用補中益氣加茯苓、半夏補脾氣而除濕熱，尋愈。

A woman suffered this condition. The sores were slightly red all around and painful. They [felt like they] were heavy and sagging and they trickled pus-water. She had inhibited chest and diaphragm, little thought of food and drink, internal heat, bitter mouth, and little sleep at night. This belonged to spleen deficiency damaged by constraint. I used *Guī Pí Tāng* F2-3 to resolve binding constraint and engender spleen blood. I used *Bŭ Zhōng Yì Qì Tāng* F2-5 adding *fú líng* and *bàn xià* to supplement spleen qì and eliminate damp heat and she recovered soon after.

**1-14-2**一婦人久不愈，色赤微熱，日晡焮腫，形體虛弱，飲食少思，勞則喘渴，惡寒發熱，此脾虛下陷，用補中益氣湯而愈。

A woman had this for a long time without recovering. The sores were red and slightly hot. They flared up and became swollen at sundown. Her body was deficient and weak with little thought of food and drink. When taxed, she panted, was thirsty, and had aversion to cold and fever. This was spleen deficiency with downward sinking. I used *Bŭ Zhōng Yì Qì Tāng* F2-5 and she recovered.

**1-14-3**一婦人三年矣，色黯腫硬，惡寒發熱，飲食少思，形體消瘦，作渴飲湯；飲食稍多，或腹脹，或泄瀉，或作嘔，或吞酸，此脾氣虛寒。用補中益氣加乾薑、肉桂，五十餘劑而愈。

For three years a woman had a dull complexion, hard swellings, aversion to cold and fever, and little thought of food and drink. Her body became emaciated and she was thirsty for hot liquids. If she ate and drank a little excessively, she would sometimes have abdominal distention, or diarrhea, or vomiting, or sour swallowing. This was deficient cold spleen qì. I used more than fifty doses of *Bŭ Zhōng Yì Qì Tāng* F2-5 adding *gān jiāng* and *ròu guì*, and she recovered.

**1-14-4**一婦人因入朝步履，惡寒發熱，倦怠懶食，瘡口出血。此勞傷元氣，不能攝血歸經，用補中益氣湯而愈。

A woman [had this type of sores] because she went for an audience to the imperial court on foot;[53] she had aversion to cold, fever, was weary, ate lazily, and the opening of the sores bled. This was taxation damaging original qì with inability to contain the blood and return it to the channel. I used *Bǔ Zhōng Yì Qì Tāng* F2-5 and she recovered.

**1-14-5**一婦人因怒，寒熱頭眩，或耳項胸脅脹痛，或小腹陰道悶墜，或小便頻數下血。此屬肝火血熱，先用小柴胡湯加炒黑山梔、川芎、當歸、車前，二劑諸症頓退；又用加味逍遙散，補其陰血而愈。後因飲食勞倦，前症復作，瘡口出血，用補中益氣湯治之而愈。

Due to anger a woman had [sensations of] cold and heat and dizzy head; she sometimes had distention and pain of her ears, nape, chest, and rib-sides; or [feelings of] oppression and sagging in her lower abdomen and vagina; or frequent urination with blood in it. This belonged to liver fire and blood heat. I first used two doses of *Xiǎo Chái Hú Tāng* F2-12 adding *zhī zǐ* that was stir-fried until black, *chuān xiōng, dāng guī,* and *chē qián zǐ* and all symptoms immediately receded; I then used *Jiā Wèi Xiāo Yáo Sǎn* F2-1 to supplement her yīn blood and she recovered. Later due to dietary indiscretions and taxation, the previous symptoms relapsed and the opening of the sores bled. I treated her with *Bǔ Zhōng Yì Qì Tāng* F2-5 and she recovered.

**1-14-6**一婦人患將兩月，焮赤腫痛，小便頻數，飲食如常，用活命飲二劑，諸症悉愈，又用八珍湯而痊。

A woman suffered this for almost two months, with scorching redness, swelling, and pain. She had frequent urination but her eating and drinking were like normal. I used two doses of *Huó Mìng Yǐn* UF-6 and all symptoms completely recovered. I then used *Bā Zhēn Tāng* F2-8 and she recuperated.

53. Thanks to Jerome Jiang for explaining the significance of this: To have an audience with the emperor was not a casual event. Any woman who was allowed an audience must have been the wife of high ranking official. Noblewomen usually had easy lives at home, but for an audience, they needed to get up before sunrise and wait outside the palace for several hours. Then they walked long distances to enter the palace (probably on bound feet), and had to kneel for a long time. This must have been quite taxing for a woman who lived in luxury.

**1-14-7**一婦人患此焮痛，惡寒發熱，用檳蘇敗毒散，而寒熱退，用仙方活命飲，而焮痛止，再用補中益氣湯，而形氣健。

A woman suffered this with scorching pain, aversion to cold, and fever. I used *Bīng Sū Bài Dú Săn* UF-5, and the [sensations of] cold and heat receded. I used *Xiān Fāng Huó Mìng Yĭn* UF-6, and the scorching pain stopped. I then used *Bŭ Zhōng Yì Qì Tāng* F2-5 and her body's qì grew strong.

## 《女科撮要·卷上·陰瘡》
## 1-15 Genital sores (yīn sores)
## （交接出血、陰挺、陰癢、陰蟲附）
## (bleeding during intercourse, vaginal protrusion, itching genitals, and genital *chóng*-worms are appended)

婦人陰瘡，乃七情鬱火，傷損肝脾，濕熱下注。其外症有陰中舒出如蛇，俗呼陰挺；有翻突如餅，俗呼陰菌；亦有如雞冠花，亦有生諸蟲，亦有腫痛濕癢，潰爛出水，脹悶脫墜者。其內症口乾，內熱，體倦，經候不調，飲食無味，晡熱發熱，胸膈不利，脅肋不調，小腹痞脹，赤白帶下，小水淋澀。

Genital sores in women are due to the seven emotions and constrained fire damaging the liver and spleen with damp heat pouring downward. As for external symptoms, there are genitals that stretch out like snakes, commonly called vaginal protrusion; there are those inverted and protruding like a pancake, commonly called genital mushroom; there are also those appearing like a cock's comb. There are also some that engender various *chóng*-worms.[54] There are also those with swelling, pain, and damp itching that burst open and discharge water, with distention, oppression, prolapse, and [a feeling of] sagging. The internal symptoms include dry mouth, internal heat, and weariness of the body. The timing of menstruation gets out of tune and food and drink are flavorless. There is late afternoon fever, fevers [of other sorts], inhibited chest and diaphragm, mal-

54. The word *chóng* 蟲 has a much broader range of meaning then worms in English. It can include snakes, bugs, reptiles, and the like (creepy-crawlies), as well as some invisible disease-causing entities. Here these are genital sores where there is evidence of some kind of *chóng*-worms, visible or invisible.

adjusted rib-sides, *pǐ*-glomus and distention of the lower abdomen, red or white vaginal discharge, and dribbling rough urination.

其治法：腫痛者，宜用四物加柴胡、山梔、丹皮、膽草；濕癢者，宜用歸脾加山梔、丹皮、柴胡；淋澀者，宜用龍膽瀉肝加白朮、丹皮；潰腐者，宜用加味逍遙散；腫悶脫墜者，宜用補中益氣加山梔、丹皮。佐以外治之法，備見治驗。

The treatment method:

- For swelling and pain, it is appropriate to use *Sì Wù Tāng* F2-51 adding *chái hú, zhī zǐ, mǔ dān pí*, and *lóng dǎn cǎo.*
- For damp itching, it is appropriate to use *Guī Pí Tāng* F2-3 adding *zhī zǐ, mǔ dān pí* and *chái hú.*
- For rough dribbling urination, it is appropriate to use *Lóng Dǎn Xiè Gān Tāng* F1-13 adding *bái zhú* and *mǔ dān pí.*
- If festering, it is appropriate to use *Jiā Wèi Xiāo Yáo Sǎn* F2-1.
- For swelling, oppression, prolapse, and [a feeling of] sagging, it is appropriate to use *Bǔ Zhōng Yì Qì Tāng* F2-5 adding *zhī zǐ* and *mǔ dān pí.*

Assist with external treatment methods, described [below] in the treatment experience.

## 治驗
## Treatment Experience

**1-15-1**一婦人胸膈不利，內熱作渴，飲食不甘，肢體倦怠，陰中悶癢，小便赤澀，此鬱怒所致，用歸脾加山梔而愈。後因怒，患處並小腹脹痛，用小柴胡加山梔、芎、歸、芍藥而愈。但內熱晡熱，用逍遙散加山梔而愈。後因勞役發熱，患處腫脹，小便仍澀，用補中益氣加山梔、茯苓、丹皮而愈。

A woman had inhibited chest and diaphragm, internal heat, and thirst. Food and drink did not taste sweet and her body was weary. She had oppression and itching in her genitals and rough red urination. This was caused by constrained anger. I used *Guī Pí Tāng* F2-3 adding *zhī zǐ* and she recovered. Later due to anger, the affected site and her lower abdomen became distended and painful. I used *Xiǎo Chái Hú Tāng* F2-12 adding *zhī zǐ, chuān xiōng, dāng guī, sháo yào* and she recovered. Only internal heat and late afternoon fever were left. I used *Xiāo Yáo Sǎn* F2-2 adding *zhī zǐ* and she recovered. Later she developed fever due to taxation, with swelling and distention of the affected site and her urination was rough. I used *Bǔ Zhōng Yì Qì Tāng* F2-5 adding *zhī zǐ, fú líng,* and *mǔ dān pí* and she recovered.

**1-15-2** 一婦人陰中突出如菌，四圍腫痛，小便頻數，內熱晡熱，似癢似痛，小腹重墜。此肝脾鬱結之症，蓋肝火濕熱而腫痛，脾虛下陷而重墜也。先以補中益氣加山梔、茯苓、車前、青皮以清肝火升脾氣，漸愈。更以歸脾湯加山梔、茯苓、川芎調理，更以生豬脂和藜蘆末，塗之而收入。

The genitals of a woman protruded like a mushroom with swelling and pain all around it. She had frequent urination, internal heat, and late afternoon fever. The sensations were similar to itching or pain. Her lower abdomen [felt like it] was heavy and sagging. This was a pattern of binding constraint of the liver and spleen. It seems that liver fire with damp heat made the swelling and pain; spleen deficiency with downward sinking made the [feeling of] heaviness and sagging. I first used *Bǔ Zhōng Yì Qì Tāng* F2-5 adding *zhī zǐ, fú líng, chē qián zǐ,* and *qīng pí* to clear liver fire and ascend spleen qì. She gradually recovered. I further used *Guī Pí Tāng* F2-3 adding *zhī zǐ, fú líng,* and *chuān xiōng* to attune and rectify. I further blended fresh pig fat with lí lú powder; she spread it on the affected site and it gathered back in.

**1-15-3** 一婦人陰中挺出一條五寸許，悶痛重墜，水出淋漓，小便澀滯，夕與龍膽瀉肝湯分利濕熱，朝與補中益氣湯升補脾氣，諸症漸愈；再與歸脾加山梔、茯苓、川芎、黃柏，間服調理而愈。後因勞役或怒氣，下部濕癢，小水不利，仍用前藥即愈。

A woman's vagina protruded straight out by about five *cùn* with oppression and pain. [It felt like] it was heavy and sagging. Water trickled out and her urination was rough and stagnant. In the evenings I gave her *Lóng Dǎn Xiè Gān Tāng* F1-13 to divide and disinhibit damp heat; in the mornings I gave her *Bǔ Zhōng Yì Qì Tāng* F2-5 to ascend and supplement spleen qì. All her symptoms gradually recovered. I also used *Guī Pí Tāng* F2-3 adding *zhī zǐ, fú líng, chuān xiōng,* and *huáng bǎi.* This was to be taken between [the other two formulas] in order to attune and rectify her. She recovered but later, due to taxation or anger, she had damp itching of her lower parts and her urination was inhibited. I still used the previous herbs and she recovered.

亦有尺許者，亦有生諸蟲物者，皆用此治 。

There are also cases [where the vagina protrudes] about a *chǐ* (31.10 cm) and cases where various things resembling *chóng*-worms are engendered; this treatment can be used for all of them.

**1-15-4**一婦人潰，膿水淋漓，腫痛寒熱，小便赤澀，內熱作渴，肢體倦怠，胸脅不利，飲食少思，三月餘矣，用補中益氣，內柴胡 、升麻各用一錢，加茯苓一錢，炒山梔二錢，數劑少愈 。又與歸脾加山梔 、川芎 、茯苓，三十餘劑，諸症悉退 。惟內熱尚在，再與逍遙散倍用山梔而愈 。

For more than three months, a woman had an open sore; pus-water trickled with swelling and pain. She had [sensations of] cold and heat, rough red urination, internal heat, and thirst. Her body was weary with inhibited chest and rib-sides and little thought of food and drink. I used several doses of *Bǔ Zhōng Yì Qì Tāng* F2-5; within the formula I used one *qián* (3.73 grams) each of *chái hú* and *shēng má*, and I added one *qián* (3.73 grams) of *fú líng* and two *qián* (7.46 grams) of stir-fried *zhī zǐ*. She recovered a little. I then gave her more than thirty doses of *Guī Pí Tāng* F2-3 adding *zhī zǐ*, *chuān xiōng*, and *fú líng*, and all her symptoms receded. Only internal heat remained. I then used *Xiāo Yáo Sǎn* F2-2 doubling the *zhī zǐ* and she recovered.

**1-15-5** 一婦人素性急，陰內或痛，小便赤澀，怒則益甚，或發熱，或寒熱 。治以芎 、歸 、炒梔 、柴胡 、苓 、朮 、丹皮 、澤瀉 、炒芍 、炒車前 、炒連 、生草，數劑漸愈；乃去黃連 、澤瀉，又數劑而痊愈 。

A woman's temperament was impatient. She sometimes had genital pain and rough red urination. This increased a lot when she was angry. Sometimes she had fever or [sensations of] cold and heat. I treated her using several doses of *chuān xiōng*, *dāng guī*, stir-fried *zhī zǐ*, *chái hú*, *fú líng*, *bái zhú*, *mǔ dān pí*, *zé xiè*, stir-fried *sháo yào*, stir-fried *chē qián zǐ*, stir-fried *huáng lián*, and *shēng gān cǎo*, and she gradually recovered. I then gave her another several doses removing the *huáng lián* and *zé xiè* and she completely recovered.

**1-15-6** 一婦人素鬱悶，陰內痛癢，不時出水，飲食少思，肢體倦怠，用歸脾加丹皮 、山梔 、芍藥 、柴胡 、生草主之而安 。

A woman usually felt constrained and oppressed [or depressed]. She had pain and itching inside her genitals and discharged water at no particular time. She had little thought of food and drink and her body was weary. I used *Guī Pí Tāng* F2-3 adding *mǔ dān pí, zhī zǐ, sháo yào, chái hú,* and *shēng gān cǎo* to govern it and she was peaceful.

**1-15-7**一婦人陰內癢痛，內熱倦怠，飲食少思，用參、耆、歸、朮、陳皮、柴胡、炒梔、炒車前、升麻、芍藥、丹皮、茯苓，治之而瘥。

A woman had itching and pain inside her genitals and internal heat. She was weary and had little thought of food and drink. I treated her with *rén shēn, huáng qí, dāng guī, bái zhú, chén pí, chái hú,* stir-fried *zhī zǐ,* stir-fried *chē qián zǐ, shēng má, sháo yào, mǔ dān pí,* and *fú líng,* and she got better.

若陰中有蟲癢痛，亦屬肝木，以桃仁研膏，和雄黃末納陰中以殺之，仍用清肝解鬱。有以雞肝納之者，乃取蟲之法也。

- If there are *chóng*-worms with itching and pain in the genitals, this also belongs to liver wood. Grind *táo rén* into a paste, blend with powdered *xióng huáng* and insert it into her genitals to kill the *chóng*-worms. Further use herbs to clear liver heat and resolve constraint.
- The insertion of chicken livers is another method to go after the *chóng*-worms.

**1-15-8** 婦人交接違理，出血作痛，發熱口乾，誤服寒涼之劑，前症益甚，不時欲嘔，飲食少思。此症屬肝經，而藥復傷脾也。先用六君子加柴胡，而脾胃漸愈；乃用加味逍遙散，而患處亦痊。

A woman had intercourse that violated the principles,[55] and then had bleeding, pain, fever, and dry mouth. She mistakenly took a cold and cool prescription, and the above symptoms increased a lot. She felt like vomiting at no particular time and had little thought of food and drink. These symptoms belong to the liver channel, and the herbs

55. Certainly one would like to know more of the details, but unfortunately we are not told which principles were violated. There are many ways to violate sexual principles. Of course rough sex or coerced sex could cause bleeding due to trauma. Other meanings are possible. For example, frequent sex might damage yīn, making heat, which in turn could cause bleeding.

again damaged her spleen. First I used *Liù Jūn Zĭ Tāng* F2-6 adding *chái hú* and the spleen and stomach gradually recovered; I then used *Jiā Wèi Xiāo Yáo Săn* F2-1, and the affected site also recuperated.

**1-15-9**一婦人每交接，輒出血作痛，敷服皆涼血止痛之劑，不時出血甚多。此肝傷而不能藏血，脾傷而不能攝血也，用補中益氣、《濟生》歸脾二湯而愈。

Every time a woman had intercourse, there was bleeding and pain. She applied prescriptions topically and took prescriptions internally to cool blood and stop pain, but then she bled a lot at no particular time. This was liver damage with inability to store blood and spleen damage with inability to contain blood. I used two decoctions, *Bŭ Zhōng Yì Qì Tāng* F2-5 and *Jì Shēng Guī Pí Tāng* F2-3 and she recovered.

若交接出血，用熟艾熱裹入陰中。若交接違理而出血，用亂髮、青布燒為末敷之，血自止。若出血過多，而見他症，但用前藥，調補肝脾，諸症自愈矣。

- If there is bleeding during intercourse, put a heated bundle of moxa floss (*shú ài*) into the vagina.
- If intercourse violates the principles and there is bleeding, apply *luàn fā* and *qīng bù* that was burned into a powder. The bleeding will automatically stop.
- If there is a lot of bleeding but you see other symptoms, just use the above herbs to attune and supplement the liver and spleen; all the other symptoms will spontaneously recover.

**1-15-10**一婦人陰腫下墜，悶痛出水，胸腹不利，小便頻數，內熱晡熱，口苦耳鳴，先用小柴胡加車前、膽草、苓、朮、升麻，二劑稍緩，又用加味逍遙加升麻，數劑稍愈；乃以加味歸脾加升麻、柴胡，並補中益氣加山梔，數劑漸愈；仍用加味逍遙、加味歸脾二藥，調理而瘥。

A woman's genitals were swollen and she felt downward pressure [a term sometimes used for tenesmus] with oppression and pain. She discharged water and had inhibited chest and abdomen, frequent urination, internal heat, late afternoon fever, bitter mouth, and tinnitus. I first used two doses of *Xiăo Chái Hú Tāng* F2-12 adding *chē qián zĭ, lóng dăn cǎo*, *fú líng*, *bái zhú*, and *shēng má*, and it moderated a little. I then used several doses of *Jiā Wèi Xiāo Yáo Sǎn* F2-1 adding *shēng má* and she recovered a little. I then used several doses of *Jiā Wèi Guī Pí Tāng* F2-4 adding *shēng má* and *chái hú* and at the same time *Bǔ Zhōng Yì Qì Tāng* F2-5 adding *zhī zǐ*, and she gradually recovered. I further used two medicines, *Jiā Wèi Xiāo Yáo Sǎn* F2-1 and *Jiā Wèi Guī Pí Tāng* F2-4, to attune and rectify her and she got better.

**1-15-11**一婦人熱痛，用寒涼敗毒，飲食不入，時欲嘔吐，小腹重墜，似欲去後。此脾胃虧損，元氣下陷，症屬虛寒，先用補中益氣加炮薑二劑，重墜若失；再用前湯加茯苓、半夏，二十餘劑而愈；乃以歸脾少加柴胡、升麻、六味地黃丸，調理兩月餘而康。

A woman had heat and pain in her genitals. She used cold and cool herbs to conquer toxins, and then she did not eat or drink. She wanted to vomit at times, her lower abdomen [felt like it] was heavy and sagging, and she felt like she was about to have a bowel movement. This was spleen and stomach debility with original qì sinking downward. The symptoms belonged to deficiency cold. I first used two doses of *Bǔ Zhōng Yì Qì Tāng* F2-5 adding *pào jiāng* and the [feeling of] heaviness and sagging was lost; I then used more than twenty doses of the previous decoction adding *fú líng* and *bàn xià* and she recovered. I then used *Guī Pí Tāng* F2-3 adding a little *chái hú* and *shēng má*, and *Liù Wèi Dì Huáng Wán* F2-16 to attune and rectify her. she was healthy after more than two months.

> **Translators note:** The recipes for formulas that were found here at the end of Volume 1 in the original text have been moved. They are now located before the formulas for Volume 2 so that all formulas are given in the same section of our translation.

## Volume 2[56]

# 《女科撮要·卷下·保胎》

## 2-1 Preventing Miscarriage

妊娠若元氣不實，發熱倦怠；或胎動不安，用當歸散。因氣惱加枳殼，胸膈痞悶再加蘇梗；或作痛加柴胡。若飲食不甘或欲嘔吐，用六君加紫蘇、枳殼。若惡阻嘔逆，頭暈體倦，用參橘散；未應，用六君子湯。若惡阻嘔吐，不食煩悶，亦用參橘散之類。若頓仆胎動，腹痛下血，用膠艾湯；未應，用八珍加膠艾。若頓仆毒藥，腰痛短氣，用阿膠散；未應，煎送知母丸。若頓仆胎傷，下血腹痛，用佛手散；未應，用八珍送知母丸。

In pregnancy:

- If her original qì is not full, with fever and weariness, or if the fetus is stirring and is not peaceful, use *Dāng Guī Sǎn* F2-54.
    - If due to sullenness, add *zhǐ qiào*.
    - For *pǐ*-glomus with oppression of the chest and diaphragm, also add *sū gěng*.
    - Or with pain, add *chái hú*.
- If food and drink do not taste sweet or she feels like vomiting, use *Liù Jūn Zǐ Tāng* F2-6 adding *zǐ sū yè* and *zhǐ qiào*.
- If there is morning sickness with vomiting, dizziness, and weariness of the body, use *Shēn Jú Sǎn* F2-28.
    - If she does not respond, use *Liù Jūn Zǐ Tāng* F2-6.
- If there is morning sickness with vomiting and she does not eat, with vexation and oppression, also use formulas like *Shēn Jú Sǎn* F2-28.
- If she suddenly collapses with stirring fetus, abdominal pain, and bleeding from below, use *Jiāo Ài Tāng* F2-31.
    - If she does not respond, use *Bā Zhēn Tāng* F2-8 adding *ē jiāo* and *ài yè*.

56. Volume two covers diseases of pregnancy and the postpartum period. While many of these formulas may still be used today, the practitioner must determine if the treatment is appropriate in the light of our modern knowledge.

- If she suddenly collapses after using toxic herbs,[57] with low back pain, and shortness of breath, use *Ē Jiāo Sǎn* F2-32.
    - If she does not respond, boil *Ē Jiāo Sǎn* F2-32 and use it to swallow *Zhī Mǔ Wán* F2-35.
- If she suddenly collapses with fetal damage, bleeding from below, and abdominal pain, use *Fó Shǒu Sǎn* F1-22.
    - If she does not respond, use *Bā Zhēn Tāng* F2-8 to swallow *Zhī Mǔ Wán* F2-35.

若心驚膽怯，煩悶不安，名子煩，用竹葉湯；未應，血虛佐以四物，氣虛佐以四君。若下血不止，名胎漏，血虛用二黃散；血去多，用八珍湯；未應，用補中益氣湯。若因事而動下血，用枳殼湯加生熟地黃；未應；或作痛，更加當歸；血不止，八珍加膠艾。若不時作痛，若小腹重墜，名胎痛，用地黃當歸湯；未應，加參、朮、陳皮；或因脾氣虛，用四君加歸、地；中氣虛，用補中益氣湯。若面目虛浮，肢體如水氣，名子腫，用《全生》白朮散；未應，用六君子湯；下部腫甚，用補中益氣倍加茯苓。

- If the heart is frightened and the gallbladder is timid, with vexation and oppression, and [the fetus] is not peaceful, this is named *child vexation*; use *Zhú Yè Tāng* F2-29.
    - If she does not respond and there is blood deficiency, assist by using *Sì Wù Tāng* F2-51.
    - If there is qì deficiency, assist by using *Sì Jūn Zǐ Tāng* F2-26.
- If bleeding from below does not stop, this is named *leaky fetus.*
    - For blood deficiency use *Èr Huáng Sǎn* F2-34.
    - If a lot of blood is lost, use *Bā Zhēn Tāng* F2-8.
    - If she does not respond use *Bǔ Zhōng Yì Qì Tāng* F2-5.
- If [the fetus] stirs and she bleeds from below due to activity, use *Zhǐ Qiào Tāng* F2-33 adding *shēng* and *shú dì huáng.*
    - If she does not respond or there is pain, further add *dāng guī.*
    - If the bleeding does not stop, use *Bā Zhēn Tāng* F2-8 adding *ē jiāo* and *ài yè.*
- If there is pain at no particular time, and if her lower abdomen [feels like it] is heavy and sagging, this is named *fetal pain*; use *Dì Huáng Dāng Guī Tāng* F2-36.

57. This statement is curious. At times 'toxic herbs' simply means herbal medicine, acknowledging that herbs may have side effects (unlike dietary therapy or acupuncture-moxibustion). Here it seems to mean something more than that. Perhaps she accidentally took herbs that were too strong or perhaps she tried to induce an abortion or even commit suicide with herbs.

- If she does not respond, add *rén shēn, bái zhú,* and *chén pí.*
- Or if it is due to spleen qì deficiency, use *Sì Jūn Zǐ Tāng* F2-26 adding *dāng guī* and *dì huáng.*
- For central qì deficiency, use *Bǔ Zhōng Yì Qì Tāng* F2-5.

- If there is deficiency puffiness of the face and eyes and the body seems llike it has water qì, this is named *child swelling;* use *Quán Shēng Bái Zhú Sǎn* UF-8.
  - If she does not respond use *Liù Jūn Zǐ Tāng* F2-6.
  - If swelling of the lower body is severe, use *Bǔ Zhōng Yì Qì Tāng* F2-5 adding a double dose of *fú líng.*

或因飲食失宜，嘔吐泄瀉，此是脾胃虧損，用六君子湯 。若足指發腫，漸至腿膝，喘悶不安；或足指縫出水，名水氣，用天仙藤散；脾胃虛弱，兼以四君子；未應，用補中益氣，兼以逍遙散 。若胎氣上攻，心腹脹滿作痛，名子懸，用紫蘇飲；飲食不甘，兼四君子；內熱晡熱，兼逍遙散 。若小便澀少；或成淋瀝，名子淋，用安榮散；不應，兼八珍湯；腿足轉筋，而小便不利，急用八味丸，緩則不救 。若項強筋攣，語澀痰盛，名子癇，用羚羊角散 。或飲食停滯，腹脹嘔吐，此是脾胃虛弱，而不能消化，用六君子湯；不應，用平胃散加參 、苓 。

- If there is vomiting and diarrhea due to inappropriate diet, this is enfeebled spleen and stomach; use *Liù Jūn Zǐ Tāng* F2-6.
- If the toes swell up, and the swelling gradually reaches the legs and knees, with panting, oppression, and [the fetus] is not peaceful, or water is discharged from the crevices of the toes, this is named *water qì*; use *Tiān Xiān Téng Sǎn* F2-38.
  - If the spleen and stomach are deficient and weak, use *Sì Jūn Zǐ Tāng* F2-26 at the same time.
  - If she does not respond, use *Bǔ Zhōng Yì Qì* F2-5 with *Xiāo Yáo Sǎn* F2-2 at the same time.
- If fetal qì attacks upward, with distention, fullness, and pain of the heart region and abdomen, this is named *child suspension*; use *Zǐ Sū Yǐn* F2-30.
  - If food and drink do not taste sweet, take *Sì Jūn Zǐ Tāng* F2-26 at the same time.
  - If there is internal heat and late afternoon fever, take *Xiāo Yáo Sǎn* F2-2 at the same time.
- If there is rough scant urination, or it becomes trickling, this is named *child lín*; use *Ān Róng Sǎn* F2-39.
  - If she does not respond, take *Bā Zhēn Tāng* F2-8 at the same time.

- If the legs and feet twitch or cramp up, and urination is inhibited, quickly use *Bā Wèi Wán* F2-17. If you are slow, you cannot save her.
- If the neck is rigid and there are convulsions, with difficult speech and abundant phlegm, this is named *child epilepsy*; use *Líng Yáng Jiǎo Sǎn* F2-40.
- Or if there is food retention, abdominal distention, and vomiting, it is deficient weak spleen and stomach with inability to disperse and transform; use *Liù Jūn Zǐ Tāng* F2-6.
    - If she does not respond use *Píng Wèi Sǎn* F2-64 adding *rén shēn* and *fú líng*.

或胎作脹；或腹作痛，此是脾胃氣虛，而不能承載，用安胎飲加升麻、白朮；不應，用補中益氣湯。或臍腹作脹；或小便淋閉，此是脾胃氣虛，胎壓尿泡，四物加二陳、參、朮，空心服後探吐，藥出氣定，又服又吐，數次必安。或因勞役所傷；或食煎炒，小便帶血，此是血得熱而流於脬中，宜清膀胱，用逍遙散。或遺尿不禁；或為頻數，此是肝火血熱，用加味逍遙散。若胸滿腹脹，小便不通，遍身浮腫，名胎水不利，用鯉魚湯；脾胃虛，佐以四君子。

- Perhaps the fetus makes distention or there is abdominal pain; this is spleen and stomach qì deficiency with inability to bear the weight [of the fetus]; use *Ān Tāi Yǐn* F2-41 adding *shēng má* and *bái zhú*.
    - If she does not respond use *Bǔ Zhōng Yì Qì Tāng* F2-5.
- Perhaps the umbilical region and abdomen are distended or urination dribbles and is blocked; this is spleen and stomach qì deficiency so the fetus presses on the urinary function; use *Sì Wù Tāng* F2-51 adding *Èr Chén Tāng* F2-42, *rén shēn* and *bái zhú*. Take it on an empty stomach and then promote vomiting [by stimulating the gag reflex]; when the herbs come back out the qì will settle. Take it again and vomit again; after several times she will be peaceful.
- Perhaps urination brings bleeding due to damage from taxation or eating stir-fried foods; this is heat in the blood so blood flows from inside the bladder. It is appropriate to clear heat from the urinary bladder; use *Xiāo Yáo Sǎn* F2-2.
- Perhaps there is urinary incontinence or frequent urination; this is liver fire with blood heat; use *Jiā Wèi Xiāo Yáo Sǎn* F2-1.
- If there is chest fullness, abdominal distention, urine does not pass, and superficial swelling of the entire body, this is named inhibited fetal water; use *Lǐ Yú Tāng* F2-44.
    - With spleen and stomach deficiency, assist with *Sì Jūn Zǐ Tāng* F2 26.

病名同而形症異，形症異而病名同，聊見本方。凡用見症之藥，不應，當分月經治之。

The names of the diseases may be the same but the physical symptoms are different, or the physical symptoms may be different but the names of the diseases are the same; rely on what you see for the root formula. Whenever the patient does not respond after you have used herbs for the symptoms you see, treat it by differentiating her menstruation.[58]

## 治驗
## Treatment Experience

**2-1-1**一妊娠三月，其經若來三五次，但不多，飲食、精神如故。此血盛有餘，兒大能飲，自不來矣，果然。

A woman was three months pregnant. It seemed like her menstrual period came three or five times, but there was not a lot [of bleeding]. Her eating, drinking, and *jīng-shén* were the same as before. This was abundant blood that had a surplus. When the fetus grows larger and is able to drink it, the bleeding will spontaneously stop. As expected, this came to pass.

**2-1-2**一妊娠六月，每怒氣便見血，甚至寒熱頭痛，脅脹腹痛，作嘔少食。余謂寒熱頭痛，肝火上沖也；脅脹腹痛，肝氣不行也；作嘔少食，肝侮脾胃也；小便見血，肝火血熱也。用小柴胡加芍藥、炒黑山梔、茯苓、白朮而愈。

A woman was six months pregnant. She bled every time she got angry. When it was severe, she had [sensations of] cold and heat, headache, rib-side distention, abdominal pain, vomiting, and reduced food intake. I said the [sensations of] cold and heat and headache were due to liver fire surging upward; rib-side distention and abdominal pain were due to non-movement of liver qì; vomiting and reduced food intake were due to liver insulting the spleen and stomach; blood in the urine was due to liver fire with blood heat. I used *Xiǎo Chái Hú Tāng* F2-12 adding *sháo yào, zhī zǐ* that was stir-fried until black, *fú líng*, and *bái zhú*. She recovered.

58. Meaning use her menstrual history before she was pregnant to see what her pattern is likely to be.

**2-1-3**一妊娠六月，體倦食少，勞役見血，用六君加當歸、熟地、升麻、柴胡而愈。

A woman who was six months pregnant had weariness of the body, reduced food intake, taxation, and bleeding. I used *Liù Jūn Zǐ Tāng* F2-6 adding *dāng guī, shú dì huáng, shēng má,* and *chái hú* and she recovered.

**2-1-4**一妊娠每三四月，胎便作痛，余用地黃當歸湯治之，不日而愈。

Every time a woman was three or four months pregnant, the fetus caused her pain. I treated her with *Dì Huáng Dāng Guī Tāng* F2-36 and she recovered within a few days.

**2-1-5**一妊娠三月，飲食後因怒患瘧，連吐三次，用藿香正氣散二劑，隨用安胎飲，一劑而愈。後因怒，痰甚狂言，發熱胸脹，手按少得，此肝脾氣滯，用加味逍遙散加川芎，二劑頓退，四劑而安。

A woman who was three months pregnant suffered *nüè*-malaria due to anger after eating and drinking. Her symptoms included vomiting three times. I used two doses of *Huò xiāng Zhèng Qì Sǎn* F2-71 followed by one dose of *Ān Tāi Yǐn* F2-41 and she recovered. Later due to anger, phlegm was extreme and she began raving, with fever and chest distention. Pressing with the hands brought some improvement. This was qì stagnation of the liver and spleen. I used two doses of *Jiā Wèi Xiāo Yáo Sǎn* F2-1 adding *chuān xiōng* and it immediately receded; she was peaceful after four more doses.

**2-1-6**一婦人每怒，發熱脅脹，小便淋澀，每月經行，旬餘未已。已受胎三月，因怒前症復作，朝用加味逍遙散，夕用安胎飲，各二劑而安。五月又怒，復作，下血如經行，四日未止，仍用前藥而愈。

Every time a woman got angry, she would have fever, rib-side distention, and rough dribbling urination. Every time her menstruation moved, it did not cease for more than ten days. She was already three months pregnant when the above symptoms relapsed due to anger. In the mornings I used *Jiā Wèi Xiāo Yáo Sǎn* F2-1; in the evenings I used *Ān Tāi Yǐn* F2-41; she was peaceful after two doses of each. She became angry again in the fifth month of pregnancy and relapsed, bleeding from below as if she were menstruating; it didn't stop for four days. I continued to use the previous herbs and she recovered.

**2-1-7**一妊娠將三月，嘔吐惡食，體倦嗜臥，此惡阻之症，用人參橘皮湯，二劑漸愈；又用六君加紫蘇，二劑而安。

A woman was almost three months pregnant. She was vomiting with aversion to food, weariness of the body, and somnolence. This was a pattern of morning sickness. I used two doses of *Rén Shēn Jú Pí Tāng* F2-28 and she gradually recovered; I then used two doses of *Liù Jūn Zǐ Tāng* F2-6 adding *zǐ sū yè* and she was peaceful.

**2-1-8**一妊娠吞酸噁心，欲作嘔吐，此飲食停滯，用六君加曲、炒黑子芩、枳殼、香附治之而愈。

A pregnant woman had sour swallowing and nausea; she was on the verge of vomiting. This was food retention. She recovered after I treated her with *Liù Jūn Zǐ Tāng* F2-6 adding *shén qū, zǐ qín* that was stir-fried until black, *zhǐ qiào,* and *xiāng fù.*

**2-1-9**一妊娠飲食後惱怒，寒熱嘔吐，頭痛惡寒，胸腹脹痛，大便不實而色青，小便頻數而有血。余曰：當清肝健脾為主。不信，乃主安胎止血，益甚。問余曰：何也?余曰：大便不實而色青，此是飲食既傷脾土而兼木侮；小便頻數而有血，此是肝火血流於胞而兼挺痿也。用六君子加枳殼、紫蘇、山梔二劑，脾胃頓醒，又用加味逍遙加紫蘇、枳殼二劑，小便頓清，更節飲食，調理而安。

After eating and drinking, a pregnant woman became infuriated, with [sensations of] cold and heat, vomiting, headache, aversion to cold, and distention and pain of the chest and abdomen. She had unformed stool that was *qīng*-green and frequent urination with blood. I said: We should take clearing heat from the liver and strengthening the spleen as governing. They did not believe me and then governed [their treatment] by pacifying the fetus and stopping bleeding, but the symptoms increased a lot. They asked me why. I said: Unformed stool that is *qīng*-green means food and drink have already damaged spleen earth while wood is insulting it at the same time; frequent urination with blood is liver fire with blood flowing into the bladder and prolapse at the same time. I used two doses of *Liù Jūn Zǐ Tāng* F2-6 adding *zhǐ qiào, zǐ sū yè,* and *zhī zǐ.* The spleen and stomach immediately woke up. I then used two doses of *Jiā Wèi Xiāo Yáo Sǎn* F2-1 adding *zǐ sū yè* and *zhǐ qiào,* and her urination immediately cleared. She further regulated her food and drink, attuned and rectified herself and was peaceful.

**2-1-10**一妊娠每至五月，肢體倦怠，飲食無味，先兩足腫，漸至遍身，後及頭面。此是脾肺氣虛，朝用補中益氣，夕用六君子加蘇梗而愈。

Every time a woman was five months pregnant, she had weariness of the body and food and drink became flavorless. At first both feet would swell up, until gradually her whole body became swollen and eventually it reached her head and face. This was spleen and lung qì deficiency. In the mornings I used *Bǔ Zhōng Yì Qì* F2-5; in the evenings I used *Liù Jūn Zǐ Tāng* F2-6 adding *sū gěng* and she recovered.

凡治妊娠，毋泥其月數，但見某經症，便用某藥為善。

Whenever treating pregnant women, do not be stuck on the number of months [of pregnancy]; but if you see symptoms of a certain channel, then it is good to use certain herbs [to treat that channel].[59]

**2-1-11** 一妊娠因怒吐血塊，四日不止，兩脅脹痛，小便淋澀。此怒而血蓄於上部，火炎而隨出也。脅脹腹痛，小便淋澀，肝經本病也。用小柴胡合四物，四劑而止；卻用六君子、安胎飲，調理而安。

Due to anger, a pregnant woman vomited blood clots for four days without stopping. She had distention and pain of both rib-sides and rough dribbling urination. This was anger depositing blood in the upper body; fire flared up and the blood followed it out. Rib-side distention, abdominal pain, and rough dribbling urination were ailments rooted in the liver channel. I used four doses of *Xiǎo Chái Hú Tāng* F2-12 combined with *Sì Wù Tāng* F2-51 and it stopped; I further used *Liù Jūn Zǐ Tāng* F2-6 and *Ān Tāi Yǐn* F2-41 to attune and rectify her and she became peaceful.

**2-1-12**一妊娠氣喘痰甚，諸藥不應，問治於余。詢之云，素有帶下，始於目下浮兩月餘，其面亦然。此氣虛有痰飲也，用六味丸料，數劑而愈。

59. In some older books, each month of pregnancy corresponded to a specific channel. The author means that the doctor should treat the patient by her symptoms, not by the corresponding channel for that month of pregnancy.

A pregnant woman was panting severely with phlegm. Various herbs had no response. She asked to be treated by me. I inquired and she said that she usually had abnormal vaginal discharge. She had puffiness that begin below the eyes for more than two months and her face was also [puffy] like this. This was qì deficiency with phlegm-rheum. I used a batch of *Liù Wèi Wán* F2-16 and she recovered after several doses.

凡婦人氣血方盛，乳房作脹；或無兒飲，痛脹寒熱，用麥芽二三兩炒熟，水煎服，立消 。其耗散血氣如此，何脾胃虛弱，飲食不消，方中多用之?一云麥芽最消腎 。若氣血虛而乳汁自出者，宜十全大補湯，其子多不育 。

- Whenever a women with abundant qì and blood has breast distention, perhaps because she does not nurse her child, she will have pain, distention, and [sensations of] cold and heat. Stir-fry two or three *liǎng* (111.9 grams) of *mài yá* until cooked, boil it in water, and have her take it. This immediately disperses the distention. If it can consume and scatter blood and qì like this, why is it often used in formulas for spleen and stomach deficiency when food and drink are not dispersed? Someone said *mài yá* mostly disperses the kidneys.[60]
- If qì and blood are deficient but milk is spontaneously discharged, it is appropriate to use *Shí Quán Dà Bǔ Tāng* F2-7 [or else] many of these children will not grow up.[61]

60. *Mài yá* reduces breast distention due to an abundance of milk because it inhibits lactation. It also disperses food stagnation and can be used in patients with spleen deficiency. The author asked how it can disperse yet be used in a patient with spleen deficiency. He answered that it is because it disperses the kidneys, not the spleen and stomach. This answer may still not satisfy the modern reader.
61. Children won't do well on milk from a deficient mother because it will not be rich and nourishing. Therefore, the mother should be supplemented.

## 《女科撮要·卷下·小產》
## 2-2 Small Birth (Abortion or Miscarriage)

小產重於大產，蓋大產如栗熟自脫，小產如生採，破其皮殼，斷自根蒂，豈不重於大產?但人輕忽致死者多矣。治法宜補形氣，生新血，去瘀血。

Small birth is more serious than large birth.[62] Now, large birth is like a ripe chestnut that disconnects [from the tree] on its own; small birth is like picking it when it is unripe. You must break open the shell and sever it from the root and stem. Isn't this more serious than large birth? But many people take it lightly and ignore it until it results in death. The appropriate treatment method is to supplement the physical body and qì, engender new blood, and remove the blood stasis.

若未足月，痛而欲產，芎歸補中湯，倍加知母止之。若產而血不止，人參黃耆湯補之。若產而心腹痛，當歸川芎湯主之。胎氣弱而小產者，八珍湯固之。若出血過多而發熱，聖愈湯。汗不止，急用獨參湯。發熱煩躁，肉筋惕，八珍湯。大渴面赤，脈洪而虛，當歸補血湯。身熱面赤，脈沉而微，四君薑附。

- If not enough months have passed, she has pain, and is about to give birth, stop it with *Xiōng Guī Bǔ Zhōng Tāng* F2-47 adding a double dose of *zhī mǔ*.
- If she gave birth [miscarried or aborted] but the bleeding does not stop, supplement her with *Rén Shēn Huáng Qí Tāng* F2-48.
- If she gave birth [miscarried or aborted] and there is pain of the heart region and abdomen, *Dāng Guī Chuān Xiōng Tāng* F2-50 governs it.
- If fetal qì is weak and there small birth [miscarriage is impending], secure it with *Bā Zhēn Tāng* F2-8.
- If she bleeds excessively and there is fever, use *Shèng Yù Tāng* F1-11.
- If sweating does not stop, quickly use *Dú Shēn Tāng* F1-9.
- If there is fever, vexation, and agitation, and the flesh and sinews are jerking, use *Bā Zhēn Tāng* F2-8.
- If there is great thirst, red face, and the pulse is surging but deficient, use *Dāng Guī Bǔ Xuè Tāng* F2-9.

62. Small birth refers to abortion or miscarriage while large birth refers to giving birth at the proper time.

- If she feels feverish with red face and sunken faint pulse, use *Sì Jūn Zǐ Tāng* F2-26 with *gān jiāng* and *fù zǐ*.

東垣云：晝發熱，而夜安靜，是陽氣自旺於陽分也。晝安靜而夜發熱躁，是陽氣下陷於陰中也；如晝夜俱發熱者，是重陽無陰也，當峻補其陰。

Lǐ Dōngyuán said[63]: When there is daytime fever but peace at night, yáng qì is at peak strength by itself in the yáng divisions. If she is peaceful in the daytime but has fever and agitation at night, yáng qì sinks down into yīn. If there is fever both day and night, this is double yáng without yīn; one should drastically supplement the yīn.

王太僕云：如大寒而甚，熱之不熱，是無火也；熱來復去，晝見夜伏，夜發晝止，時節而動，是無火也；如大熱而甚，寒之不寒，是無水也；熱動復止，倏忽往來，時動時止，是無水也。

Wáng Tàipú[64] said:

- If there is great cold and the condition is serious but using heat does not heat it up, this means fire is lacking.
- If heat comes and goes repeatedly, appearing in the day but subsiding at night, or coming out at night and ceasing in the day, stirring at regular times, this means fire is lacking.[65]
- If there is great heat and the condition is serious but using cold does not cool it down, this means water is lacking.
- If heat stirs and ceases repeatedly, swiftly coming and going, sometimes stirring and sometimes ceasing, this means water is lacking.[66]

若陽氣自旺者，補中益氣湯。陽氣陷於陰者，四物二連湯。重陽無陰者，四物湯。無火者，八味丸。無水者，六味丸。

63. The source of this quotation has not been found. Perhaps it is paraphrased or a summary of Lǐ's ideas.
64. This is another name for Wáng Bīng 王冰. He wrote this in his commentary on *Sù Wèn*, Chapter 74.
65. Wáng wrote that one should aid the heart in that case.
66. Wáng wrote that one should aid the kidneys.

- If yáng qì is at peak strength by itself, use *Bǔ Zhōng Yì Qì Tāng* F2-5.
- For yáng qì sinking into yīn, use *Sì Wù Èr Lián Tāng* F2-20.
- For double yáng without yīn, use *Sì Wù Tāng* F2-51.
- When there is no fire, use *Bā Wèi Wán* F2-17.
- When there is no water, use *Liù Wèi Wán* F2-16.

## 治驗
## Treatment Experience

**2-2-1**一妊娠五月，服剪紅丸而墮，腹中脹痛；服破血之劑，益甚，以手按之益痛。余曰：此峻藥重傷，脾胃受患。用八珍倍人參、黃耆、半夏、乳香、沒藥，二劑而痛止，數劑而痊愈。

A woman who was five months pregnant took *Jiǎn Hóng Wán* UFx-8 and miscarried,[67] with distention and pain in her abdomen. She took a prescription to break blood, and her symptoms increased a lot. Pressing with the hand increased the pain. I said: These drastic herbs caused serious damage; the spleen and stomach have received harm. I used two doses of *Bā Zhēn Tāng* F2-8 doubling the *rén shēn,* and adding *huáng qí, bàn xià, rǔ xiāng,* and *mò yào,* and the pain stopped. She completely recovered after several doses.

**2-2-2**吳江庠友史萬湖仲子室，年二十餘，疫疾墮胎，時咳，服清肺解表，喘急不寐，請治。余以為脾土虛不能生肺金，藥損益甚，先與補中益氣加茯苓、半夏、五味、炮薑，四劑漸愈。往視之，又與八珍加五味及十全大補湯痊愈。

The wife of the second son of Wújiāng school friend Shǐ Wànhú was more than twenty years old. An epidemic disease caused a miscarriage and she had an occasional cough. She took herbs to clear heat from the lungs and release the exterior, but then she had rapid breathing and inability to sleep so they invited me to treat her. I took this as deficiency of spleen earth with inability to engender lung metal. The herbs [she mistakenly took] increased the harm a lot. I first gave her four doses of *Bǔ Zhōng Yì Qì Tāng* F2-5 adding *fú*

67. This woman may have been trying to induce an abortion, or she may have mis-used this formula, which removes *chóng*-worms from the intestines and also treats vaginal discharge or dysentery.

*líng, bàn xià, wǔ wèi zǐ,* and *pào jiāng,* and she gradually recovered. I went to see her and then used *Bā Zhēn Tāng* F2-8 adding *wǔ wèi zǐ* as well as *Shí Quán Dà Bǔ Tāng* F2-7 and she completely recovered.

**2-2-3**大兒婦張氏素怯弱，嘉靖癸卯四月生女，自乳中患疥瘡，年餘不愈，遂致羸困。

My eldest son's wife, nee Zhāng, was usually weak.[68] In the fourth month of the *guǐ mǎo* year of Jiājìng's reign (1543) she gave birth to a girl. She suffered scabby sores on her breasts for more than a year without recovering. Subsequently, she became emaciated and tired.

甲辰五月，遭先母大故，以姑病勉強代執喪禮，旬月，每欲眩仆，一日感氣，忽患心脾高腫作疼，手不可按，而嘔吐不止，六脈微細之極。余以為脈雖虛而病形則實，誤認諸痛不可補氣，乃用青皮、香附、吳茱等藥而愈。

In the fifth month of the next [*jiǎ chén*] year (1544), we met with disaster when my mother died. Because my wife was sick, my daughter-in-law was compelled to substitute in the funeral rites for a whole month; each time, she became dizzy and almost fell down. One day she contracted [some kind of evil] qì and suddenly suffered high swelling of the heart and spleen with pain that refused to be pressed and vomiting that did not stop. Her six pulses were extremely faint and fine. I took this as an excess disease of the body even though her pulse was deficient. I mistakenly thought that I could not supplement qì because of all the pain. I then used herbs like *qīng pí, xiāng fù,* and *wú zhū yú* and she recovered.

繼復患瘧且墮胎，又投理氣行血之藥，病去，元氣轉脫，再投參耆補劑不應矣，六脈如絲欲絕，思非附子不能救，非立翁莫能投。

Later she relapsed, suffering *nüè*-malaria and she had a miscarriage. I then gave her herbs to rectify qì and move blood, and the disease was eliminated but her original qì began to desert. I then gave supplementing prescriptions with *rén shēn* and *huáng qí* but she did not respond. Her six pulses were like a thread and were about to expire. I thought only

68. This is another testimonial by a satisfied patient's father-in-law.

*fù zǐ* would be able to save her; only the Honored Old Man[69] (Xuē Jǐ) would be able to prescribe for her.

迎翁至，診云：皆理氣之劑，損真之誤也。連投參、耆、歸、朮、附子、薑、桂六劑，間用八味丸，五日眠食漸甘，六脈全復。翁云：心脾疼痛時，即當服此等藥，瘧亦不作矣。姑婦皆翁再造，敢述奇功，附於此門之尾，以為初知藥性者之戒。

I invited the Honored Old Man. He arrived, examined her, and said: All prescriptions to rectify qì make the mistake of harming the true. He gave her six continuous doses of *rén shēn, huáng qí, dāng guī, bái zhú, fù zǐ,* ginger and cinnamon. In between, he used *Bā Wèi Wán* F2-17. In five days she was sleeping and food gradually became sweet to her again. Her six pulses completely returned. The Honored Old Man said: At a time when there was heart and spleen pain, if she had taken this type of medicine, the *nüè*-malaria would not have appeared. The Honored Old Man gave both the girl and my wife a new lease on life. I dare to tell of his outstanding contribution and append it to the end of this section. Take this as a warning to neophytes on the nature of herbs.

制生陳遜稽顙謹識

Chén Xùn, who is still in mourning, bowing and respectfully written

69. Honored Old Man (*wēng* 翁): In Chinese, this is a term of respect for an older man. In English, Old Man does not sound respectful enough.

# 《女科撮要·卷下·保產》
## 2-3 Safeguarding Childbirth (*bǎo chǎn*)[70]

妊娠欲產之時，但覺腹內轉動，即當正身仰臥，待兒轉身，向下時作痛，試捏產母手中指中節，或本節跳動，方與臨盆，即產矣。若初覺不仰臥，以待轉胞。

At the time when a pregnant woman is about to give birth, but she feels turning movement in her abdomen, she should lie face up with her body straight and wait for the child to turn around.[71] At the time [the baby] turns downward, if it causes pain, try pinching the middle section or the base joint of the laboring woman's middle finger and shake it; then wait for the labor to progress and she will promptly give birth. If she did not initially feel [the turning of the fetus], she should lie face up and wait for it to turn in the uterus.

或未產而水頻下，此胞衣已破，血水先乾，必有逆生難產之患。

Perhaps she has not given birth yet but water has repeatedly come out; this means the amniotic sac has already broken. If blood and water dry up too early, [the fetus cannot turn so] she will have a breech birth and suffer difficult labor.

若橫生者，兒先露手臂，令母正臥，以手徐推兒臂下體，令其正直，復以中指摩其肩，勿令臍帶攀系即生。

70. Many parts of this section rely on *Fù Rén Dà Quán Liáng Fāng*《婦人大全良方》(All Inclusive Fine Formulas for Women), originally published in 1238 (Northern *Sòng*) by Chén Zìmíng 陳自明. Xuē Jǐ also revised and annotated that book, adding cases there as well. This passage is interesting as it resembles the information a midwife would use, not male scholar-physicians. *Liáng Fāng* gives much more detail; Xuē Jǐ greatly redacted it. The meaning is clearer in the earlier text, so it was used as an aid to my translation. In addition, the following dissertation was very useful: Margaret Wee Siang Ng, Male Brushstrokes and Female Touch: Medical Writings on Childbirth in Imperial China, unpublished dissertation, Department of History, Faculty of Arts, McGill University, Montreal, 2013.

71. According to Charlotte Furth in *A Flourishing Yin* (page 281), ancient Chinese people thought the fetus turned head downward just before birth.

If there is transverse presentation, the child will first present a hand or arm. Make the mother lie straight. [The midwife[72] should] use her hand to gently push the lower part of the child's arm [back in] and realign him. Again she should use her middle finger to rub the baby's shoulder, making sure that the umbilical cord will not get pulled down [by the shoulder]. Then he will be born.

逆生者，兒先露足，令母正臥，以手按推其足，仍推兒轉正即生。

In breech presentation, the child first presents a foot. Make the mother lie straight; [the midwife should] press and push on the foot with her hand. She should further push the child to turn him to the correct position and he will then be born.

偏生者，兒頭偏在一邊，亦照前法，徐正其頭即生。或見頭後骨，偏在谷道傍，徐推近上即生。

In slanting presentation, the child's head slants to one side.[73] Again, [the midwife should] slowly straighten his head according to the previous method and he will then be born. Perhaps she sees that the occiput is slanted so that it is close to the mother's grain path [anus]; [the midwife should] gently push upward and then he will then be born.

礙產者，兒頭雖正，但不能下，蓋因胎轉，臍帶攀肩所致，用中指按兒兩肩，理脫臍帶即生。

In obstructed labor, even though the child's head is straight, he is unable to descend. This must be due to the fetus turning in such a way that the umbilical cord gets pulled down around his shoulder. [The midwife should] use her middle finger to press each of the child's shoulders, putting everything in order, and removing the umbilical cord. Then he will be born.

72. An educated male doctor would not do these types of manipulations. This would be the work of a midwife. Male doctors would not be allowed to attend to the intimate details of giving birth, seeing and touching other men's wives. Besides this, scholars were averse to getting their hands dirty. Most would only touch patients to read the pulse. This type of attitude is one reason why acupuncture-moxibustion was less frequently used by scholar-doctors. These manipulations, which were first described in *Liáng Fāng*, were probably included so that the doctor or male head of the household could manage the activities of midwives.
73. Instead of the crown of the head, the side of the forehead or brow presents.

坐產者，兒將欲生，其母疲倦，久坐椅褥，抵其生路，急用巾帶高懸，令母以手攀之，輕輕屈足，良久兒順即生。

In sitting labor, the child is about to be born, but the mother has become weary. If she sits on a chair or mattress for a long time, it pushes back against the birth path. Quickly use a cloth belt suspended from [a ceiling beam] above and make the mother pull herself up with her hands. Lightly and gently bend her legs [under her so she is squatting]. After a good long time, the child will get in the proper position and will be born.

盤腸生者，臨產母腸先出，此難於收上，以蓖麻子四十九粒，研爛塗產母頭頂，待腸收上，急洗去。設或為風吹乾不能收者，以磨刀水少許，溫熱拭潤其腸，再用磁石煎湯服之即收上。磁石須陰陽家用有驗者。俗以水噀母面，皆驚而腸亦收之，蓋驚則氣散，恐反致他症，戒之。

*Coiled intestine birth* means the mother is about to give birth but her intestines emerge [prolapse] first. It is difficult to gather them back up and in. Grind forty-nine pieces of *bì má zǐ* to a pulp and spread them on the birthing mother's vertex. Wait for the intestines to gather back up and in, and quickly wash [the *bì má zǐ*] off. If the intestines dry up because of wind blowing and are unable to gather back in, use a small amount of warm knife-sharpening water to wipe her intestines in order to moisten them. Then have her take a decoction of *cí shí* and they will gather back up and in.[74] *Cí shí* that has been used by a *yīn yáng jiā* [astrologer, geomancer, etc.] should be effective. There is a custom to squirt water from the mouth into the mother's face to startle her so that her intestines will gather back in. However, qì scatters when someone is frightened, so contrary to expectations, this method risks incurring other symptoms. I warn against it.

若胎衣破而不得分娩者，用保生無憂散，以固其血，自然生息。如血已耗損，用八珍湯料一斤，益母草半斤，水數碗，煎熟不時飲之，亦有得生者。

- If amniotic sac has broken and she cannot give birth, use *Bǎo Shēng Wú Yōu Sǎn* F2-46 to secure her blood, and she will naturally survive.

74. This is a magical formula. Water in which knives have been sharpened will have small amounts of iron in it. *Cí shí* is lodestone, which would then attract the iron in the water used to wash the intestines, helping to pull them back in.

- If blood is already consumed and harmed, use a one *jīn* (596.8 grams) batch of *Bā Zhēn Tāng* F2-8, a half *jīn* (298.4 grams) of *yì mǔ cǎo,* and several cups of water. Boil until cooked and have her drink it at any time; this will also save her life.

凡孕婦只腹痛，未產也；若連腰痛甚者，將產也。蓋腎候於腰，胞係於腎故也。

Whenever a pregnant woman only has abdominal pain and the baby hasn't been born yet, if severe pain radiates to the lower back, she is about to give birth. The reason must be that kidney symptoms show up in the lower back and the uterus is connected to the kidneys.

華陀治橫逆產難，用蛇脫二條，蟬殼二十八個，胎髮二丸，各燒灰，每服二錢，酒調，連進二服，即臥片時，兒即順生。如無此藥，令產母仰面正臥，以小針刺兒手腳心三五次，用鹽塗之，手腳即縮上，待兒身轉順而生。若以蜀葵子四十九粒，白滑石三錢，順流水煎服即順生。或用好京墨濃磨服之，墨水裹兒即下。或敗筆頭一個，煅過，以藕節自然汁，溫酒和下。或紫蘇葉、當歸各三錢，長流水煎服即下。

- Huá Tuó treated a transverse presentation with difficult childbirth. He used two snake skins (*shé tuō*), twenty eight cicada shells (*chán qiào*), and two balls of fetal hair (*tāi fà*),[75] all reduced to ash. Each dose was two *qián* (7.46 grams) mixed with liquor. She swallowed two doses in a row, then lay down for a moment. The child got in the proper position and was born.
- If you don't have these herbs, make the birthing mother lie face up and straight. Prick the heart of the child's hand or foot[76] with a small needle three or five times and spread salt on it; the hand or foot will withdraw upward. Wait for the child's body to shift into the proper position and he will be born.
- If she takes forty-nine grains of *shǔ kuí zǐ* and three *qián* (11.19 grams) of *bái huá shí* boiled in properly flowing water, the fetus will move into the proper position and be born.

75. In ancient times people held a ceremony and shaved the heads of newborns (when twenty days old for girls and twenty-four days old for boys). This first shaved hair is called *fetal hair*.
76. This assumes a hand or food presentation.

- Or use densely ground *jīng mò* [a kind of ink made from pine ash] of good quality, and take it. The inky water wraps around the child and descends it.
- Or calcine one worn out writing brush, blend with the natural juice of *ǒu jié*[77] and warm liquor and swallow it.
- Or take three *qián* (11.19 grams) each of *zǐ sū yè* and *dāng guī*, boiled in long flowing water; the child will descend.

凡孕家宜預請穩婆，有仁心識見者，當施恩惠以結其心，先與說知，倘有生息不順，只說未產；或遇雙胎，只說胎衣未下，恐驚則氣散，愈難生息，余家親驗之。

Generally it is suitable for the pregnant woman's family to invite a midwife in advance. She should be kindhearted and experienced. The family should do favors for her in order to bind her heart to them. First, in giving notifications, if the baby is alive but not in proper position, she should only say the baby isn't born yet; or if she encounters twins, she should only say the placenta hasn't descended yet. Qì scatters when there is fear and fright, so it is more difficult to have a live birth.[78] My own relatives have experienced this.

大抵難產多患於鬱悶安佚富貴之家。治法雖云胎前消氣，產後補血，不可專執。若脾胃不實，氣血不充，宜預調補，不然臨產必有患難。

Generally speaking, many suffer difficult childbirth from constraint and oppression [pent-up emotions] or a leisurely life in wealthy noble families. Although the treatment methods say to disperse qì before giving birth and supplement blood after giving birth,[79] one cannot arbitrarily stick to this. If the spleen and stomach are not full and qì and blood are not ample, it is appropriate to attune and supplement before hand; otherwise there will be difficulties in giving birth.

77. This may mean the juices that are spontaneously secreted by fresh *ǒu jié* when it is cut.
78. The idea is to use comforting words for the birthing mother so she doesn't become scared. If she is frightened, the birth becomes more difficult.
79. Some editions write 胎前消氣，產後補血。*Disperse qì* before giving birth and supplement blood after giving birth. Other editions have 胎前清氣，產後補血。*Clear qì* before giving birth and supplement blood after giving birth.

如因難產，或大寒時，急以大油紙捻，徐徐燒斷其臍帶，雖兒已死，令暖氣入腹，多得復生，切不可用刀斷之。

If [the newborn is unresponsive] due to difficult childbirth or at a time of great cold, quickly burn larded twists of paper and use them to slowly and gently sever the umbilical cord. Even if the child is already dead, this makes warm qì enter his abdomen and many can can be returned to life.[80] Be sure not to use a knife to sever the cord.

## 治驗
## Treatment Experience

**2-3-1**荊婦孟冬分娩艱難，產子已死，元氣勞傷，用油紙捻燒斷臍帶，取其陽氣以補之，俄間兒啼作聲，即鵠兒也。若以刀物如常斷之，其母亦難保生。此兒嗣後一二歲間，並無傷食作瀉之症，可見前法之功。

My wife suffered difficult labor in the first month of winter. The child had already died, as taxation [from prolonged labor] had damaged original qì. We severed the umbilical cord by burning it with a rolled up piece of oil-paper. This allowed the yáng qì [of the fire] to supplement the baby. Very soon the baby cried and made sounds like the *hú* of a swan. If we had used a knife to cut it, which is a common practice, it would have also been difficult to safeguard the mother's life. Afterwards, for the first one or two years, this child never had conditions such as food damage patterns with diarrhea. We can see the achievements of the earlier methods.

其穩婆又喜平日常施少惠，得其用心，能安慰母懷，故無虞耳。此穩婆云：止有一女，分娩時，適當巡街侍御行牌取我，視其室分娩，女為此驚嚇，未產而死，後見侍御，更以威顏分付，迨視產母胎雖順，而頭偏在一邊，若以手入推正，可保順生，因畏其威，不敢施手。但回禀云，此是天生天化，非人力所能立，俟其母子俱死。

80. Ancient Chinese books often mention bringing the newly dead back to life. Of course, by modern standards, this would be reviving an unresponsive patient whose pulse and breathing were so shallow they could not be detected, or a patient whose respiration and heart beat may have stopped for a short period of time.

Midwives also like to receive small acts of kindness on ordinary days [not necessarily at the time of birth]. This can gain her motivation to comfort the mother's bosom [state of mind] so she will not be anxious. This midwife told me: I only had one daughter. While she was in labor, someone from the street patrol came to fetch me with a card from the Imperial Censor to attend to his wife when she gave birth. Because my daughter was frightened [by such a high summons], she could not give birth and died. Afterwards when I saw the Imperial Censor, he further used a threatening face when he paid my installment. I attended the laboring woman, but even though the fetus was in proper position, the head slanted to one side. If I had inserted my hand to push it straight, I could have safeguard the birth, but because I feared his threats, I did not dare to apply my hands. I only reported back to the Imperial Censor saying: "This is 'heaven giving birth and heaven transforming,'[81] it is not within the capability of human strength." So she waited while the mother and child both died.[82]

## 《女科撮要·卷下·子死腹中》
## 2-4 Fetal Death in the Abdomen

夫子死腹中者，多因驚動太早；或觸犯禁；或抱腰太重；或頻探試水，胞衣先破，血水先盡，而胎乾涸故耳。其候產母唇舌皆黑者，子母俱死。若舌黑或脹悶甚者，然其子已死矣。先以平胃散一兩，酒水各半煎，卻投朴硝半兩，即熱皮硝服；或用硝一兩，以童便調下亦妙。

A fetus dying in the abdomen is often due to fright stirring it up too early; or violating the prohibitions; or excessive interference by midwives; or frequently probing to examine the water [of the amniotic sac]. The reason for fetal death is that the amniotic sac breaks open in advance [of the birth] or blood and water are exhausted in advance, so the fetus becomes desiccated. The symptom of blackening of both the tongue and lips

81. Heaven giving birth and heaven transforming: This phrase means something is fated and there is nothing humans could do to change it.

82. This is a disturbing story. The midwife blamed the Censor for her own daughter's death. Besides that, he did not treat her well and made the midwife afraid. The Censor's wife had a difficult birth. Although the midwife thought she could help, she was afraid she would be blamed if she interfered with the process and something went wrong. In addition, her motivation was low. The author's point is to be nice to the midwife so she will do her utmost in situations of life and death.

of the woman in labor means both the child and mother will die. If the tongue is black or extremely distended and oppressed, the child is already dead.

- First use one *liǎng* (37.3 grams) of *Píng Wèi Sǎn* F2-64 boiled in a mixture of half water and half liquor. Then throw in a half *liǎng* (18.65 grams) of *pò xiāo*, which is hot *pí xiāo*, and take it;
- Or it is wonderful to mix one *liǎng* (37.3 grams) of [*pò* or *pí*] *xiāo* with child's urine to descend it.

## 治驗
## Treatment Experience

**2-4-1**一穩婆之女勤苦負重，妊娠腹中陰冷重墜，口中甚穢。余意其胎必死，令視其舌果青黑，與朴硝半兩許服之，隨下穢水而安。

A midwife's daughter worked hard and carried something heavy. She had yīn cold and a [feeling of] heaviness and sagging inside her pregnant abdomen. The inside of her mouth was extremely filthy.[83] I thought the fetus must be dead. I made [the midwife] observe her daughter's tongue which was really *qīng*-greenish black. I gave her about a half *liǎng* (18.65 grams) of *pò xiāo*. She took it, then descended filthy water, and she was peaceful.

**2-4-2**一婦人胎死，服朴硝而下穢水，肢體倦怠，氣息奄奄，用四君為主，佐以四物、薑、桂，調補而愈。

A woman's fetus died. She took *pò xiāo* and descended filthy water. Her body was weary and she gasped for breath. I used *Sì Jūn Zǐ Tāng* F2-26 as governing and assisted with *Sì Wù Tāng* F2-51 adding ginger and cinnamon. She attuned and supplemented herself and recovered.

83. Perhaps this means a dirty tongue coating; tongue diagnosis was not yet commonly used. This seems to be a case where the author did not see the patient. The midwife explained her daughter's symptoms and Xuē Jǐ prescribed based on that.

# 《女科撮要·卷下·胎衣不出》
## 2-5 Retention of Placenta

有因惡露入衣，脹而不能出；有因元氣虧損，而不能送出。其惡露流衣中者，腹中脹痛，用奪命丹或失笑散，以消瘀血，緩則不救。其元氣不能送者，腹中不脹痛，用保生無憂散，以補固元氣。或用萆麻子肉一兩，細研成膏，塗母右腳心，衣下即洗去，緩則腸亦出。如腸不上，仍用此膏塗腦頂，則腸自入，益母丸亦效。《寶慶方》胎衣未下，若欲斷臍帶，先以少物系墜，然後斷之，否則胞上掩心而死。

There are cases due to lochia entering the placenta with distention and inability for it to come out; there are cases where enfeebled original qì is unable to carry the placenta out.

- When lochia flows into the placenta, there is distention and pain within the abdomen; use *Duó Mìng Dān* F2-62 or *Shī Xiào Sǎn* F2-55 to disperse blood stasis. If you are slow, she cannot be saved.
- If her original qì is unable to carry it out, there is no distention or pain in the abdomen; use *Bǎo Shēng Wú Yōu Sǎn* F2-46 to supplement and secure original qì.
- Or finely grind one *liǎng* (37.3 grams) of *bì má zǐ* flesh into a paste and spread it onto the heart of the mother's right foot;[84] once the placenta descends, wash it off [her foot].
    - If you are slow [to wash it off], the intestines also come out [prolapse]. If the intestines do not ascend, spread this paste onto the vertex, and the intestines will spontaneously go back in. *Yì Mǔ Cǎo Wán* F2-65 is also effective.

*Bǎo Qìng Fāng*[85] says that if the placenta is retained and you are about to sever the umbilical cord, attach something small to hang down from it. Then sever the cord. Otherwise, the placenta will ascend, sneaking up to the heart, and she will die.

84. This means the region of Yǒng Quán (KI 1).
85. Various books refer to Mr. Hú's *Bǎo Qìng Fāng* 胡氏《寶慶方》(Precious Celebration Formulas) but at this time, no further information is available.

## 治驗
## Treatment Experience

**2-5-1**家人婦胞衣不出，胸腹脹痛，手不敢近，此瘀血為患，用熱酒下失笑散一劑，惡露、胎衣即並下。

A female family member retained her placenta. She had distention and pain of her chest and abdomen and could not bear for it to be touched. This suffering developed from blood stasis. She swallowed a dose of *Shī Xiào Săn* F2-55 with hot liquor and then lochia and the placenta descended together.

**2-5-2**一產婦胎衣不出，腹不脹痛，手按之痛稍緩。此是氣虛而不能送出，用無憂散而下。

A laboring woman retained her placenta. Her abdomen was not distended or painful but there was a little pain when pressed; this was qì deficiency that led to inability to expel it. I used *Băo Shēng Wú Yōu Săn* F2-46 and it descended.

前症余詢諸穩婆云：宜服益母草丸，或就以產婦頭髮，入口作嘔，胎衣自出。其不出者，必死，授與前法甚效。

I have asked various midwives about the above condition, and they said: It is appropriate to take *Yì Mŭ Căo Wán* F2-65; or if you simply put the pregnant woman's head hair into her mouth to make her vomit, the placenta will automatically come out. If the placenta is retained, she will die. I give you the above methods as they are extremely effective.

# 《女科撮要·卷下·<br>交骨不開，陰門不閉，子宮不收》

# 2-6 Failure of the Interlocking Bone to Open, Failure of the Yīn Door to Close, and Failure of the Uterus to Contract (jiāo gǔ bù kāi, yīn mén bù bì, zǐ gōng bù shōu)

三者皆元氣不足，觀諸治驗，可見。其交骨不開者，用芎歸湯加髮灰、龜板，補而開之；陰門不閉者，用十全大補加五味子，補而斂之；子宮不收者，補中益氣加醋炒芍藥、半夏，補而舉之；或助以外治之法。

These three are all due to insufficiency of original qì; this is apparent from observing all the treatment experience.

- For failure of the interlocking bone [the sacrococcygeal joint] to open, use *Xiōng Guī Tāng* F2-67 adding *fā huī* and *guī bǎn* to supplement and open it.
- For failure of the yīn door [opening of the vagina] to close, use *Shí Quán Dà Bǔ Tāng* F2-7 adding *wǔ wèi zǐ* to supplement and gather it in.
- For failure of the uterus (*zǐ gōng*) to contract, use *Bǔ Zhōng Yì Qì Tāng* F2-5 adding vinegar-fried *sháo yào* and *bàn xià* to supplement and raise it.

You can also help by using external treatment methods.

## 治驗

## Treatment Experience

**2-6-1**地官李孟卿，娶三十五歲稚女為繼室，妊娠慮其難產，與加味芎歸湯四劑備用，果產門不開，服之頓然分娩。

Government Official Lǐ Mèngqīng took a wife when he was thirty-five years old but his new wife was a young girl. During her pregnancy it was thought she would have difficult labor. I gave her four doses of *Jiā Wèi Xiōng Guī Tāng* F2-66 to keep in reserve. As expected, her birth gate [cervix] did not open. She took it and immediately gave birth.

**2-6-2**西賓費懷德之室，下血甚多，產門不開，兩日未生，服前藥一劑，實時而產。已後育胎，並無此症。懷德傳與服者，無有不效。

The wife of family tutor Fèi Huáidé bled a lot from below; her birth gate [cervix] did not open and she did not give birth for two days. She took one dose of the previous medicine, and gave birth in a short time. Afterwards when giving birth, she never had this symptom. This formula from Huáidé never failed to be effective for those who received it and took it.

**2-6-3**一婦人分娩最易，至四十妊娠，下血甚多，產門不開，亦與前湯一劑，又用無憂散斤許一劑，煎熟時時飲之，以助其血而產。

A woman had very easy childbirth until she was pregnant at forty. She bled a lot from below and her birth gate [cervix] did not open. I also gave her a dose of the previous formula, and then used about a *jīn* of *Wú Yōu Sǎn* F2-46 in one dose. It was boiled and when done she constantly drank it to assist her blood. She gave birth.

**2-6-4**一產婦陰門不閉，發熱惡寒，用十全大補加五味子數劑，而寒熱悉退，又用補中益氣加五味子，數劑而斂。

The yīn door of a laboring woman did not close, with fever and aversion to cold. I used several doses of *Shí Quán Dà Bǔ Tāng* F2-7 adding *wǔ wèi zǐ*, and all the [sensations of] cold and heat receded. I then used several doses of *Bǔ Zhōng Yì Qì Tāng* F2-5 adding *wǔ wèi zǐ* and her yīn door gathered in.

若初產腫脹，或焮痛而不閉者，當用加味逍遙散。若腫既消而不閉者，當用補中益氣湯，切忌寒涼之劑。

- If initially [after] birth there is swelling and distention or scorching pain and the yīn door does not close, one should use *Jiā Wèi Xiāo Yáo Sǎn* F2-1.
- If the swelling has already dispersed but the yīn door does not close, one should use *Bǔ Zhōng Yì Qì Tāng* F2-5.

By all means avoid cold and cool prescriptions.

**2-6-5**一婦人脾胃素弱，兼有肝火，產後陰門腫痛，寒熱作渴，嘔吐不食，敷大黄等藥，服驅利之劑，腫及於臀，虛症蜂起。此真氣虛而作，先用六君子以固脾胃，乃以補中益氣湯升舉，不數劑而消。

A woman usually had weakness of the spleen and stomach and liver fire at the same time. After giving birth, her yīn door was swollen and painful, and she had [sensations of] cold and heat, thirst, vomiting, and did not eat. They applied herbs like *dà huáng* to the site and she took a prescription to expel and disinhibit, but the swelling reached her buttocks and deficiency symptoms arose in swarms. This situation arose because of true qì deficiency. I first used *Liù Jūn Zǐ Tāng* F2-6 to secure the spleen and stomach; then I used *Bǔ Zhōng Yì Qì Tāng* F2-5 to raise upward. The swelling dispersed after not many doses.

**2-6-6**一產婦失治，腫潰不已，形體消瘦，飲食不思，朝寒暮熱，自汗盜汗半年矣。用補中益氣加茯苓、半夏以健脾胃，膿水漸少，飲食漸進；用歸脾湯以解脾鬱，共五十餘劑，元氣復而瘡亦愈矣。

A woman who gave birth lacked proper treatment. She had swellings that burst open endlessly, her body became emaciated with no thought of food and drink, cold in the mornings and hot at sunset, spontaneous sweating, and night sweating for half a year. I used *Bǔ Zhōng Yì Qì Tāng* F2-5 adding *fú líng* and *bàn xià* to strengthen the spleen and stomach. The pus-water gradually decreased and she begin eating and drinking again. I used more than fifty doses altogether of *Guī Pí Tāng* F2-3 to resolve spleen constraint. Her original qì returned and the sores also recovered.

**2-6-7**一產婦陰門不閉，小便淋瀝，腹內一物，攻動脅下，或脹或痛，用加味逍遙散加車前子而愈。

The yīn door of a laboring woman did not close. She had dribbling urination and [felt] something inside her abdomen attacking and stirring below her rib-sides; sometimes she felt distention and sometimes pain. I used *Jiā Wèi Xiāo Yáo Sǎn* F2-1 adding *chē qián zǐ* and she recovered.

**2-6-8**一婦人子宮腫大，二日方入損落一片殊類豬肝已，而面黃體倦，飲食無味，內熱晡熱，自汗盜汗，用十全大補湯二十餘劑，諸症悉愈，仍復生育。

A woman's uterus (*zǐ gōng*) was swollen and enlarged. After two days, something that looked like pork liver fell out, and then her face was yellow, her body weary, and food and drink were flavorless. She had internal heat, late afternoon fever, spontaneous sweating, and night sweating. I used more than twenty doses of *Shí Quán Dà Bǔ Tāng* F2-7 and all symptoms completely recovered. She was able to give birth again.

血滯成癰，方見後。

Blood stagnation develops into abscesses; for the formulas see below.

## 《女科撮要·卷下·產後腹痛》
## 2-7 Postpartum Abdominal Pain

產後小腹作痛，俗名兒枕塊，用失笑散行散之。若惡露既去而仍痛，用四神散調補之；若不應，用八珍湯。若痛而噁心，或欲作嘔，用六君子湯。若痛而泄瀉，用六君子湯送四神丸。若泄瀉痛而或後重，用補中益氣湯送四神丸。若胸膈飽脹，或惡食吞酸，或腹痛手不可按，此是飲食所致，當用二陳加山楂、白朮以消導。若食既消而仍痛，或按之不痛，或更加頭痛，煩熱作渴，惡寒欲嘔等症，此是中氣被傷，宜補脾胃為主。若發熱腹痛，按之痛甚，不惡食，不吞酸，此是瘀血停滯，用失笑散以消之。若止是發熱頭痛，或兼腹痛，按之卻不痛，此是血虛，用四物加炮薑、參、朮以補之。

- Postpartum lower abdominal pain is commonly named *child pillow lumps*; use *Shī Xiào Sǎn* F2-55 to move and scatter it.
- If lochia has already gone but there is still pain, use *Sì Shén Sǎn* F2-53 to attune and supplement it.
    - If she does not respond use *Bā Zhēn Tāng* F2-8.
- If there is pain and nausea or she is about to vomit, use *Liù Jūn Zǐ Tāng* F2-6.

- If there is pain and diarrhea, swallow *Sì Shén Wán* UF-19 with *Liù Jūn Zǐ Tāng* F2-6.
- If there is diarrhea, pain, and perhaps tenesmus, swallow *Sì Shén Wán* UF-19 with *Bǔ Zhōng Yì Qì Tāng* F2-5.
- If the chest and diaphragm are full and distended or there is aversion to food and sour swallowing, or abdominal pain that cannot tolerate pressing, this is caused by food and drink; one should use *Èr Chén Tāng* F2-42 adding *shān zhā* and *bái zhú* to disperse and lead it out.
    - If food has already been dispersed but there is still pain; perhaps there is no pain when pressed, or now in addition there is headache, vexation heat, thirst, aversion to cold, urge to vomit, and similar symptoms. This is central qì suffering damage, one should take supplementation of the spleen and stomach as the governing principle.
- If there is fever, abdominal pain that is severe pain when pressed, no aversion to food, and no sour swallowing, this is retained blood stasis; use *Shī Xiào Sǎn* F2-55 to disperse it.
- If there is only fever and headache, perhaps with abdominal pain at the same time, but it is not painful when pressed, this is blood deficiency; use *Sì Wù Tāng* F2-51 adding *pào jiāng*, *rén shēn*, and *bái zhú* to supplement it.

《病機要》云：胎產之病，從厥陰經論之，無犯胃氣及上二焦。為之三禁，不可汗，不可下，不可利小便。發汗者同傷寒下早之症，利大便則脈數而已動於脾，利小便則內亡津液，胃中枯燥。制藥之法，能不犯三禁，則榮衛自和，而寒熱止矣。如發渴用白虎，氣弱用黃耆，血刺痛則用當歸，腹中痛則加芍藥，宜詳察脈症而用之。

*Bìng Jī Yào*[86] says: Diseases of giving birth are discussed in regard to the juéyīn channels; do not offend stomach qì and the upper two *jiāos*. There are three prohibitions: one cannot promote sweating, one cannot promote descending [promote a bowel movement], and one cannot disinhibit urination. Promoting sweating makes the same condition as descending too early in cold damage. When the bowel movement is disinhibited, the pulse becomes rapid and the spleen becomes stirred up. When urination is disinhibited, there is internal collapse of *jīnyè*-fluids and the stomach becomes withered and dry. When the method of formulating herbs avoids offending the three prohibitions, *yíng* and *wèi* harmonize themselves and then [sensations of] cold and heat stop. If there is

86. *Jì Yīn Gāng Mù*《濟陰綱目》by Wǔ Zhīwàng 武之望 (1620, *Míng*) has a similar version of this passage that is attributed to Zhāng Jiégǔ 張潔古 (also known as Zhāng Yuánsù 張元素, *Jīn* dynasty). *Bìng Jī Yào*《病機要》seems to be a lost book written by Zhāng. *Bìng Jī*《病機》is also mentioned in Section 1-11.

thirst, use *Bái Hǔ Tāng* F2-21; when qì is weak use *huáng qí*; when there is stabbing pain due to blood, use *dāng guī*; when there is abdominal pain, add *sháo yào*. One should examine the pulse and symptoms in detail to use this.

丹溪先生云：產後當大補氣血為先，雖有雜症，從末治之。一切病多是血虛，皆不可發表。

Doctor Zhū Dānxī[87] said: After giving birth, one should first greatly supplement qì and blood. Even if there are miscellaneous symptoms, treat them at the end [after she has been supplemented]. All the many diseases are [due to] blood deficiency; one cannot describe them all.

## 治驗
## Treatment Experience

**2-7-1** 一產婦腹痛發熱，氣口脈大。余以為飲食停滯，不信，乃破血補虛，反寒熱頭痛，嘔吐涎沫；又用降火化痰理氣，四肢逆冷，泄瀉下墜，始信。謂余曰：何也?余曰：此脾胃虛之變症也，法當溫補。遂用六君加炮薑二錢，肉桂、木香一錢，四劑諸症悉退；再用補中益氣之劑，元氣悉復。

After labor, a woman had abdominal pain, fever, and her *qì kǒu* pulse was large. I took this as food retention. They did not believe me, and then they [used herbs] to break blood and supplement deficiency. Contrary to their expectations, she developed [sensations of] cold and heat, headache, and vomited saliva. Then they used herbs to descend fire, transform phlegm, and rectify qì; she developed counterflow cold of the four limbs and diarrhea with downward pressure [tenesmus]. They began to believe me. They asked me why. I said: These are mutated symptoms of spleen and stomach deficiency; the method should be to warm and supplement. I then used four doses of *Liù Jūn Zǐ Tāng* F2-6 adding two *qián* (7.46 grams) of *pào jiāng*, and one *qián* (3.73 grams) of *ròu guì* and *mù xiāng*, and all the symptoms receded. I then used *Bǔ Zhōng Yì Qì Tāng* F2-5, and her original qì completely returned.

87. This is paraphrased by Zhū Dānxī 朱丹溪 from Volume 5 of *Dān Xī Xīn Fǎ*《丹溪心法》(*Yuán*) 元.

**2-7-2**一婦人產後，腹痛後重，去痢無度，形體倦怠，飲食不甘，懷抱久鬱，患繭唇，寐而盜汗如雨，竟夜不敢寐，神思消爍。余曰：氣血虛而有熱。用當歸六黃湯，內黃芩、連、柏炒黑，一劑汗頓止，再劑全止，乃用歸脾湯、八珍散兼服，元氣漸復而愈。

A postpartum woman had abdominal pain, tenesmus, dysentery without limits, weariness of the body, and food and drink did not taste sweet. She held onto constraint for a long time. She suffered cocoon lips,[88] and when she slept, her night sweating was like rain; [it was so bad] she did not dare to sleep the whole night. Her mental state was worn out. I said: This is qì and blood deficiency with heat. I used one dose of *Dāng Guī Liù Huáng Tāng* F2-14 adding in *huáng qín, huáng lián,* and *huáng bǎi* that was stir-fried until black. The sweating immediately stopped; another dose and it completely stopped. I then used *Guī Pí Tāng* F2-3 and *Bā Zhēn Sǎn*[89] to be taken at the same time. Her original qì gradually returned and she recovered.

**2-7-3**一產婦小腹作痛，服行氣破血之藥不效，其脈洪數。此瘀血內潰為膿也，以瓜子仁湯二劑痛止，更以太乙膏下膿而愈。產後多有此病，縱非癰患，用之更效。

After labor, a woman had pain of the lower abdomen. She took herbs to move qì and break blood but they were ineffective. Her pulse was surging and rapid. This was internal blood stasis bursting out as pus. I used two doses of *Guā Zǐ Rén Tāng* UF-13 and the pain stopped. I further used *Tài Yǐ Gāo* UF-10 to descend the pus and she recovered. Many postpartum women have this disease; even if the suffering is not an abscess, using [these formulas] is more effective.

88. Cocoon lips (*jiǎn chún* 繭唇): In *Kǒu Chǐ Lèi Yào* 薛己《口齒類要》(Categorized Essentials of the Mouth and Teeth), Xuē Jǐ wrote "若唇腫起白皮皺裂如蠶繭，名曰繭唇。If the lips swell up with white skin that is wrinkled and split like silkworm cocoons, this is called *cocoon lips*."

89. *Bā Zhēn Sǎn* 八珍散 is probably a mistaken writing of *Bā Zhēn Tāng* F2-8. There appears to be the same error in *Wài Kē Fā Huī*《外科發揮》(Elucidation of External Medicine) and *Kǒu Chǐ Lèi Yào*《口齒類要》(Categorized Essentials of the Mouth and Teeth), other books by Xuē Jǐ. On the other hand, there are a number of formulas named *Bā Zhēn Sǎn*. One of them is from *Chǎn Rǔ Bèi Yào*《產乳備要》(by an unknown author and published in the *Sòng* dynasty). It has the same ingredients as *Bā Zhēn Tāng* F2-8 except it substitutes *suō shā rén* 縮砂仁 for *bái zhú*.

**2-7-4**一產婦小腹疼痛，小便不利，用薏苡仁湯，二劑痛止；更以四物加桃仁、紅花，下瘀血而愈。

After labor, a woman had lower abdominal pain and inhibited urination. I used two doses of *Yì Yĭ Rén Tāng* UF-11 and the pain stopped. I further used *Sì Wù Tāng* F2-51 adding *táo rén* and *hóng huā*. The blood stasis descended and she recovered.

大抵此症，皆因榮衛不調；或瘀血停滯所致，若脈洪數已有膿，脈但數微有膿，脈遲緊乃瘀血，下之即愈。若腹脹大，轉側作水聲；或膿從臍出；或從大便出，宜用蠟礬丸、太乙膏及托裹藥。

- Generally speaking, this symptom is always due to *yíng* and *wèi* that are out of tune or caused by retained blood stasis.
- If the pulse is surging and rapid, there is already pus; if the pulse is only rapid, there is a small amount of pus; if the pulse is slow and tight, it is blood stasis. Descend it and she will recover.
- If the abdomen is distended and large and there are watery sounds when she moves about, or if pus comes out of the umbilicus, or if it comes out with a bowel movement, it is appropriate to use *Là Fán Wán* UF-12 and *Tài Yĭ Gāo* UF-10 as well as herbs for drawing out the interior.[90]

**2-7-5**一產婦小腹作痛有塊，脈芤而澀，以四物加玄胡索、紅花、桃仁、牛膝、木香，治之而愈。

After labor, a woman had lower abdominal pain with lumps, her pulse was scallion-stalk and rough. I treated her with *Sì Wù Tāng* F2-51 adding *xuán hú suŏ, hóng huā, táo rén, niú xī,* and *mù xiāng* and she recovered.

**2-7-6**一婦人產後，小腹患痛，服瓜子仁湯，下瘀血而痊。

After labor, a woman suffered lower abdominal pain. She took *Guā Zĭ Rén Tāng* UF-13; this descended blood stasis and she recuperated.

90. Drawing out the interior (*tuō lĭ* 托裹) is also translated as internal expression. This is a treatment method of pushing toxins (including their manifestation as pus) outward from the inside of the body by supplementing right qì.

凡瘀血停滯，宜急治之，緩則腐化為膿，最難治療。若流注關節，則患骨疽，失治多為敗症。

- Whenever there is retained blood stasis, it is appropriate to treat it quickly; if slow, it putrifies and becomes pus which is most difficult to cure.
- If it flows and pools[91] into the joints, it becomes a bone abscess; in many who are not properly treated, it beomes a conquering disease.

**2-7-7**一婦人因經水多，服澀藥止之，致腹作痛，以失笑散二服而瘳。

A woman took astringing herbs to stop excessive menstruation. This resulted in abdominal pain. She took two doses of *Shī Xiào Sǎn* F2-55 and was healed.

## 《女科撮要·卷下·產後血暈並失血》
## 2-8 Postpartum Blood Clouding and Blood Loss

產後元氣虧損，惡露乘虛上攻，眼花頭暈；或心下滿悶，神昏口噤；或痰壅盛者，急用失笑散主之。若血下多而暈；或神昏煩亂者，大劑芎歸湯補之；或芸薹子散；或童子小便，有痰加二陳湯。若因勞心力而致者，宜補中益氣加香附。若因氣血虛極不省人事，用清魂散，繼以芎歸湯及大補氣血之劑。凡產可預燒秤錘令赤以器盛之，急至床前以醋沃之；或以醋塗口鼻，聞之即醒；或用破舊漆器；或乾漆燒煙熏之；或用半夏末冷水和丸，入鼻孔中，並無前患。

After giving birth, original qì is enfeebled; lochia takes advantage of the deficiency and attacks upward with blurry vision and dizziness.[92]

91. Flows and pools (*liú zhù* 流注) is also the name for streaming sores. See section 1-10 for details.
92. Lochia (*è lù* 惡露) is the discharge that occurs after giving birth. The Chinese term literally means *malign dew*. The medical thought at the time was that if it is not fully discharged, its tainted nature will harm the new mother. Modern people may or may not agree with this theory.

- Perhaps there is fullness and oppression below the heart, the *shén*-spirit is clouded, and there is lockjaw; or there is flourishing phlegm obstruction; quickly use *Shī Xiào Săn* F2-55 to govern it.
- If a lot of blood descends and there is dizziness; or the *shén*-spirit is clouded and confused, give a large dose of *Xiōng Guī Tāng* F2-67 to supplement her; or *Yún Tái Zǐ Săn* F2-49; or child's urine.
    - If there is phlegm add *Èr Chén Tāng* F2-42.
- If it is due to mental and physical taxation, use *Bŭ Zhōng Yì Qì Tāng* F2-5 adding *xiāng fù*.
- If it is due to severe qì and blood deficiency and she is not aware of human affairs [unconscious], use *Qīng Hún Săn* F2-60, followed by the use of *Xiōng Guī Tāng* F2-67 and prescriptions to greatly supplement qì and blood.
    - To be prepared whenever someone is giving birth, put the sliding weight of a scale in a vessel and heat it until red hot. Quickly take it to the bedside and pour vinegar on it. Or spread vinegar on her mouth and nose. She will wake up when she smells it. Or burn old broken laquerware or *gān qī* (laquer) and fume her with the smoke. Or blend *bàn xià* powder with cold water to make pills and put them inside her nostrils. [If you do one of these,] you will be without the above-mentioned suffering.

丹溪先生云：血暈因氣血俱虛，痰火泛上，宜以二陳導痰；或加減硃砂安神丸，以麥門冬湯下亦可 。

Doctor Zhū Dānxī said: "Blood dizziness is due to deficiency of both qì and blood or phlegm fire floating upward."

- It is appropriate to use *Èr Chén Tāng* F2-42 to lead out phlegm; or modified (*Jiā Jiăn*) *Zhū Shā Ān Shén Wán* F2-61; you can also use *Mài Mén Dōng Tāng* F2-43 to descend [the floating fire].

大凡產後口眼喎斜等症，當大補氣血為主，而兼以治痰 。若脾胃虛而不能固者，用六君子湯；至五七個月，宜服安胎飲；至八九個月，再加大腹皮 、黃楊腦 。如臨產時，更宜服保生無憂散，庶無前患 。

- In most cases, postpartum symptoms that are similar to deviation of the mouth and eyes should be governed by strong supplementation of qì and blood, and phlegm should be treated at the same time.

- If the spleen and stomach are deficient with inability to secure, use *Liù Jūn Zǐ Tāng* F2-6.
    - Up until the fifth month of pregnancy, it is appropriate to take *Ān Tāi Yǐn* F2-41.
    - Up until the eighth or ninth month [out of ten lunar months of pregnancy], also add *dà fù pí* and *huáng yáng nǎo*.
    - When about to give birth, it is further appropriate to take *Bǎo Shēng Wú Yōu Sǎn* F2-46, and many patient will not have the above-mentioned suffering.

## 治驗
## Treatment Experience

**2-8-1**一產婦月餘矣，因怒兩脅脹痛，忽吐血甚多，發熱惡寒，胸腹脹滿，用八珍加柴胡、丹皮、炮薑而安；卻用十全大補，仍加炮薑而愈。前症因脾肺氣血虧損，而胸腹虛痞，雖投大補，若非薑桂辛溫助其脾肺，以行藥勢，亦無以施其功，而反助其脹耳。

More than five months after giving birth, a woman had distention and pain of both rib-sides due to anger. She suddenly vomited a lot of blood, had fever and aversion to cold, and distention and fullness of the chest and abdomen. I used *Bā Zhēn Tāng* F2-8 adding *chái hú, mǔ dān pí,* and *pào jiāng* and she was peaceful; I further used *Shí Quán Dà Bǔ Tāng* F2-7, still adding *pào jiāng* and she recovered. The earlier pattern was due to enfeebled qì and blood of the spleen and lungs, and deficiency in the chest and abdomen with *pǐ*-glomus. Even if I had given her herbs to strongly supplement, they would be unable to carry out the results unless the spleen and lungs were assisted by the acrid warmth of ginger and cinnamon to move the herbal influence around; contrary to expectations they would have assisted her distention.

**2-8-2**家人婦產後，小腹作痛，忽牙關緊急，灌以失笑散良久而蘇，又用四物加炮薑、白朮、陳皮而愈。

After childbirth, a family member had lower abdominal pain and clenched jaw. I poured in[93] *Shī Xiào Sǎn* F2-55 and she revived after a good long while. I then used *Sì Wù Tāng* F2-51 adding *pào jiāng, bái zhú,* and *chén pí* and she recovered.

**2-8-3**一產婦筋攣臂軟，肌肉掣動，此氣血俱虛，用十全大補湯而愈。

After labor, a woman suffered sinew spasms, weak arms, and pulling and stirring of the muscles and flesh. This was deficiency of both qì and blood. I used *Shí Quán Dà Bǔ Tāng* F2-7 and she recovered.

**2-8-4**一產婦兩手麻木，服愈風丹、天麻丸，遍身皆麻，神思倦怠，晡熱作渴，自汗盜汗。此氣血俱虛也，用十全大補加炮薑數劑，諸症悉退；卻去炮薑，又數劑而愈。但內熱，此血虛也，用逍遙散而痊。

After labor, a woman suffered numbness of both hands. She took *Yù Fēng Dān* UFx-9 and *Tiān má* Wán UFx-10. Her entire body became numb. Her mental state became weary, and she had late afternoon fever, thirst, spontaneous sweating, and night sweating. This was deficiency of both qì and blood. I used several doses of *Shí Quán Dà Bǔ Tāng* F2-7 adding *pào jiāng* and all her symptoms receded; I gave her another several doses removing *pào jiāng,* and she recovered. Only internal heat remained; this was blood deficiency. I used *Xiāo Yáo Sǎn* F2-2 and she recuperated.

93. Pouring in (*guàn* 灌) is used in an unconscious patient. The herbal powder or decoction is poured into the person's mouth or maybe into the nose. See case 2-9-2, below.

## 《女科撮要·卷下·產後發痓》（痓當作痙）
## 2-9 Postpartum Tetany (痓 chì should be written as 痙 jìng[94])

產後發痓因去血過多，元氣虧極；或外邪相搏，其形牙關緊急，四肢勁強；或腰背反張，肢體抽搐。若有汗而不惡寒者，曰柔痓。若無汗而惡寒者，曰剛痓。然產後患之，實由亡血過多，筋無所養而致。故傷寒汗下過多，潰瘍膿血大泄，多患之，乃敗症也。若大補血氣，多保無虞。若攻風邪，死無疑矣。

Postpartum tetany is due to excessive loss of blood and extreme lack of original qì or due to external evils wrestling with each other. It takes the form of clenched jaw and powerful rigidity of the four limbs; or arched-back rigidity with twitching of the body. If there is sweating and no aversion to cold, it is called *soft tetany*. If there is no sweating and aversion to cold, it is called *hard tetany*. However, when postpartum women suffer this, it is really from blood collapse and excessive [bleeding]; the reason is that the sinews have nothing to nourish them. Thus people with cold damage who are excessively made to sweat or descend [inducing a bowel movement], or with open sores that discharge a lot of pus and blood often suffer this; it is a conquering pattern. If one greatly supplements blood and qì, many can be protected from the unpredictable. If one attacks wind evils, there is no doubt they will die.

### 治驗
### Treatment Experience

**2-9-1**一產婦牙關緊急，腰背反張，四肢抽搐，兩目連札，余以為去血過多，元氣虧損，陰火熾盛，用十全大補加炮薑一劑而蘇，又數劑而安。

After labor, a woman suffered clenched jaw, arched-back rigidity, twitching of the four limbs, and both eyes continuously [moved as if] reading. I took this as excessive blood loss, enfeebled original qì, and yīn fire blazing and flourishing. I used one dose of *Shí*

94. This note correcting a character must have been written by a later editor.

*Quán Dà Bǔ Tāng* F2-7 adding *pào jiāng* and she revived; she was peaceful after several more doses.

**2-9-2**余在吴江史萬湖第，將入更時，聞喧嚷云：某家人婦，忽仆牙關緊急，已死矣。詢云是新產婦出直廚，余意其勞傷血氣而發痙也。急用十全大補加附子煎滾，令人推正其身，一人以手夾正其面，卻挖開其口，將藥灌之，不咽，藥已冷，令側其面出之，仍正其面復灌以熱藥，又冷又灌，如此五次，方嚥下，隨灌以熱藥遂蘇。

I was in Wújiāng, in the residence of Shǐ Wànhú. It was about to enter the evening hours when I heard a clamor. They were saying: In a certain household a woman suddenly fell down [collapsed] with clenched jaws; she is already dead. I inquired and they said the new mother had gone directly to the kitchen [to work without recovering first]. I thought it was taxation damaging blood and qì that then erupted in tetany. I quickly boiled *Shí Quán Dà Bǔ Tāng* F2-7 adding *fù zǐ*. I made people push her body straight. Someone manually pressed her face straight and pried her mouth open. I poured the herbs in. She did not swallow and the herbs got cold, so we turned her face to the side to let them out. We again straightened her face and again poured in the hot herbs. They got cold again and we poured them in again. We did this five times. She finally swallowed some down. We followed up using the hot herbs and she then revived.

# 《女科撮要·卷下·產後便血》
## 2-10 Postpartum Blood in the Stool

產後便血；或飲食起居；或六淫七情，以致元氣虧損，陽絡外傷。治法：若因膏粱積熱，用加味清胃散；若因醇酒濕毒，葛花解酲湯；若因怒動肝火，六君加柴、芍、芎、歸；若因鬱結傷脾，加味歸脾湯；若因思慮傷心，妙香散；若因大腸風熱，四物加側柏、荊、防、枳殼、槐花；若因大腸血熱，四物加芩、連；若因腸胃虛弱，六君加升麻、柴胡；若因腸胃虛寒，六君加肉蔻、木香；若因元氣下陷，補中益氣加茯苓、半夏；若因氣虛，用六君、升麻；若因血虛，用四物；氣血俱虛，用八珍，俱加柴胡、升麻。

Postpartum blood in the stool: Perhaps [improper] food and drink or rising and dwelling, or the six excesses [external evils] and seven emotions result in enfeebled original qì and external damage to the yáng *luò*-networks. The treatment method:

- If it is due to rich foods accumulating heat, use *Jiā Wèi Qīng Wèi Sǎn* F2-11.
- If it is due to damp toxins from fine liquor, use *Gé Huā Jiě Chéng Tāng* F2-70.
- If it is due to anger stirring up liver fire, use *Liù Jūn Zǐ Tāng* F2-6 adding *chái hú, sháo yào, chuān xiōng,* and *dāng guī.*
- If it is due to binding constraint damaging the spleen, use *Jiā Wèi Guī Pí Tāng* F2-4.
- If it is due to excessive thought and consideration damaging the heart, use *Miào Xiāng Sǎn* F2-79.
- If it is due to wind heat of the large intestine, use *Sì Wù Tāng* F2-51 adding *cè bǎi yè, jīng jiè, fáng fēng, zhǐ qiào,* and *huái huā.*
- If it is due to blood heat in the large intestine, use *Sì Wù Tāng* F2-51 adding *huáng qín* and *huáng lián.*
- If it is due to deficient weak intestines and stomach, use *Liù Jūn Zǐ Tāng* F2-6 adding *shēng má* and *chái hú.*
- If it is due to deficient cold intestines and stomach, use *Liù Jūn Zǐ Tāng* F2-6 adding *ròu kòu* and *mù xiāng.*
- If it is due to original qì sinking downward, use *Bǔ Zhōng Yì Qì Tāng* F2-5 adding *fú líng* and *bàn xià.*
- If it is due to qì deficiency, use *Liù Jūn Zǐ Tāng* F2-6 adding *shēng má.*
- If it is due to blood deficiency, use *Sì Wù Tāng* F2-51.
    - For deficiency of both qì and blood, use *Bā Zhēn Tāng* F2-8, for both of these add *chái hú* and *shēng má.*

大凡病久，或元氣虛弱；見病百端，皆因脾胃虧損，內真寒而外假熱，但用六君子，或補中益氣加炮薑溫補脾氣，諸症悉退。若四肢畏冷，屬陽氣虛寒，急加附子。病因多端，當臨症制宜，庶無誤矣。

In most cases, when the disease lasts a long time, perhaps original qì is deficient and weak. The disease appears in many ways, but all are due to enfeebled spleen and stomach with true cold on the interior and false heat on the exterior. Only use *Liù Jūn Zǐ Tāng* F2-6, or *Bǔ Zhōng Yì Qì Tāng* F2-5 adding *pào jiāng* to warm and supplement spleen qì, and all the symptoms will recede. If the four limbs fear cold, it belongs to deficient cold yáng qì; quickly add *fù zǐ*. There are many disease causes; in clinic you should suit the treatment to the pattern and there will be no mistake.

## 治驗
## Treatment Experience

**2-10-1**一產婦糞後下血，諸藥不應，飲食少思，肢體倦怠，此中氣虛弱，用補中益氣加茱炒黃連五分，四劑頓止。但怔忡少寐，盜汗未止，用歸脾湯治之而痊。

A postpartum woman suffered bleeding after defecation and did not respond to various herbs. She had little thought of food and drink and her body was weary. This was deficient weak central qì. I used four doses of *Bǔ Zhōng Yì Qì Tāng* F2-5 adding five *fēn* (1.85 grams) of *huáng lián* stir-fried with *wú zhū yú*[95] and it immediately stopped. Only fright palpitations, decreased sleep, and night sweating had not stopped. I treated her with *Guī Pí Tāng* F2-3 and she recuperated.

**2-10-2**一婦人但怒便血，寒熱口苦；或胸脅脹痛；或小腹痞悶。此木乘土，用六君加山梔、柴胡而愈，用補中益氣、加味逍遙二藥，而不復作。

A woman had blood in the stool only when she was angry, with [sensations of] cold and heat and bitter mouth. She sometimes had chest and rib-side distention and pain

95. While it is not the same recipe used here, *Xiāng Lián Wán* UF-14 (*Mù Xiāng* and *Huáng Lián* Pill) explains how to make *huáng lián* stir-fired with *wú zhū yú*.

or *pǐ*-glomus of the lower abdomen with oppression. This was wood taking advantage of earth. I used *Liù Jūn Zǐ Tāng* F2-6 adding *zhī zǐ* and *chái hú* and she recovered. I used two decoctions: *Bǔ Zhōng Yì Qì Tāng* F2-5 and *Jiā Wèi Xiāo Yáo Sǎn* F2-1, and she did not relapse.

**2-10-3**一婦人久下血在糞前，屬脾胃虛寒，元氣下陷。用補中益氣加連炒吳茱一錢，數劑稍緩；乃加生吳茱五分，數劑而愈。

For a long time, a woman bled before she had a bowel movement. This belonged to deficient cold spleen and stomach with original qì sinking downward. I used several doses of *Bǔ Zhōng Yì Qì Tāng* F2-5 adding one *qián* (3.73 grams) of *wú zhū yú* stir-fried with *huáng lián*.[96] It moderated somewhat. I then added five *fēn* (1.85 grams) of unprocessed *wú zhū yú*, and she recovered after several doses.

**2-10-4**一婦人產後便血，口乾飲湯，胸脅膨滿，小腹悶墜，內熱晡熱，飲食不甘，體倦面黃，日晡則赤，灑淅惡寒。此脾肺氣虛，先用六君加炮薑、木香，諸症漸愈；用補中益氣將愈；用歸脾湯痊愈。後飲食失節，勞役兼怒氣，發熱血崩，夜間熱甚，譫語不絕。此熱入血室，用加味小柴胡，二劑而熱退；用補中益氣而血止；用逍遙散、歸脾湯，調理而康。

A postpartum woman had blood in her stool and dry mouth. She drank hot drinks, and had fullness and inflation in her chest and rib-sides, [a feeling of] oppression and sagging in her lower abdomen, internal heat, and late afternoon fever. Food and drink did not taste sweet to her. She had weariness of the body, yellow face that turned red around sunset, and aversion to cold as if after a soaking. This was qì deficiency of the spleen and lungs. I first used *Liù Jūn Zǐ Tāng* F2-6 adding *pào jiāng* and *mù xiāng*; all her symptoms gradually began to recover. I used *Bǔ Zhōng Yì Qì Tāng* F2-5 and she had almost recovered. I used *Guī Pí Tāng* F2-3 and she completely recovered. Later due to loss of regulation in her diet at the same time as taxation and anger, she developed fever with flooding of blood. The fever was quite high at night and she had unceasing delirious speech. This was heat entering the blood chamber. I used two doses of *Jiā Wèi Xiǎo Chái Hú Tāng* F2-13 and the fever receded. I used *Bǔ Zhōng Yì Qì Tāng* F2-5 and the bleeding stopped. I used *Xiāo Yáo Sǎn* F2-2 and *Guī Pí Tāng* F2-3 to attune and rectify her and she became healthy.

96. If you were wondering the author did with the discarded *wú zhū yú* that was stir-fried with *huáng lián* in case 2-10-1, the author made use of it in this case.

# 《女科撮要·卷下·產後大便不通》
## 2-11 Postpartum Constipation

產後大便不通，因去血過多，大腸乾涸；或血虛火燥乾涸，不可計其日期，飲食數，多用藥通之潤之。必待腹滿覺脹，自欲去而不能者，乃結在直腸，宜用豬膽汁潤之。若服苦寒藥潤通，反傷中焦元氣；或愈加難通；或通而瀉不能止，必成敗症。若屬血虛火燥，用加味逍遙散；氣血俱虛，八珍湯。慎不可用麻子、杏仁、枳殼之類。

Postpartum constipation is due to excessive blood loss making the large intestine desiccated; or blood deficiency with fire-dryness desiccating it. One cannot calculate how many days it will last. If there is frequent eating and drinking, many use herbs to free and moisten [the stool]. One must wait for abdominal fullness and the feeling of distention, for the spontaneous desire but inability to go; then it is bound up in the straight intestine [rectum]. [At that point] it is appropriate to moisten it with pig bile.[97] If one takes bitter cold herbs to moisten and free it, contrary to expectations it will damage the middle *jiāo* and original qì. This will either make freeing it more difficult or it will flow but become diarrhea that cannot be stopped. These can become conquering patterns.

- If it belongs to blood deficiency with fire-dryness, use *Jiā Wèi Xiāo Yáo Sǎn* F2-1.
- If both qì and blood are deficient, use *Bā Zhēn Tāng* F2-8.

Be careful not to use the likes of *má zǐ, xìng rén,* and *zhǐ qiào.*

97. Pig bile clears heat, moistens dryness, and is used to treat constipation as well as internal heat diseases, jaundice, cough red eyes, and so forth. Pig bile may be taken internally in decoctions, pills, or with powders. Externally, it can be spread on a site, used in eye drops, or as an enema. Xuē tended to use it for constipation, often as an enema, although recipes exist for decocting pig bile with honey and taking it internally for bound up dry stool.

## 治驗
## Treatment Experience

**2-11-1**一產婦大便不通七日矣，飲食如常，腹中如故。余曰：飲食所入，雖倍常數，腹不滿脹，用八珍加桃、杏二仁。至二十一日，腹滿，欲去，用豬膽汁潤之，先去乾糞五七塊，後皆常糞而安。

A postpartum woman suffered constipation for seven days. Her eating and drinking were like normal and her abdomen was like normal. I said: Although double the normal food and drink have entered, her abdomen is not full or distended. I used *Bā Zhēn Tāng* F2-8 adding *táo rén* and *xìng rén*. Reaching twenty-one days, she had abdominal fullness and the desire to go. I used pig bile to moisten it. At first five or seven lumps of dry stool came out. Then all the normal stool came out and she was peaceful.

**2-11-2**一產婦大便八日不通，用通利之藥，中脘作痛，飲食甚少。或云：通則不痛，痛則不通。乃用蜜導之，大便不禁，吃逆不食。余曰：此脾腎復傷，用六君加吳茱、肉果、骨脂、五味數劑。喜其年壯，不然，多致不起。

A postpartum woman suffered constipation for eight days. She used herbs to free and disinhibit it. Zhōng Wǎn [the region of Rèn 12] became painful and she ate and drank very little. Someone said: When there is free flow there is no pain; when there is pain, there is no free flow. They then used honey to lead it out, but it became incontinence of stool, hiccups, and she did not eat. I said: This is repeated damage to the spleen and kidneys. I used several doses of *Liù Jūn Zǐ Tāng* F2-6 adding *wú zhū yú, ròu guǒ,*[98] *bǔ gǔ zhī,* and *wǔ wèi zǐ*. I was pleased she was in her prime; otherwise, many cases result in death.

98. *Ròu guǒ* 肉果 is an alternate name for *ròu dòu kòu* 肉豆蔻.

## 《女科撮要·卷下·產後寒熱》
## 2-12 Postpartum [Sensations of] Cold and Heat

產後寒熱，因氣血虛弱，或脾胃虧損，乃不足之症。經云：陰虛則發熱，陽虛則惡寒。若兼大便不通，尤屬氣血虛弱，切不可用發表降火。若寸口脈微，名陽氣不足。陰氣上入於陽中則惡寒，用補中益氣湯。尺部脈弱，名陰氣不足。陽氣下陷於陰中則發熱，用六味地黄丸。大抵陰不足，陽往從之，則陽內陷而發熱；陽不足，陰往從之，則陰上入而惡寒。此陰陽不歸其分，以致寒熱交爭，故惡寒而發熱也，當用八珍湯。若病後四肢發熱；或形氣倦怠，此元氣未復，濕熱乘之耳，宜補中益氣湯。若肌熱大渴引飲，目赤面紅，此血虛發熱，用當歸補血湯，若認為寒則誤矣。

Postpartum [sensations of] cold and heat are due to deficient weak qì and blood or enfeebled spleen and stomach; this is an insufficiency pattern. The Classic says: When yīn is deficient, there is fever; when yáng is deficient, there is aversion to cold.[99] If there is constipation at the same time, it especially belongs to deficient weak qì and blood; be sure not to use herbs to effuse the exterior or descend fire.

- If the *cùn kǒu* pulse is faint, it is named *insufficient yáng qì*. Yīn qì has ascended and entered into yáng so there is aversion to cold; use *Bǔ Zhōng Yì Qì Tāng* F2-5.
- If the *chǐ* section of the pulse is weak, it is named *insufficient yīn qì*. When yáng qì has descended and sunken into yīn there is fever; use *Liù Wèi Dì Huáng Wán* F2-16.
- Generally speaking, when yīn is insufficient, yáng frequently follows it, so yáng sinks inside and becomes fever. When yáng is insufficient, yīn frequently follows it, so yīn ascends and enters, becoming aversion to cold. This is yīn and yáng failing to return to their own divisions; it results in cold and heat interacting contentiously, so there is aversion to cold and fever. One should use *Bā Zhēn Tāng* F2-8.
- If after being ill, the four limbs are feverish; or the physical-body and qì are weary, this means original qì has not returned and damp heat is taking advantage of it; use *Bǔ Zhōng Yì Qì Tāng* F2-5.
- If the muscles are hot, there is great thirst with desire to drink, and the eyes and face are red, this is blood deficiency fever; use *Dāng Guī Bǔ Xuè Tāng* F2-9. If you believe it is cold, you are mistaken.

99. This is similar to a statement in *Sù Wèn • Tiáo Jīng Lùn*, Chapter 62《素問·調經論篇第六十二》. It must be a paraphrase of this or from some other unknown source.

## 治驗
## Treatment Experience

**2-12-1**一產婦惡寒發熱，用十全大補加炮薑治之而愈。但飲食不甘，肢體倦怠，用補中益氣而安。又飲食後犯怒，惡寒發熱，抽搐咬牙，難候其脈，視其面色，青中隱黃，欲按其腹，以手護之。此肝木侮脾土，飲食停滯而作，用六君加木香，一劑而安。

After labor, a woman suffered aversion to cold and fever. I treated her with *Shí Quán Dà Bǔ Tāng* F2-7 adding *pào jiāng* and she recovered. Only food and drink did not taste sweet and her body was weary. I used *Bǔ Zhōng Yì Qì Tāng* F2-5 and she was peaceful. Later, she became angry after eating and drinking, with aversion to cold, fever, twitching, and clenching her teeth. It was difficult to read her pulse [because of her movements]. In observing her facial color, there was yellow hidden within *qīng*-green. I wanted to press her abdomen, but she guarded it with her hands. This arose from liver wood insulting spleen earth with food retention. I used one dose of *Liù Jūn Zǐ Tāng* F2-6 adding *mù xiāng* and she was peaceful.

**2-12-2**一產婦惡寒發熱，余欲用八珍加炮薑治之，其家知醫，以為風寒，用小柴胡湯。余曰：寒熱不時，乃氣血虛。不信，仍服一劑，汗出不止，譫語不絕，煩熱作渴，肢體抽搐，余用十全大補，二劑益甚，脈洪大，重按如無，仍以前湯加附子，四劑稍緩，數劑而安。

After labor, a woman suffered aversion to cold and fever. I was about to treat her with *Bā Zhēn Tāng* F2-8 adding *pào jiāng*, but her family knew a doctor who took it as wind cold. They used *Xiǎo Chái Hú Tāng* F2-12. I said: [Sensations of] cold and heat at at no particular time means qì and blood deficiency. They did not believe me and she took a dose. She began sweating incessantly with non-stop delirious speech, vexation heat, thirst, and twitching of her body. I used two doses of *Shí Quán Dà Bǔ Tāng* F2-7 and it increased a lot. Her pulse was surging and large, but when heavily pressed it felt like nothing was there. I still used four [more] doses of the above decoction adding *fù zǐ*, and it moderated a little. She was peaceful after several doses.

# 《女科撮要·卷下·產後咳嗽》
## 2-13 Postpartum Cough

產後咳嗽；或因陰血耗損；或因肺氣虧傷；或陰火上炎；或風寒所感。主治之法：若陰血虛者，用芎、歸、熟地、參、朮。肺氣傷者，用四君、芎、歸、桔梗。陰火上炎者，六味地黃加參朮。風寒所感者，補中益氣加桔梗、紫蘇。若瘀血入肺發喘，急用二味參蘇飲，多有得生者。若兼口鼻起黑；或鼻出血，急用前散，亦有得生者。然而，所患悉因胃氣不足，蓋胃為五臟之根本，人身之根蒂，胃氣一虛，五臟失所，百病生焉。但患者多謂腠理不密所致，殊不知肺屬辛金，生於己土，亦因土虛不能生金，而腠理不密，外邪所感。只陰火上炎亦壯土，金生腎水以制火為善。若徑治其病，則誤矣。

Postpartum cough is due to consumption of yīn and blood, or due to damage to lung qì, or yīn fire flaring upward, or contraction of wind cold. The governing treatment method:

- If yīn and blood are deficient, use *chuān xiōng, dāng guī, shú dì huáng, rén shēn,* and *bái zhú.*
- For damage to lung qì, use *Sì Jūn Zǐ Tāng* F2-26 adding *chuān xiōng, dāng guī,* and *jié gěng.*
- For yīn fire flaring upward, use *Liù Wèi Dì Huáng Wán* F2-16 adding *rén shēn* and *bái zhú.*
- For contraction of wind cold, use *Bǔ Zhōng Yì Qì Tāng* F2-5 adding *jié gěng* and *zǐ sū yè.*
- If blood stasis enters the lungs with panting, quickly use *Èr Wèi Shēn Sū Yǐn* F2-59 and you can save many lives.
- If the mouth and nose turn black at the same time or blood comes from the nose, quickly use the previous powder [*Èr Wèi Shēn Sū Yǐn*[100] F2-59] and you can also save many lives.

Even so, what is suffered is completely due to insufficient stomach qì. Now, the stomach is the root of the five *zàng*-organs, the stem of the human body. Once stomach qì is deficient, the five *zàng*-organs lose their place and the hundred diseases are engendered. But

100. *Èr Wèi Shēn Sū Yǐn* F2-59 lists these indications, but it is not a powder.

sufferers often say it is caused by unclosed *còu lǐ*,[101] hardly realizing that the lungs belong to *xīn*-metal and are engendered by *jǐ*-earth;[102] this is also due to deficiency of earth with inability to engender metal so the *còu lǐ* do not close and external evils are contracted. In yīn fire flaring upward, also simply invigorate earth; metal engenders kidney water which then controls fire, so it does good. One who treats the disease directly will be mistaken.

## 治驗
## Treatment Experience

**2-13-1**一產婦咳嗽聲重，鼻塞流涕。此風寒所感，用參蘇飲一鍾，頓愈六七；乃與補中益氣加桔梗、茯苓、半夏，一劑而痊；又與六君加黃耆，以實其腠理而安。

After labor, a woman suffered a loud cough and a stuffy runny nose. This was contraction of wind cold. I used a cup of *Shēn Sū Yǐn* F2-59 and she immediately recovered sixty or seventy percent. I then gave her a dose of *Bǔ Zhōng Yì Qì Tāng* F2-5 adding *jié gěng*, *fú líng*, and *bàn xià* and she recuperated. I then gave her *Liù Jūn Zǐ Tāng* F2-6 adding *huáng qí* to fill up her *còu lǐ* and she was peaceful.

**2-13-2**一產婦朝吐痰，夜發熱，兼之無寐，泥用清痰降火，肌體日瘦，飲食日少，前症愈甚。余曰：早間吐痰，脾氣虛也；夜間發熱，肝血虛也；晝夜無寐，脾血耗也。遂用六君子湯、加味逍遙散、加味歸脾湯以次調補，不月而痊。

After labor, a woman spit phlegm in the mornings and had fever at night. Furthermore she could not sleep. She stubbornly used herbs to clear phlegm and descend fire; her flesh and body became thinner by the day and her food intake decreased by the day. The previous pattern increased a lot. I said: Spitting phlegm in the morning is spleen qì deficiency and fever at night is liver blood deficiency. Not sleeping day or night is consump-

101. *Còu lǐ* 腠理 is often translated as pores. Wiseman glosses it as interstices. This is the anatomical entity within the skin that opens to allow sweating but is held closed by *wèi* qì most of the time to prevent invasion by exterior evils.
102. *Xīn*-metal, *jǐ*-earth: *Xīn* 辛 and *jǐ* 己 are two of the ten heavenly stems. *Xīn* corresponds to yīn metal and therefore the lungs; *jǐ* corresponds to yīn earth and the spleen.

tion of spleen blood. I then used *Liù Jūn Zǐ Tāng* F2-6, *Jiā Wèi Xiāo Yáo Sǎn* F2-1, and *Jiā Wèi Guī Pí Tāng* F2-4 in proper order to attune and supplement her and she recuperated in less than a month.

**2-13-3**一產婦咳嗽痰盛，面赤口乾，內熱晡熱，徹作無時。此陰火上炎，當補脾腎，遂用補中益氣湯、六味地黃丸而愈。

After labor, a woman suffered cough with copious phlegm. She also had red face, dry mouth, internal heat, and late afternoon fever that occured at any time. This was yīn fire flaring upward. We should supplement the spleen and kidneys. I then used used *Bǔ Zhōng Yì Qì Tāng* F2-5 and *Liù Wèi Dì Huáng Wán* F2-16 and she recovered.

**2-13-4**一產婦咳而腹滿，不食涕唾，面腫氣逆。此病在胃，關於肺，用異功散而愈。

After labor, a woman suffered cough with abdominal fullness. She did not eat and had nasal mucus and saliva, swollen face, and qì counterflow. This disease was located in the stomach and connected to the lungs. I used *Yì Gōng Sǎn* F2-27 and she recovered.

時疫墮胎咳嗽見小產。

If seasonal epidemic induces a miscarriage with cough, see Section 2-2 on Small Birth (Abortion or Miscarriage).

## 《女科撮要·卷下·產後瘧疾》
## 2-14 Postpartum Malaria

產後瘧疾，因脾胃虛弱，飲食停滯；或因外邪所感；或鬱怒傷脾；或暑邪所伏。審系飲食，用六君加桔梗、蒼朮、藿香。如外邪多而飲食少，用藿香正氣散。如外邪少而飲食多，用人參養胃湯。飲食勞役，用補中益氣湯。氣血虛弱，用十全大補加炮薑。虛寒用六君加薑、桂。元氣脫陷，急加附子。大凡久瘧，多屬元氣虛寒。

Postpartum *nüè*-malarial disease is due to deficient weak spleen and stomach and food retention; or due to contraction of external evils; or constrained anger damaging the spleen; or summerheat evils that remain latent.

- When it is related to food and drink, use *Liù Jūn Zǐ Tāng* F2-6 adding *jié gěng, cāng zhú,* and *huò xiāng.*
- If external evils are the greater problem and food and drink are less of a factor, use *Huò Xiāng Zhèng Qì Sǎn* F2-71.
- If external evils are less of a factor and food and drink are the greater problem, use *Rén Shēn Yǎng Wèi Tāng* F2-73.
- If it is due to food and drink and taxation, use *Bǔ Zhōng Yì Qì Tāng* F2-5.
- For deficient weak qì and blood, use *Shí Quán Dà Bǔ Tāng* F2-7 adding *pào jiāng.*
- For deficiency coldness, use *Liù Jūn Zǐ Tāng* F2-6 adding ginger and cinnamon.
    - If original qì deserts and sinks, quickly add *fù zǐ*. Many cases of *nüè*-malaria that last a long time belong to deficient cold original qì.

蓋氣虛則寒，血虛則熱，胃虛則惡寒，陰火下流則寒熱交作。或吐瀉不食，腹痛煩渴，發熱譫語；或手足逆冷，寒戰如栗。雖見百症，當峻溫補，其病自退；若誤用清脾、截瘧之類，多致不起。

Now, when there is qì deficiency there is coldness; when there is blood deficiency there is heat; when there is stomach deficiency there is aversion to cold; when yīn fire flows downward, cold and heat interact contentiously. Perhaps there is vomiting and diarrhea, no food intake, abdominal pain, vexation, thirst, fever, and delirious speech; or counterflow cold of the hands and feet, and cold shivering that resembles trembling. Even if you see a hundred symptoms, you should drastically warm and supplement, and then the disease will spontaneously recede. If you mistakenly use herbs in the category of clearing heat from the spleen and interrupting *nüè*-malaria, it will result in many deaths.

# 治驗
## Treatment Experience

**2-14-1**一產婦患瘧，發熱作渴，胸膈脹滿，遍身作痛，三日不食，咽酸噯氣。此是飲食所傷，脾胃不能消化，用六君加神曲、山楂，四劑而不作酸；乃去神曲、山楂，又數劑而飲食進，其大便不通。至三十五日，計進飲食七十餘碗，腹始悶，令用豬膽汁導而通之，其糞且不甚燥。

After labor, a woman suffered *nüè*-malaria, with fever, thirst, distention and fullness of the chest and diaphragm, and pain of the entire body. She did not eat for three days and suffered sour swallowing and belching. This was damage by food and drink with inability of the spleen and stomach to disperse and transform [inability to digest]. After I used four doses of *Liù Jūn Zĭ Tāng* F2-6 adding *shén qū* and *shān zhā*, there was no more sour swallowing. Then I removed the *shén qū* and *shān zhā*; after another several doses she could eat and drink but she had constipation. Reaching the thirty-fifth day, we counted that she had eaten and drank more than seventy bowls [of food without a bowel movement] and she began to have abdominal oppression. I made her use pig bile as an enema and it passed through,[103] but her stool was not extremely dry.

**2-14-2**一產婦患瘧久不愈，百病蜂起，其脈或洪大；或微細；或弦緊；或沉伏，難以名狀。用六君加炮薑二十餘劑，脈症稍得；又用參朮煎膏，佐以歸脾湯，百餘劑而瘥。

After labor, a woman suffered *nüè*-malaria for a long time without recovering; a hundred diseases arose in swarms, her pulse was sometimes surging and large; or faint and fine; or bowstring and tight; or sunken and hidden. It was difficult to name the condition. I used more than twenty doses of *Liù Jūn Zĭ Tāng* F2-6 adding *pào jiāng* and her pulse and disease improved a little. I also used *rén shēn* and *bái zhú* boiled into a paste and assisted using *Guī Pí Tāng* F2-3. She got better after more than a hundred doses.

103. For pig bile was used as an enema, see section 2-11 on postpartum constipation.

**2-14-3**一產婦朝寒暮熱；或不時寒熱，久不愈，用六君子、補中益氣兼服，百餘劑而尋愈。

After labor, a woman suffered cold in the morning and heat in the evening or [sensations of] cold and heat at no particular time. She did not recover after a long while. I had her take *Liù Jūn Zǐ Tāng* F2-6 and *Bǔ Zhōng Yì Qì Tāng* F2-5 at the same time. She recovered after more than a hundred doses.

產後瘧疾心脾痛見小產。

For postpartum *nüè*-malarial disease with heart and spleen pain, see Section 2-2 on Small Birth (Abortion or Miscarriage).

## 《女科撮要·卷下·產後瀉痢》(二症治同兼呕吐)

## 2-15 Postpartum Diarrhea and Dysentery

(These two diseases can be treated the same way as vomiting.)

產後瀉痢；或因飲食傷損脾土；或脾土虛不能消食，當審而治之。若米食所傷，用六君加穀蘗。若麵食所傷，用六君加麥蘗。若肉食所傷，用六君加山楂、神曲。凡兼嘔吐，皆加藿香。若兼咽酸或嘔吐，用前藥送越鞠丸。若肝木來侮脾土，用六君加柴胡、炮薑。若寒水反來侮土，用錢氏益黃散。若久瀉；或元氣下陷，兼補中益氣湯以升發陽氣。若瀉痢色黃，乃脾土真氣，宜加木香、肉果。若屬脾土虛寒，當用六君加木香、薑、桂。若脾腎虛寒，用補中益氣及四神丸。若屬命門火衰，而脾土虛寒，用八味丸以補土母。若小便澀滯，肢體漸腫；或兼喘咳，用《金匱》腎氣丸以補脾腎，利水道。若胃氣虛弱，而四肢浮腫，治須補胃為主。

Postpartum diarrhea and dysentery are sometimes due to food and drink damaging spleen earth or inability of deficient spleen earth to disperse food. You should examine and treat it.

- If damaged by eating rice, use *Liù Jūn Zǐ Tāng* F2-6 adding *gǔ niè*.[104]
- If if damaged by eating wheat, use *Liù Jūn Zǐ Tāng* F2-6 adding *mài niè*.[105]
- If damaged by eating meat, use *Liù Jūn Zǐ Tāng* F2-6 adding *shān zhā* and *shén qū*.
- Whenever there is vomiting at the same time, add *huò xiāng* to all [the above].
- If there is sour swallowing or vomiting at the same time, use the previous herbs to swallow *Yuè Jū Wán* F1-2.
- If liver wood comes to insult spleen earth, use *Liù Jūn Zǐ Tāng* F2-6 adding *chái hú* and *pào jiāng*.
- If cold water contrarily comes to insult earth, use *Qián Shì Yì Huáng Sǎn* F2-22.
- If diarrhea lasts a long time or original qì sinks downward, use *Bǔ Zhōng Yì Qì Tāng* F2-5 at the same time to ascend and send out yáng qì.
- If the diarrhea or dysentery are yellow-colored, true qì of spleen earth [is affected]; it is appropriate to add *mù xiāng* and *ròu guǒ*.
- If it belongs to deficient cold spleen earth, you should use *Liù Jūn Zǐ Tāng* F2-6 adding *mù xiāng*, ginger, and cinnamon.
- If the spleen and kidneys are deficient and cold, use *Bǔ Zhōng Yì Qì Tāng* F2-5 and *Sì Shén Sǎn* F2-53.
- If it belongs to debility of *mìng mén* fire and deficient cold spleen earth, use *Bā Wèi Wán* F2-17 to supplement the mother of earth.
- If urination is rough and stagnant and the body gradually swells up or if there is panting and cough at the same time, use *Jīn Guì Shèn Qì Wán* F2-17 to supplement the spleen and kidneys and disinhibit the waterways.
- If it is due to deficient weak stomach qì and the four limbs have superficial swelling, the treatment must take supplementing the stomach as governing the treatment.

若久而不愈；或非飲食所傷而致，乃屬腎氣虧損。蓋胞胎主於任而係於腎，況九月十月，乃腎與膀胱所養，必用四神、六味、八味三藥以補腎。若用分利導水之劑，是虛其虛也。

If it lasts a long time without recovery or if it is not caused by damage from food and drink, it belongs to enfeebled kidney qì. Now, the uterus and fetus are governed by the rèn vessel and are attached to the kidneys; moreover the ninth months and tenth months [of pregnancy] are nourished by the kidneys and urinary bladder. You must use three medicines, *Sì Shén Sǎn* F2-53, *Liù Wèi Wán* F2-16, and *Bā Wèi Wán* F2-17 to supplement the kidneys. If you use prescriptions to divide, disinhibit, and lead out water, this is adding deficit to deficiency.

104. *Gǔ niè* 穀糵 is an alternate name for *gǔ yá* 穀芽.
105. *Mài niè* 麥糵 is an alternate name for *mài yá* 麥芽.

## 治驗
## Treatment Experience

**2-15-1**一產婦瀉痢，發熱作渴，吐痰甚多，肌體消瘦，飲食少思；或胸膈痞滿；或小腹脹墜年餘矣。余以為脾胃瀉，朝用二神丸，夕用六君子湯，三月餘而痊。

For more than a year after giving birth, a woman suffered diarrhea and dysentery with fever and thirst, and she spat a lot of phlegm. Her body became emaciated with little though of food and drink. Sometimes she had *pǐ*-glomus and fullness of the chest and diaphragm and sometimes her lower abdomen felt distended and sagging. I took this as spleen and stomach diarrhea. In the mornings I used *Èr Shén Wán* F2-23; in the evenings I used *Liù Jūn Zǐ Tāng* F2-6 and she recuperated after more than three months.

**2-15-2**一婦人產後泄瀉，兼嘔吐咽酸，面目浮腫，此脾氣虛寒，先用六君加炮薑為主，佐以越鞠丸而咽酸愈；又用補中益氣加茯苓、半夏而脾胃康。

A postpartum woman had diarrhea and vomiting at the same time with sour swallowing and puffy swelling of the face and eyes. This was deficient cold spleen qì. I first used *Liù Jūn Zǐ Tāng* F2-6 adding *pào jiāng* as governing; I assisted it with *Yuè Jū Wán* F1-2 and the sour swallowing recovered. I then used *Bǔ Zhōng Yì Qì Tāng* F2-5 adding *fú líng* and *bàn xià* and her spleen and stomach grew healthy.

**2-15-3**一產婦瀉痢年餘，形體骨立，內熱晡熱，自汗盜汗，口舌糜爛，日吐痰三碗許，脈洪大，重按全無。此命門火衰，脾土虛寒而假熱，然痰者乃脾虛不能統攝歸源也，用八味丸補火以生土，用補中益氣湯兼補肺金而脾胃健。

For more than a year after giving birth, a woman suffered diarrhea and dysentery. Her body was skin and bones, with internal heat, late afternoon fever, spontaneous sweating, and night sweating. Her mouth and tongue had erosions and every day she spat out about three bowls of phlegm. Her pulse was surging and large but nothing was there when it was pressed. This was debility of mìng mén fire, deficient cold spleen earth, and false heat. Although there was phlegm, it was from inability of her deficient spleen to control [fluids] and return them to the source. I used *Bā Wèi Wán* F2-17 to supplement fire in order to engender earth. I used *Bǔ Zhōng Yì Qì Tāng* F2-5 at the same time to supplement lung metal and her spleen and stomach grew stronger.

**2-15-4**一產婦腹痛後重，去痢無度，形體倦怠，飲食不進，與死為鄰。此脾腎俱虛，用四神丸、十全大補湯而愈。但飲食難化，肢體倦怠，用補益湯調理而康。

After labor, a woman suffered abdominal pain, tenesmus, incessant dysentery, and weariness of the body. She did not eat or drink and her death was approaching. This was deficiency of both spleen and kidneys. I used *Sì Shén Sǎn* F2-53 and *Shí Quán Dà Bǔ Tāng* F2-7 and she recovered. The only remaining symptoms were difficulty transforming food and drink and weariness of the body. I used supplementing and boosting decoctions to attune and rectify her and she became healthy.

**2-15-5**一婦人五月患痢，日夜無度，小腹墜痛，發熱惡寒，用六君子湯送香連丸，二服漸愈；仍以前湯送四神丸，四服痊愈。至七月終，怠惰嗜臥，四肢不收，體重節痛，口舌乾燥，飲食無味，大便不實，小便頻數，灑淅惡寒，凄慘不樂，此肺之脾胃虛，而陽氣寒不伸也，用升陽益胃湯而痊。

A woman suffered dysentery during the fifth lunar month, incessant day and night. Her lower abdomen [felt like it was] sagging and was painful. She had fever and aversion to cold. I used two doses of *Liù Jūn Zǐ Tāng* F2-6 to swallow *Xiāng Lián Wán* UF-14 and she gradually recovered. She continued to use the previous decoction to swallow four doses of *Sì Shén Sǎn* F2-53 and she completely recovered. Reaching the end of the seventh lunar month, she became lazy and somnolent, with loss of use of the four limbs, heavy body, joint pain, and dry mouth and tongue. Food and drink were flavorless, she had unformed stool, frequent urination, and aversion to cold as if after a soaking. She felt wretched and unhappy. This was lung, spleen, and stomach deficiency with cold yáng qì failing to extend. I used *Shēng Yáng Yì Wèi Tāng* UF-15 and she recuperated

## 《女科撮要·卷上·附方并注》
## Attached Formulas and Notes for Volume 1[1]

### Bǎo Hé Wán 保和丸
### Harmony-Preserving Pill F1-1

治飲食停滯，胸膈痞滿；或作呑酸等症 。

Treats retention and stagnation of food and drink, *pǐ*-glomus and fullness of the chest and diaphragm, sometimes accompanied by sour swallowing and similar symptoms.

山楂( 取肉，二兩，蒸 )神曲( 炒 )半夏茯苓( 各一兩 )蘿蔔子( 炒 )陳皮翹( 各五錢 )

| shān zhā | 山楂 | select the flesh, steamed | two *liǎng* | 74.6g |
|---|---|---|---|---|
| shén qū | 神曲 | stir-fried | one *liǎng* of each | 37.3g |
| bàn xià | 半夏 | | | |
| fú líng | 茯苓 | | | |
| luó bo zǐ | 蘿蔔子 | stir-fried | five *qián* of each | 18.65g |
| chén pí | 陳皮 | | | |
| lián qiáo | 連翹 | | | |

上為末，粥丸 。加白朮二兩，名大安丸 。

Powder the above and make it into pills with rice porridge. When two *liǎng* (74.6 grams) of *bái zhú* are added, it is named *Dà Ān Wán* F1-1a (Great Peace Pill).

1. These formulas were originally placed at the end of Volume 1, but have been moved to the end of the book for the convenience of the reader.

## Yuè Jū Wán 越鞠丸
## Constraint-Overcoming Pill F1-2

治六鬱，胸膈痞滿，嘔吐吞酸；或濕熱腹脹，腿腳酸疼等症。

Treats the six constraints, *pǐ*-glomus and fullness of the chest and diaphragm, vomiting, and sour swallowing. Perhaps it is accompanied by damp heat that makes abdominal distention, painful aching legs, and similar symptoms.

蒼朮（炒）神曲（炒）香附山楂山梔（炒）撫芎麥芽（炒。各等分）

| | | | |
|---|---|---|---|
| cāng zhú | 蒼朮 | stir-fried | equal portions of each |
| shén qū | 神曲 | stir-fried | |
| xiāng fù | 香附 | | |
| shān zhā | 山楂 | | |
| shān zhī zǐ | 山梔 | stir-fried | |
| fǔ xiōng | 撫芎 | | |
| mài yá | 麥芽 | stir-fried | |

上各另為末，水調炒曲麵糊為丸，桐子大。每服五七十丸，白滾湯下。

Powder each of the above separately. Make it into pills the size of *wú tóng zǐ* (about 0.6-0.9 centimeters in diameter) by mixing with a paste of water and stir-fried leavened flour. Each dose is fifty or seventy pills, swallowed with boiled water.

## Zuǒ Jīn Wán 左金丸
## Left-Running Metal Pill F1-3
### also named Huí Lìng Wán 回令丸
### Command-Returning Pill

治肝火胸脅刺痛；或發寒熱；或頭目作痛，小便淋秘；或小腹疼痛，一切肝火之症。

Treats liver fire with pricking pain in the chest and rib-sides, perhaps with fever and chills, or pain in the head and eyes and dribbling urination, or pain of the lower abdomen. All are symptoms of liver fire.

黃連（ 六兩 ）吳茱萸（ 一兩，湯煮片時用 ）

| huáng lián | 黃連 | | six *liǎng* | 223.8g |
|---|---|---|---|---|
| wú zhū yú | 吳茱萸 | boiled for a moment | one *liǎng* | 37.3g |

上為末，粥丸，白朮陳皮湯下 。

Powder the above. Make it into pills with rice porridge. Swallow with a decoction of *bái zhú* and *chén pí*.

## Jiāo Rén Wán 椒仁丸
## Jiāo Rén Pill[2] F1-4

治先因經水斷絕，後至四肢浮腫，小便不通，血化為水 。

Treats inability of urine to pass when blood has transformed into water. This occurs when menstrual flow is cut off first and superficial swelling of the four limbs develops afterwards.

椒仁甘遂續隨子（ 去皮研 ）附子（ 炮 ）鬱李仁黑牽牛五靈脂（ 研碎 ）當歸吳茱萸延胡索（ 各五錢 ）芫花（ 醋浸，一錢 ）石膏蚖青（ 十枚，去頭翅足同糯米炒黃，去米不用 ）斑蝥（ 十個，糯米炒黃，去米不用 ）膽礬人言（ 各一錢 ）

| jiāo rén | 椒仁 | | five *qián* of each | 18.65g |
|---|---|---|---|---|
| gān suì | 甘遂 | | | |
| xù suí zǐ | 續隨子 | remove the skin, ground | | |
| fù zǐ | 附子 | blast-fried | | |
| yù lǐ rén | 郁李仁 | | | |
| hēi qiān niú | 黑牽牛 | | | |

2. Due to toxicity, this formula should not be used today.

| | | | | |
|---|---|---|---|---|
| wǔ líng zhī | 五靈脂 | ground to pieces | | |
| dāng guī | 當歸 | | | |
| wú zhū yú | 吳茱萸 | | | |
| yán hú suǒ | 延胡索 | | | |
| yuán huā | 芫花 | vinegar-soaked | one *qián* | 3.73g |
| shí gāo | 石膏 | | [unstated] | |
| yuán qīng | 蚖青 | remove the head, wings, and feet; stir-fry with glutinous rice until yellow; remove the rice and do not use it | 10 *méi* | 10 pcs |
| bān máo | 斑蝥 | stir-fry with glutinous rice until yellow; remove the rice and do not use it | 10 *méi* | 10 pcs |
| dǎn fán | 膽礬 | | one *qián* of each | 3.73g |
| rén yán | 人言 | | | |

上為末，麵糊為丸，如豌豆大。每服一丸，橘皮湯下。

Powder the above and make it into pills the size of garden peas (*wān dòu*) with flour paste. Each dose is one pill swallowed with a decoction of *jú pí*.

此方藥雖峻利，所用不多。若畏而不服，有養病害身之患。常治虛弱之人，亦未見其有誤也。

Although the herbs in this formula drastically disinhibit [promote urination and defecation], it is not used often. If someone fears it and refuses to take it, there is the peril of nourishing the disease and harming the body. I have often treated deficient weak people with it and I have never seen there be a mistake.

## Xuè Fēn Tíng Lì Wán 血分葶藶丸
## Blood Division Tíng Lì Pill [F1-5]

治先因小便不利，後至身面浮腫，經水不通，水化為血。

Treats inability of menstrual fluids to pass when water has transformed into blood. This occurs when urination is inhibited first and superficial swelling of the body and face develops afterwards.

葶藶（研、炒）續隨子（去殼。各半兩，研）乾筍末（一兩）

| tíng lì | 葶藶 | ground and stir-fried | a half *liǎng* of each | 18.65g |
|---|---|---|---|---|
| xù suí zǐ | 續隨子 | remove the husk, ground | | |
| gàn sǔn mò | 乾筍末 | | one *liǎng* | 37.3g |

上為末，棗肉丸，如桐子大。每服七丸，煎萹竹湯下。如大便利者，減續隨子、葶藶各一錢，加白朮五錢。

Powder the above and make it into pills the size of *wú tóng zǐ* (about 0.6-0.9 centimeters in diameter) with *zǎo-date* flesh. Each dose is seven pills swallowed with a decoction of *biǎn zhú*. If it makes loose stool, decrease the *xù suí zǐ* and tíng lì each by one *qián* (3.73 grams) and add five *qián* (18.65 grams) of *bái zhú*.

## Rén Shēn Wán 人參丸
### Rén Shēn Pill F1-6

治經脈不利，化為水流走四肢，悉皆腫滿，名曰血分。其候與水相類，若作水治之非也，宜用此。

Treats inhibition of the menstrual vessel that transform into water flowing into the four limbs, all of which are swollen and full. This is named the blood division. The symptoms are similar to the water division but it is a mistake to treat this as water; it is appropriate to use this instead.

人參當歸大黃（濕紙裹，飯上蒸熟，去紙，切、炒）桂心瞿麥穗赤芍藥白茯苓（各半兩）葶藶（炒，另研一錢）

| rén shēn | 人參 | | a half *liǎng* of each | 18.65g |
|---|---|---|---|---|
| dāng guī | 當歸 | | | |
| dà huáng | 大黃 | wrap in moist paper, place on rice and steam until cooked, remove the paper, slice and stir-fry it | | |
| guì xīn | 桂心 | | | |
| qú mài suì | 瞿麥穗 | | | |

| chì sháo yào | 赤芍藥 | | | |
|---|---|---|---|---|
| bái fú líng | 白茯苓 | | | |
| tíng lì | 葶藶 | stir-fried, ground separately | one *qián* | 3.73g |

上為末，煉蜜丸，桐子大。每服十五丸，至二三十丸，空心飲湯下。

Powder the above and make it into pills the size of *wú tóng zǐ* (about 0.6-0.9 centimeters in diameter) using processed honey. Each dose is fifteen pills up to twenty or thirty pills. Take on an empty stomach and swallow with hot water.

## Bǎi Zǐ Rén Wán 柏子仁丸
### Bǎi Zǐ Rén Pill F1-7

治血虛有火，月經耗損，漸至不通，日漸羸瘦，而生潮熱。慎毋以毒藥通之，宜柏子仁丸、澤蘭湯主之。

Treats blood deficiency with fire that gradually consumes menstruation until it does not flow. She becomes more emaciated each day and this engenders tidal fevers. Be careful not to use toxic herbs to make menstruation flow. *Bǎi Zǐ Rén Wán* F1-7 and *Zé Lán Tāng* F1-8 are appropriately indicated for this.

柏子仁（炒砂）牛膝（酒拌）卷柏（各半兩）澤蘭葉續斷（各二兩）熟地黃（用生者，三兩，酒拌蒸半日，忌鐵器，杵膏）

| bǎi zǐ rén | 柏子仁 | stir-fried in sand | a half *liǎng* of each | 18.65g |
|---|---|---|---|---|
| niú xī | 牛膝 | mixed with liquor | | |
| juǎn bǎi | 卷柏 | | | |
| zé lán yè | 澤蘭葉 | | two *liǎng* of each | 74.6g |
| xù duàn | 續斷 | | | |
| shú dì huáng | 熟地黃 | use the fresh, mix with liquor and steam for half a day,* avoid iron utensils, pestle into a paste | three *liǎng* | 111.9g |

* This word for *day* means a twenty-four hour period (not daytime). So one would steam it for about twelve hours.

上為末，入地黃膏，加煉蜜丸，桐子大。每服三十丸，空心米飲下。

Powder the above. Add the *dì huáng* paste and honey and make into pills the size of *wú tóng zǐ* (about 0.6-0.9 centimeters in diameter). Each dose is thirty pills taken on an empty stomach and swallowed with rice drink.

## Zé Lán Tāng 澤蘭湯
## Zé Lán Decoction [F1-8]

治症同前。

Treats the same conditions as the previous formula (*Bǎi Zǐ Rén Wán* [F1-7]).

澤蘭葉（三兩）當歸（酒拌）芍藥（炒。各一兩）甘草（五錢）

| | | | | |
|---|---|---|---|---|
| zé lán yè | 澤蘭葉 | stir-fried in sand | three *liǎng* | 111.9g |
| dāng guī | 當歸 | mixed with liquor | one *liǎng* of each | 37.3g |
| sháo yào | 芍藥 | stir-fried | | |
| gān cǎo | 甘草 | | five *qián* | 18.65g |

上為粗末，每服五錢，水二鐘，煎至一鍾，去渣溫服。

Make the above into a coarse powder. Each dose is five *qián* (18.65 grams) boiled in two cups of water down to one cup. Remove the dregs and drink it warm.

## Dú Shēn Tāng 獨參湯
## Pure Rén Shēn Decoction [F1-9]

治一切失血，惡寒發熱，作渴煩躁，並宜此藥補氣，蓋血生於氣，陽生陰長之理也。

Treats all types of blood loss with aversion to cold, fever, thirst, vexation, and agitation. At the same time these herbs are appropriate to supplement qì. Blood is engendered by qì; this is the theory that yáng engenders and yīn grows.

用人參二兩，棗十枚，水煎服。

Use two *liǎng* (74.6 grams) of *rén shēn* and ten *zǎo*-dates; boil in water and take it.

## Yù Lù Sǎn 玉露散
## Jade Dew Powder [F1-10]

治乳脈不行，身體壯熱，頭目昏痛，大便澀滯等症。

Treats non-movement of the milk vessels with vigorous heat in the body, cloudy painful head and eyes, rough stagnant bowel movement, and similar symptoms.

人參白茯苓桔梗炒川芎白朮當歸芍藥（各一錢）甘草（五分）

| rén shēn | 人參 | | one *qián* of each | 3.73g |
|---|---|---|---|---|
| bái fú líng | 白茯苓 | | | |
| jié gěng | 桔梗 | stir-fried | | |
| chuān xiōng | 川芎 | | | |
| bái zhǐ | 白芷 | | | |
| dāng guī | 當歸 | | | |
| sháo yào | 芍藥 | | | |
| gān cǎo | 甘草 | | five *fēn* | 1.85 g |

上水煎服。若熱甚，大便秘，量加炒大黃。

Boil the above and take them. If fever is high and there is constipation, consider adding stir-fried *dà huáng*.

## Shèng Yù Tāng 聖愈湯
## Sagacious Cure Decoction F1-11

治血虛心煩，睡眠不寧；或五心煩熱。

Treats blood deficiency with heart vexation when sleep is not peaceful, or five heart vexation heat.

地黃（酒拌，蒸半日）生地黃（酒拌）川芎人參（各五錢）當歸（酒拌）黃耆（炒。各一錢）

| dì huáng | 地黃 | mix with liquor, steam for half a day | five *qián* | 18.65g |
|---|---|---|---|---|
| shēng dì huáng | 生地黃 | mix with liquor | | |
| chuān xiōng | 川芎 | | | |
| rén shēn | 人參 | | | |
| dāng guī | 當歸 | mix with liquor | one *qián* | 3.73g |
| huáng qí | 黃耆 | stir-fry | | |

上水煎服。

Boil the above in water and take it.

## Dāng Guī Yǐn 當歸飲
## Dāng Guī Drink F1-12

治血熱，癮疹痛，膿水淋漓，發熱等症。

Treats heat in the blood, hidden rash [*yǐn zhěn* – usually urticaria] with pain, trickling pus-water, fever, and similar symptoms.

當歸白芍藥川芎生地黃白蒺藜（各一錢）防風荊芥（各五分）黃耆（一錢）何首烏甘草（各五分）

| dāng guī | 當歸 | one *qián* of each | 3.73g |
|---|---|---|---|
| bái sháo yào | 白芍藥 | | |
| chuān xiōng | 川芎 | | |
| shēng dì huáng | 生地黃 | | |
| bái jí lí | 白蒺藜 | | |
| fáng fēng | 防風 | five *fēn* of each | 1.85g |
| jīng jiè | 荊芥 | | |
| huáng qí | 黃耆 | one *qián* | 3.73g |
| hé shǒu wū | 何首烏 | five *fēn* of each | 1.85g |
| gān cǎo | 甘草 | | |

上水煎服。

Boil the above in water and take it.

## Lóng Dǎn Xiè Gān Tāng 龍膽瀉肝湯
## Lóng Dǎn Cǎo Liver-Draining Decoction F1-13

治肝經濕熱，下部腫焮作痛，小便澀滯，陰挺如菌；或出物如蟲等症。

Treats damp heat of the liver channel, painful swelling and flaring-heat of the lower body, rough stagnant urination, vaginal prolapse that looks like a mushroom, or something resembling *chóng*-worms coming out, and similar patterns.

龍膽草（酒拌，炒黃）澤瀉（各一錢）車前子（炒）木通生地黃（酒拌）當歸尾（酒拌）山梔（炒）黃芩生甘草（各五分）

| lóng dǎn cǎo | 龍膽草 | mix with liquor, stir-fry until yellow | one *qián* of each | 3.73g |
|---|---|---|---|---|
| zé xiè | 澤瀉 | | | |
| chē qián zǐ | 車前子 | stir-fry | five *fēn* of each | 1.85g |
| mù tōng | 木通 | | | |
| shēng dì huáng | 生地黃 | mix with liquor | | |
| dāng guī wěi | 當歸尾 | mix with liquor | | |

| shān zhī zǐ | 山梔 | stir-fry | | |
|---|---|---|---|---|
| huáng qín | 黃芩 | | | |
| shēng gān cǎo | 生甘草 | | | |

上水煎服。

Boil the above in water and take it.

## Wū Zéi Yú Gǔ Wán 烏賊魚骨丸
## Cuttlefish Bone Pill F1-14

治婦人血枯，胸膈四肢滿，妨於食飲，病至聞腥、臊臭氣先唾血出清液；或前後泄血，目眩轉，月事衰少不來。

Treats withered blood in women with fullness of the chest, diaphragm, and four limbs that impedes eating and drinking. The patient ends up with a fishy (*xīng*) or urine (*sāo*) odor before spitting blood and clear *yè*-fluids, or bleeding from the front or rear [two lower orifices], with dizzy vision when turning [the head] and menstruation that decreases until it does not come.

烏賊魚骨（去甲，四兩）閭茹（一兩）

| wū zéi yú gǔ | 烏賊魚骨 | remove the shell | four *liǎng* | 149.2g |
|---|---|---|---|---|
| lú rú | 閭茹 | | one *liǎng* | 37.3g |

上為末，以雀卵和成劑，丸如小豆大。每服五丸，加至十丸，以鮑魚煎湯下，以飯壓之。

Powder the above. Blend a sparrow egg into the prescription and make pills the size of adzuki beans (*xiǎo dòu* - about 6 mm indiameter). Each dose is five to ten pills. Swallow them with abalone (*bào yú*) soup and press it down with rice.[3]

3. This means to eat rice after taking the pills with the soup. The rice helps push the medicine down to its target.

## Qīng Zhōu Bái Wán Zǐ 青州白丸子
## Qīngzhōu White Pill F1-15

治風痰咳嗽；或牙關緊急，不知人事；或痰滯作麻。

Treats wind phlegm cough, or clenched jaw with inability to recognize human affairs [unconsciousness], or phlegm stagnation that causes numbness.

南星（三兩）半夏（七兩）白附子（二兩）川烏（半兩。各生用）

| tiān nán xīng | 南星 | use each fresh | three *liǎng* | 111.9g |
|---|---|---|---|---|
| bàn xià | 半夏 | | seven *liǎng* | 261.1g |
| bái fù zǐ | 白附子 | | two *liǎng* | 74.6g |
| chuān wū | 川烏 | | a half *liǎng* | 18.65g |

上為末，絹袋盛，井水擺浸，仍換水浸三五日，曬乾糯米粉丸。如急用，以薑汁糊丸亦可。

Powder the above. Fill a rough silk bag with it and wave it around in well water. Then change the water and soak it for three or five days. Dry the powder in the sun and make pills with glutinous rice powder. If you need to use it quickly, you can also make pills with a wheat paste made with ginger juice.

## Sì Qī Tāng 四七湯
## Four-Seven Decoction F1-16

治七情鬱結，咽間如有一核，吞吐不利；或中脘痞滿，痰涎壅喘；或噁心少食。

Treats binding constraint from the seven emotions, with a feeling like a pit is in the throat that cannot be swallowed or spit out; or *pǐ*-glomus and fullness at Zhōng Wǎn [the region of Rèn 12] with phlegm drool obstruction and panting; or nausea and reduced food intake.

紫蘇葉（一錢）濃樸（一錢五分）茯苓（一錢）半夏（薑製，七分）

| zǐ sū yè | 紫蘇葉 | | one *qián* | 3.73g |
|---|---|---|---|---|
| nóng pǔ | 濃樸 | | 1.5 *qián* | 5.6g |
| fú líng | 茯苓 | | one *qián* | 3.73g |
| bàn xià | 半夏 | prepared with ginger | seven *fēn* | 2.59g |

上薑棗水煎服。若白帶，以此湯送前丸，其效如神。

Boil the above in water with ginger and *zǎo*-dates and take it. If there is white vaginal discharge, use this decoction to swallow the previous pill [*Qīng Zhōu Bái Wán Zǐ* F1-15]. Its effectiveness is miraculous.

## Dāng Guī Lóng Huì Wán 當歸龍薈丸
## Dāng Guī, Lóng Dǎn Cǎo, and Lú Huì Pill F1-17

治肝經症，脅下作痛；或有積塊；或下疳便癰，小便淋澀；或瘀血凝滯，小腹作痛。

Treats liver channel symptoms with pain below the rib-sides, or accumulations and lumps, or lower body *gān*-erosions that become abscesses and dribbling urination, or blood stasis and stagnation with pain of the lower abdomen.

當歸（酒拌）龍膽草（酒拌炒）梔子仁（炒）黃連青皮黃芩（各一兩）大黃（酒拌炒）蘆薈青黛柴胡（各五錢）木香（二錢五分）麝香（五分，另研）

| dāng guī | 當歸 | mix with liquor | one *liǎng* of each | 37.3g |
|---|---|---|---|---|
| lóng dǎn cǎo | 龍膽草 | mix with liquor, stir-fry | | |
| zhī zǐ rén | 梔子仁 | stir-fry | | |
| huáng lián | 黃連 | | | |
| qīng pí | 青皮 | | | |
| huáng qín | 黃芩 | | | |

| dà huáng | 大黃 | mix with liquor, stir-fry | five *qián* of each | 18.65g |
|---|---|---|---|---|
| lú huì | 蘆薈 | | | |
| qīng dài | 青黛 | | | |
| chái hú | 柴胡 | | | |
| mù xiāng | 木香 | | 2.5 *qián* | 9.33g |
| shè xiāng | 麝香 | grind separately | five *fēn* | 1.85g |

上為末，炒神曲糊丸。每服二三十丸，薑湯下。

Powder the above and make it into pills with a paste of stir-fried *shén qū*. Each dose is 20 or 30 pills, swallowed with a decoction of ginger.

## Ā Wèi Gāo 阿魏膏
## Ā Wèi Plaster F1-18

治一切痞塊。

Treats all types of *pǐ*-glomus lumps.

羌活獨活玄參官桂赤芍藥川山甲生地黃兩頭尖大黃白芷天麻（各五錢）紅花（四錢）槐柳桃枝（各三錢）木鱉子（三十枚，去殼）亂發（如雞子大一塊）

| qiāng huó | 羌活 | | five *qián* of each | 18.65g |
|---|---|---|---|---|
| dú huó | 獨活 | | | |
| xuán shēn | 玄參 | | | |
| guān guì | 官桂 | | | |
| chì sháo yào | 赤芍藥 | | | |
| chuān shān jiǎ | 穿山甲 | | | |
| shēng dì huáng | 生地黃 | | | |
| liǎng tóu jiān | 兩頭尖 | | | |
| dà huáng | 大黃 | | | |
| bái zhǐ | 白芷 | | | |
| tiān má | 天麻 | | | |

| | | | | |
|---|---|---|---|---|
| hóng huā | 紅花 | | four *qián* | 14.92g |
| huái, liǔ, and táo zhī | 槐、柳、桃枝 | | three *qián* of each | 11.9g |
| mù biē zǐ | 木鱉子 | remove the shell | thirty *méi* | 30 pcs |
| luàn fā | 亂髮 | | a lump the size of a chicken egg | |

上用香油二斤四兩，煎黑去渣，入髮再煎化，仍去渣，徐下黃丹，煎軟硬得中，方入芒硝、阿魏、蘇合油、乳香、沒藥五錢，麝香三錢，調勻成膏矣。

Boil the above in two *jīn* and four *liǎng* (1342.8 grams) of sesame oil until black and remove the dregs. Add in the hair and boil again until it dissolves; as before remove the dregs. Gradually add in *huáng dān*[4] and boil until the proper degree of viscosity is obtained. Then add in five *qián* (18.65 grams) [each] of *máng xiāo, ā wèi, sū hé yóu, rǔ xiāng,* and *mò yào,* and three *qián* (11.19 grams) of *shè xiāng.* Mix evenly to make it into a paste.

攤貼患處。內服蘆薈丸等。黃丹須真正者效。凡貼膏藥，先用朴硝隨患處鋪半指濃，以紙蓋，用熱熨斗熨良久，如消耗，再加熨之，熨二時許方貼膏藥。若是肝積，加蘆薈末同熨。

Spread it and apply it onto the affected site.[5] Internally take *Lú Huì Wán* F1-19 and so forth. *Huáng dān* must be genuine to be effective. Whenever applying the plaster, first spread *pò xiāo* a half finger thick over the affected site and cover it with paper; iron it with a hot iron for a good long time. If the *pò xiāo* evaporates, add more and iron it. Iron for about two double-hours before applying the plaster. If this is a liver accumulation, add *lú huì* powder and iron it together [with the *pò xiāo*].

## Lú Huì Wán 蘆薈丸
### Lú Huì Pill F1-19

治肝疳口舌生瘡，牙齦腐爛；或遍身生瘡等症。

Treats liver *gān*-erosion that engenders sores on the mouth and tongue with rotten teeth, or sores on the entire body and similar conditions.

4. *Huáng dān* is red lead oxide or minium, It is toxic if inhaled, ingested, or is absorbed through the skin. Therefore, we cannot use it medicinally today.
5. It is probably spread on cloth which is then applied to the effective site.

大皂角青黛蘆薈（ 研 ）朱砂（ 研 ）麝香（ 研 。各一錢 ）乾蝦蟆（ 用皂角各等分，燒存性為末，一兩入前項藥 ）

| dà zào jiǎo | 大皂角 | | [see below] | |
|---|---|---|---|---|
| qīng dài | 青黛 | | one *qián* of each | 3.73g |
| lú huì | 蘆薈 | ground | | |
| zhū shā | 硃砂 | ground | | |
| shè xiāng | 麝香 | ground | | |
| gān há má | 乾蝦蟆 | use the same amount as for zào jiǎo, roast preserving its nature and powder, add to the previous herbs | one *liǎng* | 37.3g |

上為末，蒸餅糊丸，麻子大 。每服五七十丸，米飲下 。

Powder the above, steam as cakes and make pills the size of *má zǐ* (about 4 mm in diameter) with wheat paste. Each dose is fifty or seventy pills swallowed with rice drink.

## Jú Fāng Xiǎo Xù Mìng Tāng 《局方》小續命湯
## Minor Life-Prolonging Decocotion from Jú Fāng[6] F1-20

治歷節痛風，痰盛口噤，背反張等症 。

Treats joint-running painful wind, phlegm exuberance with lockjaw, arched back rigidity, and similar conditions.

防己肉桂（ 去粗皮 ）杏仁（ 去皮尖，炒黃 ）黃芩白芍甘草川芎麻黃（ 去節 ）人參（ 去蘆，各一兩 ）防風（ 一兩五錢 ）附子（ 炮去皮臍，半兩 ）

| fang jǐ | 防己 | | one *liǎng* of each | 37.3g |
|---|---|---|---|---|
| ròu guì | 肉桂 | remove the coarse bark | | |
| xìng rén | 杏仁 | remove the skin and tip, stir-fry until yellow | | |
| huáng qín | 黃芩 | | | |

6. *Jú Fāng* refers to *Tài Píng Huì Mín Hé Jì Jú Fāng*《 太平惠民和劑局方 》, the official *Sòng* dynasty formulary.

| | | | | |
|---|---|---|---|---|
| bái sháo | 白芍 | | | |
| gān cǎo | 甘草 | | | |
| chuān xiōng | 川芎 | | | |
| má huáng | 麻黄 | renove the joints | | |
| rén shēn | 人參 | remove the stem | | |
| fáng fēng | 防風 | | 1.5 *liǎng* | 55.95g |
| fù zǐ | 附子 | blast-fry, remove the skin and umbilicus | a half *liǎng* | 18.65g |

上為粗末，每服三錢，薑棗水煎服。

Make the above into a coarse powder. Each dose is three *qián* (11.19 grams); boil in water with ginger and *zǎo*-dates and take it.

## Tiáo Zhōng Yì Qì Tāng 調中益氣湯<br>Center-Attuning Qì-Boosting Decoction F1-21

治體怠嗜臥，不思飲食；或痰嗽泄瀉等症。

Treats body fatigue with somnolence with no thought of food or drink, or phlegm cough, diarrhea, and similar conditions.

黃耆（一錢）人參（去蘆頭）甘草蒼朮（各五分）柴胡橘皮升麻木香（各二分）

| | | | | |
|---|---|---|---|---|
| huáng qí | 黃耆 | | one *qián* | 3.73g |
| rén shēn | 人參 | remove the stem and head | one *fēn* of each | 1.85g |
| gān cǎo | 甘草 | | | |
| cāng zhú | 蒼朮 | | | |
| chái hú | 柴胡 | | two *fēn* of each | 0.74g |
| jú pí | 橘皮 | | | |
| shēng má | 升麻 | | | |
| mù xiang | 木香 | | | |

上薑棗水煎，空心服。

Boil the above in water with ginger and *zǎo*-dates and take it on an empty stomach.

## Fó Shǒu Sǎn 佛手散
## Hand-of-Buddha Powder F1-22

治妊娠，傷胎下血。

Treats fetal damage with bleeding in pregnancy.

當歸（三錢）川芎（二錢）

| dāng guī | 當歸 | three *qián* | 11.19g |
|---|---|---|---|
| chuān xiōng | 川芎 | two *qián* | 7.46g |

上水煎，食前服。

Boil the above in water and take it before meals.

## Mù Xiāng Bǐng 木香餅
## Mù Xiāng Cakes F1-23

治一切氣滯結腫；或痛或閃肭，及風寒所傷作痛并效。

Treats all types of qì stagnation with bindings and swellings; or pain, or wrenching sprains, as well as pain after damage by wind cold. It is equally effective for all.

木香（五錢）生地黃（一兩）

| mù xiāng | 木香 | five *qián* | 18.65g |
|---|---|---|---|
| shēng dì huáng | 生地黃 | one *liǎng* | 37.3g |

上木香為末，地黄杵膏和匀，量患處大小作餅置患處，以熱熨斗熨之。

Powder the *mù xiāng*. Pestle the *dì huáng* into a paste and blend evenly. Make cakes based on the size of the affected site. Place one on the affected site. Iron it with a hot iron.

## Gé Suàn Jiǔ Fǎ 隔蒜灸法
## Garlic-Isolated Moxibustion F1-24

治一切瘡毒，大痛或不痛；或麻木如痛者，灸至不痛，不痛者灸至痛，其毒隨火而散。蓋火以暢達，拔引鬱毒，此從治之法也，有回生之功。

Treats all types of sores with toxins. They may have strong pain or no pain, or there may be numbness and tingling similar to pain: Apply moxibustion [on garlic] until it is not painful. If it is not painful apply moxibustion until it becomes painful. The toxins follow the fire and scatter. It must be that fire uses its nature of unimpeded outward spreading to uproot and pull out the constrained toxins. This is a following method of treatment.[7] It has the results of returning life.

用大蒜頭去皮，切三文錢濃，安瘡頭上，用艾壯于蒜上，灸之三壯，換蒜復灸，未成者即消，已成者亦殺其大勢，不能為害。

Remove the peel from a head of garlic (*dà suàn*). Slice it to the thickness of three coins and set one on top of the sore. Place mugwort cones on top of the garlic and burn three cones on it. Change the garlic and apply moxibustion again. If the sore has not formed yet, it will disperse. If it has already formed, this treatment will still fight the general trend; it is unable to do harm.

如瘡大，用蒜搗爛攤患處，將艾鋪上燒之，蒜敗再換。

If the sore is large, mash garlic into a pulp and spread it on the affected site. Spread mugwort on top and burn it. When the garlic is withered [dried out], change it again.

7. A *following treatment* means paradoxically using heat to treat a hot disease or cold against a cold disease.

如不痛；或不作膿，及不起發，或陰瘡尤宜多灸，灸而仍不痛，不作膿，不起發者不治，此氣血虛極也 。

If it is not painful, or if the sore does not make pus, or the pus does not exude, or if there are yīn sores, it is especially appropriate to apply a lot of moxibustion. If you apply moxibustion but it is still not painful, does not make pus, or the pus does not exude, do not treat it [further];[8] this is extreme qì and blood deficiency.

## Shén Xiào Cōng Yùn Fǎ 神效蔥熨法
## Wondrously Effective Ironing Method with Scallions [F1-25]

治虛怯人，肢體患腫塊；或作痛；或不痛；或風襲於經絡，肢體疼痛；或四肢筋攣骨痛 。又治流注，跌撲傷損腫痛 。

Treats deficient weak people whose body suffers swollen lumps. Some are painful, some are not painful. Sometimes wind makes a surprise attack on the channels and *luò*-networks so the body is painful, or there are sinew spasms and bone pain of the four limbs. This also treats streaming sores (*liú zhù*) and injuries from knocks and falls with swelling and pain.

用蔥頭細切，杵爛炒熱敷患處，冷易之再熨，腫痛即止，其效如神 。

Pestle thinly sliced scallions (*cōng tóu*) to a pulp, stir-fry them until hot, and apply them to the affected site. Change them when they become cold and iron again. The swelling and pain will then stop; its effectiveness is miraculous.

8. This implies that it is a hopeless case and the patient will die anyway, so there is no point to continue treatment. Before antibiotics, people often died of septicaemia from such sores.

## Dòu Chǐ Bǐng 豆豉餅
## Fermented Soybean Cakes F1-26

治瘡瘍腫硬不潰，及潰而不斂，並一切頑瘡惡瘡。

Treats sores that are swollen and hard and have not burst open, as well as those that have burst open but do not close up, and all types of stubborn or malign sores.

用江西豆豉為末，唾津和作餅子，如錢大，厚如三文，置患處，以艾壯于餅上，灸之，乾則易之。如背瘡，用漱口水調作餅覆患處，以艾鋪餅上灸之。如未成者即消，已成者能消其毒。如有不效，氣血虛敗也。

Powder *dòu chǐ* from Jiāngxī and blend it with saliva. Make it into cakes the diameter of a coin and as thick as a stack of three coins. Place it on the affected site. Put mugwort cones on top of the cakes and apply moxibustion. When the cake is dry, change it. If the sores are on the back, mix the powder with water from rinsing the mouth,[9] make cakes, and put them on the affected site. Spread mugwort on the cakes and apply moxibustion to them. If the sores have not yet developed, they will then disperse; if they have already developed, this is able to disperse their toxins. If this is ineffective, qì and blood deficiency will conquer [the patient].

## Yì Qì Yǎng Róng Tāng 益氣養榮湯
## Qì-Boosting Yíng-Construction Nourishing Decoction F1-27

治抑鬱瘰癧；或四肢患腫，肉色不變；或日晡發熱；或潰而不斂。

Treats restraint and constraint with scrofula. Perhaps there are swellings on the four limbs with unchanged color of the flesh; or with fevers at sunset; or they have burst open but do not close up.

9. Sores on the back generally cover a larger area, so to make cakes, more liquid is needed. The two types of saliva (drool and spittle) belong to the spleen and kidneys. So while we will not use saliva today, there was a reason for using it as a medicinal substance.

人參茯苓陳皮貝母香附當歸（酒拌）川芎黃耆（鹽水拌，炒）熟地黃（酒拌）芍藥（炒。各一錢）甘草（炙）桔梗（炒。各五分）白朮（炒，二錢）

| rén shēn | 人參 | | one *qián* of each | 3.73g |
|---|---|---|---|---|
| fú líng | 茯苓 | | | |
| chén pí | 陳皮 | | | |
| bèi mǔ | 貝母 | | | |
| xiāng fù | 香附 | | | |
| dāng guī | 當歸 | mixed with liquor | | |
| chuān xiōng | 川芎 | | | |
| huáng qí | 黃耆 | mixed with brine, stir-fried | | |
| shú dì huáng | 熟地黃 | mixed with liquor | | |
| sháo yào | 芍藥 | stir-fried | | |
| gān cǎo | 甘草 | | five *fēn* of each | 1.85g |
| jié gěng | 桔梗 | stir-fried | | |
| bái zhú | 白朮 | stir-fried | two *qián* | 7.46g |

上薑水煎服。

Boil the above in water with ginger and take it.

## Rén Shēn Yǎng Róng Tāng 人參養榮湯
## Rén Shēn Yíng-Construction Nourishing Decoction [F1-28]

治潰瘍發熱惡寒，四肢倦怠，體瘦少食，面黃短氣，不能收斂。若大瘡愈後，多服之，不變他病。

Treats sores that have burst open with fever and aversion to cold, fatigued limbs, thin body, decreased food intake, yellow face, shortness of breath, and inability [of the sores] to close up. If this formula is taken often after large sores recover, it will not mutate into another disease.

白芍藥（ 一錢五分 ）人參陳皮黃耆（ 蜜炙 ）桂心當歸（ 酒拌 ）白朮甘草（ 炙 。各一錢 ）熟地黃（ 酒拌 ）五味子（ 炒 ）茯苓（ 各七分半 ）遠志（ 去心 ， 炒 。五分 ）

| bái sháo yào | 白芍藥 | | 1.5 *qián* | 5.6g |
|---|---|---|---|---|
| rén shēn | 人參 | | one *qián* of each | 3.73g |
| chén pí | 陳皮 | | | |
| huáng qí | 黃耆 | honey-fried | | |
| guì xīn | 桂心 | | | |
| dāng guī | 當歸 | mixed with liquor | | |
| bái zhú | 白朮 | | | |
| gān cǎo | 甘草 | mix-fried | | |
| shú dì huáng | 熟地黃 | mixed with liquor | 7.5 *fēn* of each | 2.78g |
| wǔ wèi zǐ | 五味子 | stir-fried | | |
| fú líng | 茯苓 | | | |
| yuǎn zhì | 遠志 | remove the heart, stir-fried | five *fēn* | 1.85g |

上薑棗水煎服 。

Boil the above in water with ginger and *zǎo*-dates and take it.

## Fāng Mài Liú Qì Yǐn Zǐ 方脈流氣飲子
## Qì-Flowing Drink for Miscellaneous Diseases F1-29

治惱怒胸膈脹滿；或肢體作痛；或結壅腫，血氣無虧者 。

Treats anger with distention and fullness of the chest and diaphragm, or painful body, or bindings, obstructions, and swellings without any lack of blood and qì.

紫蘇葉青皮苦梗半夏（ 煨 ）當歸芍藥烏藥茯苓川芎黃耆枳殼（ 去穰，麸炒 ）防風（ 各半兩 ）甘草橘皮（ 各五分 ）大腹皮木香（ 各三分 ）

| zǐ sū yè | 紫蘇葉 | | a half *liǎng* of each | 18.65g |
|---|---|---|---|---|
| qīng pí | 青皮 | | | |
| kǔ gěng | 苦梗 | | | |
| bàn xià | 半夏 | roasted | | |
| dāng guī | 當歸 | | | |
| sháo yào | 芍藥 | | | |
| wū yào | 烏藥 | | | |
| fú líng | 茯苓 | | | |
| chuān xiōng | 川芎 | | | |
| huáng qí | 黄耆 | | | |
| zhǐ qiào | 枳殼 | remove the pulp, stir-fry with wheat bran | | |
| fáng fēng | 防風 | | | |
| gān cǎo | 甘草 | | five *fēn* of each | 1.85g |
| jú pí | 橘皮 | | | |
| dà fù pí | 大腹皮 | | three *fēn* of each | 1.12g |
| mù xiāng | 木香 | | | |

上薑棗水煎服 。

Boil the above in water with ginger and *zǎo*-dates and take it.

## Xiè Qīng Wán 瀉青丸
## Green-Blue Draining Pill F1-30

治肝經鬱火實熱，脅乳作痛，大便秘結，及肝經一切實火症 。

Treats constrained fire and excess heat of the liver channel, with pain in the rib-sides and breasts, and constipation, as well as all types of excess fire patterns of the liver channel.

當歸龍膽草川芎山梔大黃羌活防風（ 各等分 ）

| dāng guī | 當歸 | equal portions of each |
|---|---|---|
| lóng dǎn cǎo | 龍膽草 | |

| | | |
|---|---|---|
| chuān xiōng | 川芎 | |
| shān zhī zǐ | 山梔 | |
| dà huáng | 大黃 | |
| qiāng huó | 羌活 | |
| fáng fēng | 防風 | |

上為末，蜜丸，雞子大，每服一二丸 。

Powder the above and make honey pills the size of chicken eggs. Each dose is one or two pills.

## Rén Shēn Bài Dú Sǎn 人參敗毒散
## Rén Shēn Toxin-Conquering Powder F1-31

治瘡瘍焮痛，發寒熱；或拘急頭痛等症 。

Treats sores and skin diseases with scorching pain and [sensations of] cold and heat, or hypertonicity with headache and similar patterns.

人參羌活獨活前胡柴胡桔梗枳殼茯苓川芎甘草（ 各一錢 ）

| | | | |
|---|---|---|---|
| rén shēn | 人參 | one *qián* of each | 3.73g |
| qiāng huó | 羌活 | | |
| dú huó | 獨活 | | |
| qián hú | 前胡 | | |
| chái hú | 柴胡 | | |
| jié gěng | 桔梗 | | |
| zhǐ qiào | 枳殼 | | |
| fú líng | 茯苓 | | |
| chuān xiōng | 川芎 | | |
| gān cǎo | 甘草 | | |

上水煎服 。

Boil the above in water and take it.

## **Shēng Dì Huáng Wán 生地黃丸**
## **Shēng Dì Huáng Pill** F1-32

治師尼寡婦，乍寒乍熱，肝脈弦長，而出魚際。

Treats nuns and widows who have alternating chills and fever; the liver pulse is bow-string and long, going out as far as Yú Jì [the region of LU 10].

生地黃（一兩，酒拌，杵膏）秦艽黃芩硬柴胡（各五錢）赤芍藥（一兩）

| shēng dì huáng | 生地黃 | mix with liquor, pestle into a paste | one *liǎng* | 37.3g |
|---|---|---|---|---|
| qín jiāo | 秦艽 | | five *qián* of each | 18.65g |
| huáng qín | 黃芩 | | | |
| yìng chái hú | 硬柴胡 | | | |
| chì sháo yào | 赤芍藥 | | one *liǎng* | 37.3g |

上為細末，入地黃膏，加煉蜜少許，丸桐子大。每服三十丸，烏梅煎湯下，日進二服，亦治室女患此。

Make the above into a fine powder. Add in the *dì huáng* paste, add a little processed honey, and make pills the size of *wú tóng zǐ* (about 0.6-0.9 centimeters in diameter). Each dose is thirty pills swallowed with a decoction of *wū méi*. Take two doses per day. This also treats unmarried girls who suffer this condition.

## **Lián Qiáo Yǐn Zǐ 連翹飲子**
## **Lián Qiáo Drink** F1-33

治乳內結核。

Treats bound nodules within the breasts.

連翹川芎栝蔞仁（研）皂角刺（炒）橘葉青皮（去白）甘草節桃仁（各一錢半）

| | | | | |
|---|---|---|---|---|
| lián qiáo | 連翹 | | 1.5 *qián* of each | 5.6g |
| chuān xiōng | 川芎 | | | |
| guā lóu rén | 栝蔞仁 | grind | | |
| zào jiǎo cì | 皂角刺 | stir-fry | | |
| jú yè | 橘葉 | | | |
| qīng pí | 青皮 | remove the white | | |
| gān cǎo jié | 甘草節 | | | |
| táo rén | 桃仁 | | | |

上水煎服。

Boil the above in water and take it.

## Bì Xiào Sǎn 必效散
## Sure Effect Powder[10] F1-34

治瘰癧，未成膿者自消，已潰者自斂。

Treats scrofula. If it has not developed pus yet, it will spontaneously disperse; if it has already burst open, it will spontaneously close up.

南硼砂（二錢五分）輕粉（一錢）斑蝥（四十個，糯米同炒熟，去頭翅）麝香（五分）巴豆（五粒，去殼心膜）白檳榔（一個）

| | | | | |
|---|---|---|---|---|
| nán péng shā | 南硼砂 | | 2.5 *qián* | 9.33g |
| qīng fěn | 輕粉 | | one *qián* | 3.73g |
| bān máo | 斑蝥 | stir-fry with glutinous rice until cooked, remove the head and wings | | 40 pcs |
| shè xiāng | 麝香 | | five *fēn* | 1.85g |
| bā dòu | 巴豆 | remove the shell, heart, and membrane | | 5 pcs |
| bái bīng láng | 白檳榔 | | | 1 pc |

10. Due to toxicity, this formula is inappropriate today.

上為細末，每服一錢，五更用滾湯調下 。

Make the above into a fine powder. Each dose is one *qián* (3.73 grams), mix it with boiled water and swallow it during the fifth watch (3 – 5 a.m.).

如小水澀滯或微痛，此瘰毒欲下也，進益元散一服即下 。

If urination is rough or there is mild pain, the scrofula toxins are about to descend; take one dose of *Yì Yuán Săn* UF-7 and they will descend.

此方斑蝥 、巴豆似為峻厲，然用巴豆乃解斑蝥之毒，用者勿畏 。

This formula with *bān máo* and *bā dòu* seems drastic, but using *bā dòu* like this resolves the toxins of *bān máo*; do not fear its use.

## Hŭ Pò Gāo 琥珀膏
**Hŭ Pò Ointment** F1-35

治頸項瘰癧及腋下，初如梅子腫結硬強，漸如連珠，不消不潰；或潰而膿水不絕，經久不瘥，漸成漏症 。

Treats scrofula on the nape and neck as well as below the axilla. Initially they appear like plums (*méi zĭ*), swollen, bound up, hard, and rigid. They gradually develop until they look like a string of pearls, not dispersing and not bursting open. Or they burst open and pus-water flows ceaselessly for a long time without recovery; it gradually becomes a *lòu*-leaking disease.

琥珀（ 一兩 ）木通桂心當歸白芷防風松脂朱砂（ 研 ）木鱉子肉（ 各五錢 ）麻油（ 二斤 ）丁香木香（ 各三錢 ）

| | | | | |
|---|---|---|---|---|
| hŭ pò | 琥珀 | | one *liăng* | 37.3g |
| mù tōng | 木通 | | five *qián* of each | 18.65g |
| guì xīn | 桂心 | | | |
| dāng guī | 當歸 | | | |
| bái zhĭ | 白芷 | | | |

| fáng fēng | 防風 | | | |
|---|---|---|---|---|
| sōng zhī | 松脂 | | | |
| zhū shā | 硃砂 | ground | | |
| mù biē zǐ ròu | 木鱉子肉 | | | |
| má yóu | 麻油 | | two *jīn* | 1193.6g |
| dīng xiāng | 丁香 | | three *qián* of each | 11.19g |
| mù xiāng | 木香 | | | |

上先用琥珀、丁香、桂心、硃砂、木香為細末，其餘藥入油內，煎焦黑濾去渣，徐徐入黃丹，再煎軟硬得中，即成膏矣。

In the above, first make a fine powder with *hǔ pò, dīng xiāng, guì xīn, zhū shā,* and *mù xiāng.*[11] Add the rest of the herbs into the oil, boil until the herbs are burnt black and filter to remove the dregs. Add *huáng dān*[12] little by little, boil it again until it is the appropriate viscosity and it becomes an ointment.

## Shén Xiào Guā Lóu Sǎn 神效栝蔞散
## Wondrously Effective Guā Lóu Powder [F1-36]

治乳癰初起腫痛，及一切癰疽；或膿出後餘毒，亦宜用之。

Treats initial onset of breast abscess with swelling and pain, as well as all types of abscesses; or it is also appropriate to use this for residual toxins after pus is discharged.

黃栝蔞（子多者一個）當歸（半兩）生甘草（半兩）沒藥（一錢，另研）乳香（一錢）

11. The text does not state how these powdered herbs are used, but they must be added at the end, after the huáng dān was stirred in and the oil becomes the appropriate viscosity. Some of the powdered herbs, such as *zhū shā*, should not be exposed to heat, so it must be added after the cooking is complete. The ointment is applied to the affective site.
12. *Huáng dān* is red lead oxide or minium. It is toxic if inhaled, ingested, or is absorbed through the skin. Therefore, we cannot use it medicinally today.

| huáng guā lóu | 黃栝蔞 | with a lot of seeds | | 1 pc |
|---|---|---|---|---|
| dāng guī | 當歸 | | a half *liǎng* | 18.65g |
| shēng gān cǎo | 生甘草 | | a half *liǎng* | 18.65g |
| mò yào | 沒藥 | grind separately | one *qián* | 3.73g |
| rǔ xiāng | 乳香 | | one *qián* | 3.73g |

上酒水煎服 。

Boil the above in liquor and water and take it.

餘方見下卷 。

For the rest of the formulas, see Volume 2.

# 《女科撮要·卷下·附方并注》
# Attached Formulas and Notes for Volume 2

## Jiā Wèi Xiāo Yáo Sǎn 加味逍遙散
## Supplemented Free Wanderer Powder [F2-1]

治血虛有熱，遍身瘙癢；或口燥咽乾，發熱盜汗，食少嗜臥，小便澀滯等症。

Treats blood deficiency with heat and itching of the entire body; or dry throat and mouth, fever, night sweating, decreased food intake, somnolence, rough stagnant bowel movement, and similar conditions.

甘草（炙）當歸（炒）芍藥（酒炒）茯苓白朮（炒）柴胡（各一錢）牡丹皮山梔（炒。各五分）

| gān cǎo | 甘草 | mix-fried | one *qián* of each | 3.73g |
|---|---|---|---|---|
| dāng guī | 當歸 | stir-fried | | |
| sháo yào | 芍藥 | stir-fried with liquor | | |
| fú líng | 茯苓 | | | |
| bái zhú | 白朮 | stir-fried | | |
| chái hú | 柴胡 | | | |
| mǔ dān pí | 牡丹皮 | | five *fēn* of each | 1.85g |
| shān zhī zǐ | 山梔 | stir-fried | | |

上水煎服。

Boil the above in water and take it.

## Xiāo Yáo Sǎn 逍遙散
## Free Wanderer Powder [F2-2]

即前方去丹皮、山梔。

This means the previous formula [*Jiā Wèi Xiāo Yáo Sǎn* [F2-1]] removing *mǔ dān pí* and *zhī zǐ*.

## Guī Pí Tāng 歸脾湯
## Spleen-Returning Decoction [F2-3]

治脾經失血，少寐發熱，盜汗；或思慮傷脾，不能攝血妄行；或健忘怔忡，驚悸不寐；或心脾傷痛，怠惰嗜臥，飲食不思。

Treats blood loss of the spleen channel with reduced sleep, fever, and night sweating; or contemplation damaging the spleen with inability to contain the blood and reckless movement; or forgetfulness, fearful throbbing, fright palpitations, and insomnia; or heart and spleen damage with pain, laziness, somnolence, and no thought of food and drink.

人參白朮白茯苓黃耆（炒）當歸龍眼肉遠志酸棗仁（炒。各一錢）木香（五分）甘草（五分）

| rén shēn | 人參 | | one *qián* of each | 3.73g |
|---|---|---|---|---|
| bái zhú | 白朮 | | | |
| bái fú líng | 白茯苓 | | | |
| huáng qí | 黃耆 | stir-fried | | |
| dāng guī | 當歸 | | | |
| long yǎn ròu | 龍眼肉 | | | |
| yuǎn zhì | 遠志 | | | |
| suān zǎo rén | 酸棗仁 | stir-fried | | |
| mù xiāng | 木香 | | five *fēn* | 1.85g |
| gān cǎo | 甘草 | mix-fried | five *fēn* | 1.85g |

上薑棗水煎服。

Boil the above in water with ginger and *zǎo*-dates and take it.

## Jiā Wèi Guī Pí Tāng 加味歸脾湯
## Supplemented Spleen-Returning Decoction F2-4

即前方加柴胡、山梔。

This means the previous formula [*Guī Pí Tāng* F2-3] adding *chái hú* and *zhī zǐ*.

## Bǔ Zhōng Yì Qì Tāng 補中益氣湯
## Center-Supplementng Qì-Boosting Decoction F2-5

治元氣不足，四肢倦怠，口乾發熱，飲食無味；或飲食失節，勞倦身熱，脈洪大而無力；或頭痛發熱；或惡寒自汗；或氣高而喘，身熱而煩。

Treats insufficient original qì with fatigue of the four limbs, dry mouth, fever, food and drink are flavorless; or lost regularity of eating and drinking with fatigue, feverish feeling, and surging large but forceless pulse; or headache and fever; or aversion to cold with spontaneous sweating; or shallow breathing, panting, feverish feeling, and vexation.

黃耆（炙，一錢五分）甘草（炙）人參當歸（酒拌）白朮（炒。各一錢）升麻柴胡（各三分）陳皮（一錢）

| huáng qí | 黃耆 | mix-fried | 1.5 *qián* | 5.6g |
|---|---|---|---|---|
| gān cǎo | 甘草 | mix-fried | one *qián* of each | 3.73g |
| rén shēn | 人參 | | | |
| dāng guī | 當歸 | mixed with liquor | | |
| bái zhú | 白朮 | stir-fried | | |

| | | | | |
|---|---|---|---|---|
| shēng má | 升麻 | | three *fēn* of each | 1.12g |
| chái hú | 柴胡 | | | |
| chén pí | 陳皮 | | one *qián* | 3.73g |

上薑棗水煎服。

Boil the above in water with ginger and *zǎo*-dates and take it.

## Liù Jūn Zǐ Tāng 六君子湯
## Six Gentlemen Decoction F2-6

即異功散加半夏。

This means *Yì Gōng Sǎn* F2-27 adding *bàn xià*.

## Shí Quán Dà Bǔ Tāng 十全大補湯
## Perfect Major Supplementation Decoction F2-7

治諸臟虧損，氣血俱虛，惡寒發熱；或自汗盜汗，便血吐血；或大便不實，飲食少思；或胸腹作痛，口舌生瘡；或耳目不明，牙齒不固。

Treats debility of all the *zàng*-organs, deficiency of both qì and blood, aversion to cold and fever; or spontaneous sweating, night sweating, blood in the stool, and vomiting blood; or unformed stool with little thought of food and drink; or pain of the chest and abdomen and sores engendered on the mouth and tongue; or dimness of the ears and eyes and the teeth are not firm.

人參白朮白茯苓黃耆當歸熟地黃（酒洗，蒸，焙）川芎白芍藥（炒。各一錢）肉桂甘草（炙。五分）

| | | | | |
|---|---|---|---|---|
| rén shēn | 人參 | | one *qián* of each | 3.73g |
| bái zhú | 白朮 | | | |
| bái fú líng | 白茯苓 | | | |
| huáng qí | 黃耆 | | | |
| dāng guī | 當歸 | | | |
| shú dì huáng | 熟地黃 | alcohol washed, steamed, and baked | | |
| chuān xiōng | 川芎 | | | |
| bái sháo yào | 白芍藥 | stir-fried | | |
| ròu guì | 肉桂 | | [unstated] | |
| gān cǎo | 甘草 | mix-fried | five *fēn* | 1.85g |

上薑棗水煎服。

Boil the above in water with ginger and *zǎo*-dates and take it.

## Bā Zhēn Tāng 八珍湯
## Eight Gem Decoction F2-8

治脾胃虧損，氣血俱虛，乃內傷之症。蓋人之生，以脾胃為主，脾胃一虛，諸臟失所，百病生焉。

Treats debility of the spleen and stomach with deficiency of both qì and blood. This is a pattern of internal damage. It seems that a person's life is governed by the spleen and stomach, so if the spleen and stomach are both deficient, all the *zàng* organs lose their place and the hundred diseases are engendered.

即前方大補湯，去黃耆、肉桂。

This means the previous formula, *Shí Quán Dà Bǔ Tāng* F2-7, removing the *huáng qí* and *ròu guì*.

## Dāng Guī Bǔ Xuè Tāng 當歸補血湯<br>Dāng Guī Blood-Supplementing Decoction F2-9

治肌熱躁熱，目赤面紅，煩渴引飲，晝夜不息，脈洪大而虛，重按全無。此脈虛血虛也，若誤服白虎湯必死。

Treats heat of the muscles with agitation and heat, red eyes and face, vexation thirst with desire to drink, and inability to rest day and night. The pulse is surging and large but deficient; when pressed hard there is absolutely nothing. This pulse is deficient so deficiency of blood. If *Bái Hǔ Tāng* is mistakenly given, the patient will die.

當歸（三錢）黃耆（炙，一兩）

| | | | | |
|---|---|---|---|---|
| dāng guī | 當歸 | | three *qián* | 11.19g |
| huáng qí | 黃耆 | mix-fried | one *liǎng* | 37.3g |

上水煎服。

Boil the above in water and take it.

## Qīng Wèi Sǎn 清胃散<br>Stomach-Clearing Powder F2-10

治胃經濕熱，牙齒或牙根腫痛；或牽引頭腦；或面發熱。

Treats damp heat in the stomach channel with swollen painful teeth and gums; perhaps pain radiates to the head and brain or the face feels feverish.

當歸身（酒拌，一錢）黃連生地黃（酒拌）升麻（各二錢）牡丹皮（一錢五分）

| | | | | |
|---|---|---|---|---|
| dāng guī shēn | 當歸身 | mixed with liquor | one *qián* | 3.73g |
| huáng lián | 黃連 | | two *qián* of each | 7.46g |

| shēng dì huáng | 生地黄 | mixed with liquor | | |
|---|---|---|---|---|
| shēng má | 升麻 | | | |
| mǔ dān pí | 牡丹皮 | | 1.5 *qián* | 5.6g |

上水煎服。

Boil the above in water and take it.

## Jiā Wèi Qīng Wèi Sǎn 加味清胃散
## Supplemented Stomach-Clearing Powder F2-11

治脾胃有熱，口內生瘡；或齒作痛；或齦腐爛。

Treats heat of the spleen and stomach with sores in the mouth, perhaps with toothache or rotting gums.

即前方加犀角、連翹、甘草。

This means the previous formula [*Qīng Wèi Sǎn* F2-10] adding *xī jiǎo,*[13] *lián qiáo,* and *gān cǎo.*

## Xiǎo Chái Hú Tāng 小柴胡湯
## Minor Chái Hú Decoction F2-12

治肝膽經症，寒熱往來；或晡熱潮熱，不欲飲食；或口苦耳聾，咳嗽發熱；或脅痛胠滿，轉側不便；或瀉痢咳嗽，嘔吐酸水。

Treats liver-gallbladder channel patterns with [sensations of] cold and heat that come and go; or late afternoon fevers, tidal fevers, and no desire to eat or drink; or bitter mouth, tinnitus, cough, and fever; or rib-side pain, fullness of the flanks, and discomfort moving about; or diarrhea, cough, and vomiting of sour fluids.

13. This comes from an endangered species and cannot be used.

柴胡（ 二錢 ）黃芩（ 一錢五分 ）半夏（ 一錢 ）人參（ 一錢 ）甘草（炙，五分 ）

| chái hú | 柴胡 | | two *qián* | 7.46g |
|---|---|---|---|---|
| huáng qín | 黃芩 | | 1.5 *qián* | 5.6g |
| bàn xià | 半夏 | | one *qián* | 3.73g |
| rén shēn | 人參 | | one *qián* | 3.73g |
| gān cǎo | 甘草 | mixed-fried | five *fēn* | 1.85g |

上薑棗水煎服。

Boil the above in water with ginger and *zǎo*-dates and take it.

## Jiā Wèi Xiǎo Chái Hú Tāng 加味小柴胡湯
## Supplemented Minor Chái Hú Decoction F2-13

治婦女經行，感冒發熱，熱入血室，寒熱如瘧，晝則安靜，夜則發熱妄語；或素血虛，大勞大怒火動，熱入血室亦能致。

Treats menstruating women with external contraction and fever. Heat enters the blood chamber with [sensations of] cold and heat like *nüè*-malaria. She is peaceful in the daytime but has fever and delirious speech at night. Or heat entering the blood chamber can also occur in those who are usually blood deficient with great taxation or great anger stirring up fire.

此即前方加生地黃。

This means the previous formula [*Xiǎo Chái Hú Tāng* F2-12] adding *shēng dì huáng*.

## Dāng Guī Liù Huáng Tāng 當歸六黃湯
## Dāng Guī plus Six Yellows Decoction F2-14

治氣血虛，而發熱盜汗等症 。

Treats qì and blood deficiency with fever, night sweating, and similar conditions.

當歸（ 二錢 ）黃耆（ 炒 ）生地黄熟地黄（ 各一錢 ）黃連（ 炒焦 ）黃芩（ 炒焦 ）黃柏（ 炒焦 。各五分 ）

| dāng guī | 當歸 | | two *qián* | 7.46g |
|---|---|---|---|---|
| huáng qí | 黃耆 | stir-fried | 1 *qián* of each | 3.73g |
| shēng dì huáng | 生地黄 | | | |
| shú dì huáng | 熟地黄 | | | |
| huáng lián | 黃連 | stir-fry until burnt | five *fēn* of each | 1.85g |
| huáng qín | 黃芩 | stir-fry until burnt | | |
| huáng bǎi | 黃柏 | stir-fry until burnt | | |

上水煎服 。

Boil the above in water and take it.

## Huáng Qín Qīng Fèi Yǐn 黃芩清肺飲
## Huáng Qín Lung-Clearing Decoction F2-15

治肺熱而小便不利 。

Treats lung heat and inhibited urination.

黃芩山梔（ 各一錢 ）

| huáng qín | 黃芩 | 1 *qián* of each | 3.73g |
|---|---|---|---|
| shān zhī zǐ | 山梔 | | |

上水煎服。不利，加鹽豉二十粒。

Boil the above in water and take it. If [urination] is inhibited, add twenty grains of *yán chǐ*.

## Liù Wèi Wán 六味丸
## Six Ingredient Pill [F2-16]

一名地黃丸。

Also named *Dì Huáng Wán* [F2-16] (Dì Huáng Pill).

加肉桂一兩，名加減八味丸。

Adding one *liǎng* (37.3 grams) of *ròu guì* is named *Jiā Jiǎn Bā Wèi Wán* [F2-18] (Eight Ingredient Variant Pill).

治腎虛發熱，作渴唾痰，小便淋瀝，頭暈眼花，咽燥唇裂，齒不堅固，腰腿酸軟，自汗盜汗，便血諸血，失喑，水氾為痰之聖藥，血虛發熱之神劑。

Treats kidney deficiency with fever, thirst, spitting phlegm, dribbling urination, dizziness with flowery vision, dry throat, cracked lips, teeth not hard and firm, aching weak low back and legs, spontaneous sweating, night sweating, blood in the stool, various bleeding disorders, and loss of voice. This is the medicine of the sages for overflowing water that becomes phlegm; it is a miraculous prescription for blood deficiency fevers.

熟地黃（半斤，杵膏）山茱萸肉乾山藥（各四兩）牡丹皮白茯苓澤瀉（各三兩）

| | | | | |
|---|---|---|---|---|
| shú dì huáng | 熟地黃 | pestle into a paste | a half *jīn* | 298.4g |
| shān zhū yú ròu | 山茱萸肉 | | four *liǎng* of each | 149.2g |
| gān shān yào | 乾山藥 | | | |
| mǔ dān pí | 牡丹皮 | | three *liǎng* of each | 111.9g |
| bái fú líng | 白茯苓 | | | |
| zé xiè | 澤瀉 | | | |

上各另為末，和地黄加煉蜜丸桐子大。每服七八十丸，空心食前白滾湯下。地黄須自製。

Powder each of the above separately [from the *dì huáng*], blend in the *dì huáng* and add processed honey to make pills the size of *wú tóng zǐ* (about 0.6-0.9 centimeters in diameter). Each dose is seventy or eighty pills taken on an empty stomach before meals, swallowed with boiled water while still hot. You must process the *dì huáng* yourself.

## Bā Wèi Wán 八味丸
## Eight Ingredient Pill[14] F2-17

治命門火衰，不能生土，以致脾胃虛寒，飲食少思；或臍腹疼痛；或多漩溺。

Treats debility of *mìng mén* fire with inability to engender earth; this results in deficient cold spleen and stomach with little thought of food and drink; or pain of the umbilicus and abdomen; or frequent urination.

即前方加桂、附各一兩。

This means the previous formula [*Liù Wèi Wán* F2-16] adding one *liǎng* (37.3 grams) each of cinnamon and *fù zǐ*.

14. This formula has a few names and a few variations. While it is called *Bā Wèi Wán* here, in the text it is more often called *Shèn Qì Wán* (Kidney Qì Pill) or *Jīn Guì Jiā Jiǎn Shèn Qì Wán* 《金匱》加減腎氣丸 (Kidney Qì Variant Pill from *Jīn Guì Yào Lüè*). (*Jīn Guì Yào Lüè* was written by Zhāng Zhòngjǐng 張仲景《金匱要略》 during the late *Hàn* dynasty). In addition, *Jiā Jiǎn Bā Wèi Wán* F2-18 and *Jiā Jiǎn Jì Shēng Shèn Qì Wán* F2-19 are variations of *Bā Wèi Wán*.

## Jiā Jiǎn Bā Wèi Wán 加減八味丸
## Eight Ingredient Variant Pill[F2-18]

即六味丸加肉桂一兩。

This means *Liù Wèi Wán*[F2-16] adding one *liǎng* (37.3 grams) of *ròu guì*.

## Jiā Jiǎn Jì Shēng Shèn Qì Wán 加減《濟生》腎氣丸
## Kidney Qì Variant Pill from Jì Shēng[15] [F2-19]

治脾腎虛，腰重脚腫，濕飲留積，小便不利；或肚腹腫脹，四肢浮腫，氣喘痰甚，或已成水症。其效如神。

Treats spleen and kidney deficiency, heaviness of the lower back, swollen legs, lingering accumulations of damp rheum, and inhibited urination; or swelling and distention of the belly, superficial swelling of the four limbs, and severe panting with phlegm; perhaps it has already become a water condition. Its effects are like a miracle.

白茯苓（三兩）附子（半兩）川牛膝桂心澤瀉車前子山茱萸山藥牡丹皮（各一兩）熟地黃（四兩，掐碎，酒拌，杵膏）

| | | | | |
|---|---|---|---|---|
| bái fú líng | 白茯苓 | | three *liǎng* | 111.9g |
| fù zǐ | 附子 | | a half *liǎng* | 18.65g |
| chuān niú xī | 川牛膝 | | one *liǎng* of each | 37.3g |
| guì xīn | 桂心 | | | |
| zé xiè | 澤瀉 | | | |
| chē qián zǐ | 車前子 | | | |
| shān zhū yú | 山茱萸 | | | |
| shān yào | 山藥 | | | |
| mǔ dān pí | 牡丹皮 | | | |

15. *Jì Shēng Fāng*《濟生方》(Formulas to Aid Life) was written by Yán Yònghé 嚴用和 and was published in 1253 (*Sòng*).

| shú dì huáng | 熟地黄 | break into pieces, mix with liquor, pestle into a paste | four *liǎng* | 149.2g |
|---|---|---|---|---|

上為末，和地黃膏，加煉蜜丸，桐子大。每服七八十丸，空心米飲下。

Powder the above, blend with the *dì huáng* paste, and add processed honey to make pills the size of *wú tóng zǐ* (about 0.6-0.9 centimeters in diameter). Each dose is seventy or eighty pills swallowed with rice drink on an empty stomach.

## Sì Wù Èr Lián Tāng 四物二連湯<br>Four Agents plus Two Lián Decoction F2-20

治血虛發熱；或口舌生瘡；或晝安夜熱。

Treats blood deficiency with fevers; or sores engendered on the mouth and tongue; or peaceful in the daytime but feverish at night.

當歸川芎芍藥熟地黃胡黃連宣黃連（各一錢）

| dāng guī | 當歸 | one *qián* of each | 3.73g |
|---|---|---|---|
| chuān xiōng | 川芎 | | |
| sháo yào | 芍藥 | | |
| shú dì huáng | 熟地黄 | | |
| hú huáng lián | 胡黃連 | | |
| xuān huáng lián | 宣黃連 | | |

上作一劑，水煎服。

The above makes one dose. Boil in water and take it.

## **Bái Hǔ Tāng 白虎湯**
## **White Tiger Decoction** F2-21

治胃熱作渴，暑熱尤效。

Treats stomach heat with thirst; it is especially effective in hot summer weather.

知母（一錢五分）石膏（四錢）粳米（一合）

| zhī mǔ | 知母 | 1.5 *qián* of each | 5.6g |
|---|---|---|---|
| shí gāo | 石膏 | four *qián* | 14.92g |
| jīng mǐ | 粳米 | one gě | 59.68g |

上作一劑，水煎服。

The above makes one dose; boil in water and take it.

## **Qián Shì Yì Huáng Sǎn 錢氏益黃散**
## **Qián's Yellow-Boosting Powder** F2-22

治脾土虛寒，寒水反來侮土，而嘔吐不食；或肚腹作痛；或大便不實，手足逆冷等症。

Treats deficient cold spleen earth with cold water contrarily insulting earth. This leads to vomiting and not eating; or belly pain; or unformed stool, counterflow cold of the hands and feet, and similar conditions.

陳皮（一兩）青皮訶子肉甘草（炙）丁香（二錢）

| chén pí | 陳皮 | | one *liǎng* | 37.3g |
|---|---|---|---|---|
| qīng pí | 青皮 | | [unstated] | |
| hē zǐ ròu | 訶子肉 | | [unstated] | |
| gān cǎo | 甘草 | mix-fried | [unstated] | |
| dīng xiāng | 丁香 | | four *qián* | 7.46g |

上為粗末，每服四錢，水煎服。

Make the above into a coarse powder; each dose is four *qián* (14.92 grams) boiled in water and taken.

## Èr Shén Wán 二神丸
## Two Spirits Pill F2-23

治脾腎虛弱，侵晨五更作瀉；或全不思食；或食而不化，大便不實，神效。

Treats deficient weak spleen and kidneys with diarrhea around dawn in the fifth watch (3 – 5 a.m.); or absolutely no thought of food; or eating but food is not transformed [digested] with unformed stool. This is wondrously effective.

破故紙（四兩，炒）肉豆蔻（二兩，生用）

| pò gù zhǐ | 破故紙 | stir-fried | four *liǎng* | 149.2g |
|---|---|---|---|---|
| ròu dòu kòu | 肉荳蔻 | use the fresh | two *liǎng* | 74.6g |

上為末，用大紅棗四十九枚，生薑四兩，切碎同棗用水煮熟，去薑取棗肉，和藥丸桐子大。每服五十丸，空心鹽湯下。

Powder the above. Use forty-nine pieces of *dà hóng zǎo* with four *liǎng* (149.2 grams) of *shēng jiāng*. Slice and smash the *shēng jiāng* together with the *zǎo*-dates. Boil in water until cooked, remove the ginger and keep the flesh of the *zǎo*-dates. Blend the *zǎo*-date flesh with the powdered herbs to make pills the size of *wú tóng zǐ* (about 0.6-0.9 centimeters in diameter). Each dose is fifty pills, swallowed with boiled salt water on an empty stomach.

## Rén Shēn Lǐ Zhōng Tāng 人參理中湯
## Rén Shēn Center-Rectifying Decoction F2-24

治脾胃虛寒，嘔吐泄瀉，飲食少思，肚腹膨脹。

Treats deficient cold spleen and stomach with vomiting, diarrhea, little thought of food and drink, and inflated distended belly.

人參白朮乾薑（炮）甘草（炙。各一錢）

| rén shēn | 人參 | | one *qián* of each | 3.73g |
|---|---|---|---|---|
| bái zhú | 白朮 | | | |
| gān jiāng | 乾薑 | blast-fried | | |
| gān cǎo | 甘草 | mix-fried | | |

上薑棗水煎服。

Boil the above in water with ginger and *zǎo*-dates and take it.

## Fù Zǐ Lǐ Zhōng Tāng 附子理中湯
## Fù Zǐ Center-Rectifying Decoction F2-25

治脾胃虛寒，手足俱冷，飲食不入；或腸鳴切痛，嘔逆吐瀉。

Treats deficient cold spleen and stomach with cold hands and feet and not eating or drinking; or intestinal gurgling with cutting pain, vomiting counterflow, vomiting and diarrhea.

即前方加附子一錢。

This means the previous formula [*Rén Shēn Lǐ Zhōng Tāng* F2-24] adding one *qián* (3.73 grams) of *fù zǐ*.

## Sì Jūn Zǐ Tāng 四君子湯
## Four Gentlemen Decoction F2-26

治脾胃虛損，飲食少思；或大便不實，肢體消瘦；或胸膈虛痞，痰嗽吞酸；或脾胃虛弱，停食而患瘧痢；或瘧痢因脾胃虛而不能愈。

Treats spleen and stomach deficiency with little thought of food and drink; or unformed stool while the body beomes emaciated; or deficiency and *pǐ*-glomus of the chest and diaphragm, phlegmy cough, and sour swallowing; or deficient weak spleen and stomach with food retention and then suffering *nüè*-malarial dysentery; or *nüè*-malarial dysentery due to spleen and stomach deficiency with inability to recover.

人參白朮茯苓（各二錢）甘草（各一錢）

| rén shēn | 人參 | | two *qián* of each | 7.46g |
|---|---|---|---|---|
| bái zhú | 白朮 | | | |
| fú líng | 茯苓 | | | |
| gān cǎo | 甘草 | mix-fried | one *qián* | 3.73g |

上薑棗水煎服。

Boil the above in water with ginger and *zǎo*-dates and take it.

若因肝木剋脾土而致，宜加柴胡、芍藥。若命門火衰而患，宜兼八味丸。

If it is due to liver wood controlling spleen earth, it is appropriate to add *chái hú* and *sháo yào.* If the suffering is from debility of *mìng mén* fire, it is appropriate take *Bā Wèi Wán* F2-17 at the same time.

## Yì Gōng Sǎn 異功散
## Special Achievement Powder [F2-27]

即前湯加陳皮，治脾胃虛弱，飲食少思；或久患咳嗽；或腹滿不食，面浮氣逆等症 。

This means the previous decoction [*Sì Jūn Zǐ Tāng* [F2-26]] adding *chén pí* to treat deficient weak spleen and stomach with little thought of food and drink; or suffering cough for a long time; or abdominal fullness, not eating, facial superficial [edema] with qì counterflow, and similar conditions.

## Rén Shēn Jú Pí Tāng 人參橘皮湯
## Rén Shēn and Jú Pí Decoction [F2-28]

治脾胃虛弱，氣滯惡阻，嘔吐痰水 。

Treats deficient weak spleen and stomach, with qì stagnation, morning sickness, and vomiting phlegmy water.

人參陳皮白朮麥門（ 去心 。各一錢 ）甘草（ 三分 ）濃樸（ 製 ）白茯苓（ 去皮 。各五分 ）

| | | | | |
|---|---|---|---|---|
| rén shēn | 人參 | | one *qián* of each | 3.73g |
| chén pí | 陳皮 | | | |
| bái zhú | 白朮 | | | |
| mài mén dōng | 麥門 | remove the heart | | |
| gān cǎo | 甘草 | | three *fēn* | 1.12g |
| nóng pǔ | 濃樸 | processed | five *fēn* of each | 1.85g |
| bái fú líng | 白茯苓 | remove the peel | | |

上用淡竹茹一塊，薑水煎溫服 。

Boil ginger and a lump of *dàn zhú rú* with the above in water and take it warm.

若因中脘停痰，宜用二陳、枳殼。若因飲食停滯，宜用六君子加枳殼。若因脾胃虛，宜用異功散。

If the condition is due to abiding phlegm at Zhōng Wǎn [the region of Rèn 12], it is appropriate to use *Èr Chén Tāng* F2-42 and *zhǐ qiào*. If it is due to food retention, it is appropriate to use *Liù Jūn Zǐ Tāng* F2-6 adding *zhǐ qiào*. If it is due to spleen and stomach deficiency, it is appropriate to use *Yì Gōng Sǎn* F2-27.

## Zhú Yè Tāng 竹葉湯
## Zhú Yè Decoction F2-29

治妊娠心驚膽怯，煩悶不安，名曰子煩。

Treats pregnant women with heart fright, gallbladder timidity, vexation, and oppression. [The fetus] is not peaceful. This is named *child vexation*.

白茯苓麥門黃芩（各三兩）

| bái fú líng | 白茯苓 | three *liǎng* of each | 111.9g |
|---|---|---|---|
| mài mén dōng | 麥門 | | |
| huáng qín | 黃芩 | | |

上每服四錢，竹葉五片，水煎服。

Each dose of the above is four *qián* (14.92 grams); boil in water with five bamboo leaves (*zhú yè*) and take.

若因血虛煩熱，宜兼用四物。若因中氣虛弱，宜兼四君。

If the condition is due to blood deficiency with vexation heat, it is appropriate to use *Sì Wù Tāng* F2-51 at the same time. If it is due to deficient weak central qì, it is appropriate to use *Sì Jūn Zǐ Tāng* F2-26 at the same time.

## Zǐ Sū Yǐn 紫蘇飲
### Zǐ Sū Drink F2-30

治妊娠失調，胎氣不安，上疞作痛，名子懸。

Treats a pregnant women who is out of tune, with fetal qì that is not peaceful and her upper body is colicky and painful. This is called *fetal suspension.*

大腹皮川芎白芍陳皮蘇葉當歸（各一兩）人參甘草（各半兩）

| dà fù pí | 大腹皮 | one *liǎng* of each | 37.5g |
|---|---|---|---|
| chuān xiōng | 川芎 | | |
| bái sháo | 白芍 | | |
| chén pí | 陳皮 | | |
| zǐ sū yè | 蘇葉 | | |
| dāng guī | 當歸 | | |
| rén shēn | 人參 | a half *liǎng* of each | 18.65g |
| gān cǎo | 甘草 | | |

上薑蔥水煎服。

Boil the above in water with ginger and scallions and take it.

若肝脾氣血虛而有火不安，宜兼逍遙散。若脾氣虛弱而不安，宜用四君、芎、歸。

If there is liver-spleen qì-blood deficiency with fire and [the fetus] is not peaceful, it is appropriate to use *Xiāo Yáo Sǎn* F2-2 at the same time. If spleen qì is deficient and weak and [the fetus] is not peaceful, it is appropriate to use *Sì Jūn Zǐ Tāng* F2-26 adding *chuān xiōng* and *dāng guī.*

## Jiāo Ài Tāng 膠艾湯
## Ē Jiāo and Ài Yè Decoction F2-31

治妊娠頓仆，胎動不安，腰腹疼痛；或胎上搶；或去血腹痛。

Treats sudden falling down [collapse] of pregnant women with stirring fetus that is not peaceful, and pain of the lower back and abdomen; or the fetus rushes upward; or bleeding with abdominal pain.

阿膠（一兩，炙）艾葉（數莖）

| ē jiāo | 阿膠 | mix-fried | one *liǎng* | 37.3g |
|---|---|---|---|---|
| ài yè | 艾葉 | | several stalks | |

上二味，以水五升煮二升，分三服。

Use five *shēng* (5368.5 mililiters) of water to boil the above two herbs down to two *shēng* (2147.4 mililiters); divide into three doses.

## Ē Jiāo Sǎn 阿膠散
## Ē Jiāo Powder F2-32

或頓仆；或因毒藥，胎動不安；或脅肋痛腹痛，上搶短氣。

Perhaps there is sudden falling down [collapse]; or the fetus stirs and is not peaceful because of herb toxins; or rib-side pain and abdominal pain with [a sensation of] rushing upward and shortness of breath.

熟地黃艾葉白芍川芎黃耆阿膠當歸甘草（炙，各一兩）

| shú dì huáng | 熟地黃 | | one *liǎng* of each | 37.3g |
|---|---|---|---|---|
| ài yè | 艾葉 | | | |
| bái sháo | 白芍 | | | |
| chuān xiōng | 川芎 | | | |

| huáng qí | 黃耆 | | | |
|---|---|---|---|---|
| ē jiāo | 阿膠 | | | |
| dāng guī | 當歸 | | | |
| gān cǎo | 甘草 | mix-fried | | |

上每服四錢，薑棗水煎 。

[Powder] the above. Each dose is four *qián* (14.92 grams) boiled in water with ginger and *zǎo*-dates.

## Zhǐ Qiào Tāng 枳殼湯
## Zhǐ Qiào Decoction F2-33

治胎漏下血；或因事下血 。

Treats fetal spotting with lower bleeding; or lower bleeding due to activity.

枳殼( 炒 )黃芩( 炙，半兩 )白朮( 一兩 )

| zhǐ qiào | 枳殼 | stir-fried | [unstated] | |
|---|---|---|---|---|
| huáng qín | 黃芩 | mix-fried | a half *liǎng* | 18.65g |
| bái zhú | 白朮 | | one *liǎng* | 37.3g |

上為末，每服一錢，白湯調下 。

Powder the above; each dose is one *qián* (3.73 grams) mixed with clear soup and swallowed.

# Èr Huáng Sǎn 二黃散
## Two Yellows Powder F2-34

治胎漏下血，或內熱晡熱；或頭痛頭暈；或煩躁作渴；或脅肋脹痛等症。

Treats fetal spotting with lower bleeding, perhaps with internal heat and late afternoon fevers; or headache and dizziness; or vexation and agitation making thirst; or distention and pain of the rib-sides and similar conditions.

生地黃熟地黃

| shēng dì huáng | 生地黃 |
|---|---|
| shú dì huáng | 熟地黃 |

上為末，每服三錢，煎白朮、枳殼湯下。

Powder the above; each dose is three *qián* (11.19 grams) boiled in a decoction of *bái zhú* and *zhǐ qiào* and swallowed.

前四症若因脾胃虛弱，宜用補中益氣湯加五味。若因脾胃虛陷，宜用前湯，倍用升麻、柴胡。若因晡熱內熱，宜用逍遙散。

If the above four conditions [described for this formula] are due to deficient weak spleen and stomach, it is appropriate to use *Bǔ Zhōng Yì Qì Tāng* F2-5 adding *wǔ wèi zǐ*. If due to spleen and stomach deficiency with sinking, it is appropriate to use the previous formula [*Bǔ Zhōng Yì Qì Tāng* F2-5], doubling the dose of *shēng má* and *chái hú*. If due to late afternoon fever with internal heat, it is appropriate to use *Xiāo Yáo Sǎn* F2-2.

## Zhī Mǔ Wán 知母丸
## Zhī Mǔ Pill F2-35

治妊娠頓仆胎動不安，或欲墮產 。

Treats sudden falling down [collapse] in pregnant women with stirring fetus that is not peaceful or threatened miscarriage.

用知母一味，炒為末，丸梧桐子大 。每服二十丸，白湯下；或嚼咽之 。

Stir-fry and powder *zhī mǔ* alone and make pills the size of *wú tóng zǐ* (about 0.6-0.9 centimeters in diameter). Each dose is twenty pills swallowed with clear soup, or chew and swallow it.

## Dì Huáng Dāng Guī Tāng 地黃當歸湯
## Dì Huáng and Dāng Guī Decoction F2-36

治血虛胎動 。

Treats blood deficiency with stirring fetus.

當歸（ 一兩 ）熟地黃（ 二兩 ）

| | | | |
|---|---|---|---|
| dāng guī | 當歸 | one *liǎng* | 37.3g |
| shú dì huáng | 熟地黃 | two *liǎng* | 74.6g |

上每服五錢，水煎 。

Each dose of the above is five *qián* (18.65 grams) boiled in water.

若因脾胃弱而血虛者，宜用四君 、芎 、歸 。氣血俱虛者，宜用八珍湯 。

If this is due to weak spleen and stomach with blood deficiency, it is appropriate to use *Sì Jūn Zǐ Tāng*[F2-26] adding *chuān xiōng* and *dāng guī*. For deficiency of both qì and blood, it is appropriate to use *Bā Zhēn Tāng*[F2-8].

## Jīn Shēng Bái Zhú Sǎn 金生白朮散
## Metal-Engendering Bái Zhú Powder[F2-37]

治妊娠，面目虛浮，四肢腫如水氣，名曰胎腫。

Treats pregnant women with deficiency puffiness of the face and eyes and swelling of the four limbs as if there were water qì; this is named *fetal swelling*.

白朮（一兩）生薑皮大腹皮陳皮白茯苓（各半兩）

| bái zhú | 白朮 | one *liǎng* | 37.3g |
|---|---|---|---|
| shēng jiāng pí | 生薑皮 | a half *liǎng* of each | 18.65g |
| dà fù pí | 大腹皮 | | |
| chén pí | 陳皮 | | |
| bái fú líng | 白茯苓 | | |

上各為末，每服二錢，米飲下。

Powder each of the above; each dose is two *qián* (7.46 grams) swallowed with rice drink.

若未應，佐以四君子湯。

If she does not respond, use *Sì Jūn Zǐ Tāng*[F2-26] as an assistant.

## Tiān Xiān Téng Sǎn 天仙藤散
## Tiān Xiān Téng Powder [F2-38]

治妊娠自三月之後，足指發腫，漸至腿膝，飲食不甘，狀似水氣；或腳指間出黃水，名曰子氣 。

Treats women pregnant more than three months when the toes become swollen and the swelling gradually rises up the legs to the knees. Food and drink do not taste sweet. This condition is similar to water qì. Perhaps yellow fluid comes out from between the toes. This is named *child qì*.

天仙藤（ 洗略炒 ）香附（ 炒 ）陳皮甘草烏藥（ 各等分 ）

| | | | |
|---|---|---|---|
| tiān xiān téng | 天仙藤 | wash and briefly stir-fry | equal portions of each |
| xiāng fù | 香附 | stir-fried | |
| chén pí | 陳皮 | | |
| gān cǎo | 甘草 | | |
| wū yào | 烏藥 | | |

上每服三五錢，生薑 、木瓜各三片，紫蘇三葉，水煎，食前日進三服 。

Each dose of the above is three or five *qián* (18.65 grams) boiled in water with three slices each of *shēng jiāng* and *mù guā,* and three leaves of *zǐ sū yè*. Take it before meals, three doses per day.

若因脾胃虛弱，宜兼六君子 。中氣下陷，須用補中益氣湯 。

If this is due to deficient weak spleen and stomach, it is appropriate to take *Liù Jūn Zǐ Tāng* [F2-6] at the same time. If central qì sinks downward, you must use *Bǔ Zhōng Yì Qì Tāng* [F2-5].

# Ān Róng Sǎn 安榮散
## Quiet Yíng-Construction Powder [F2-39]

治妊娠，小便澀少，遂成淋瀝，名曰子淋 。

Treats pregnant women with rough scant urination that becomes dribbling; this is named *child lín-dribbling*.

麥門冬（ 去心 ）通草滑石（ 各二錢 ）當歸燈心甘草（ 各五錢 ）人參細辛（ 各一兩 ）

| | | | | |
|---|---|---|---|---|
| mài mén dōng | 麥門冬 | remove the heart | two *qián* of each | 7.46g |
| tōng cǎo | 通草 | | | |
| huá shí | 滑石 | | | |
| dāng guī | 當歸 | | five *qián* of each | 18.65g |
| dēng xīn | 燈心 | | | |
| gān cǎo | 甘草 | | | |
| rén shēn | 人參 | | one *liǎng* of each | 37.3g |
| xì xīn | 細辛 | | | |

上為末，每服二錢，煎麥門湯調下 。

Powder the above. Each dose is two *qián* (7.46 grams). Boil a decoction of *mài mén dōng*, mix, and swallow it.

若因肺經蘊熱，宜用黃芩清肺飲 。若因膏粱濃味，宜用清胃散 。若因肝經濕熱，宜用加味逍遙散 。

If this is due to heat accumulating in the lung channel, it is appropriate to use *Huáng Qín Qīng Fèi Yǐn* [F2-15]. If it is due to rich foods with concentrated flavors, it is appropriate to use *Qīng Wèi Sǎn* [F2-10]. If it is due to damp heat of the liver channel, it is appropriate to use *Jiā Wèi Xiāo Yáo Sǎn* [F2-1].

## Líng Yáng Jiǎo Sǎn 羚羊角散
## Líng Yáng Jiǎo Powder F2-40

治妊娠虛風，頸項強直，筋脈攣急，語言蹇塞，痰涎不利；或時發搐；或不省人事，名曰子癇 。

Treats pregnant women with deficiency wind, neck rigidity, tension of the sinews, difficulty speaking, and inhibited phlegm drool; or occasional convulsions; or not recognizing human affairs [unconsciousness]. This is named *child epilepsy*.

羚羊角( 鎊 )川獨活酸棗仁( 炒 )五加皮( 各五錢 )薏苡仁防風當歸川芎茯神杏仁( 各四分 )木香甘草( 各二分半 )

| líng yáng jiǎo | 羚羊角 | filed | five *qián* of each | 18.65g |
|---|---|---|---|---|
| chuān dú huó | 川獨活 | | | |
| suān zǎo rén | 酸棗仁 | stir-fried | | |
| wǔ jiā pí | 五加皮 | | | |
| yì yǐ rén | 薏苡仁 | | four *fēn* of each | 1.48g |
| fáng fēng | 防風 | | | |
| dāng guī | 當歸 | | | |
| chuān xiōng | 川芎 | | | |
| fú shén | 茯神 | | | |
| xìng rén | 杏仁 | | | |
| mù xiāng | 木香 | | 2.5 *fēn* of each | 0.93g |
| gān cǎo | 甘草 | | | |

上每服五注，薑水煎 。

Each dose of the above is five *zhù*,[16] boiled in water with ginger.

若因肝經風熱；或怒火所致，須用加味逍遙散 。

If this is due to wind heat in the liver channel or caused by fiery anger, you must use *Jiā Wèi Xiāo Yáo Sǎn* F2-1.

16. There is no known measurement of *zhù* 注 so this must be a typographical error. It is likely that each dose is five *qián*.

# Ān Tāi Yǐn 安胎飲
## Fetus-Quieting Powder F2-41

治妊娠五七個月，用數服可保全產。

Treats women pregnant for five or seven months; using several doses can safeguard pregnancy and childbirth.

白朮人參當歸川芎熟地黃白芍陳皮甘草紫蘇炙黃芩（各一錢）

| | | | | |
|---|---|---|---|---|
| bái zhú | 白朮 | | one *qián* of each | 3.73g |
| rén shēn | 人參 | | | |
| dāng guī | 當歸 | | | |
| chuān xiōng | 川芎 | | | |
| shú dì huáng | 熟地黃 | | | |
| bái sháo | 白芍 | | | |
| chén pí | 陳皮 | | | |
| gān cǎo | 甘草 | | | |
| zǐ sū yè | 紫蘇 | | | |
| huáng qín | 黃芩 | mix-fried | | |

上用薑水煎服。

Boil the above in water with ginger and take it.

若因中氣虛弱，須用四君子加陳皮、紫蘇。若陰虛內熱，宜用四物、黃芩、白朮。

If this is due to deficient weak central qì, you must use *Sì Jūn Zǐ Tāng* F2-26 adding *chén pí* and *zǐ sū yè*. If it is yīn deficiency with internal heat, it is appropriate to use *Sì Wù Tāng* F2-51 with *huáng qín* and *bái zhú*.

## Èr Chén Tāng 二陳湯
## Two Matured Ingredients Decoction F2-42

治妊娠失調，脾胃不和，嘔吐痰涎；或飲食不思。

Treats pregnant women who are out of tune, with disharmony of spleen and stomach and vomiting of phlegm drool or no thought of food and drink.

陳皮茯苓（各一錢五分）半夏（一錢）甘草（五分）

| chén pí | 陳皮 | 1.5 *qián* of each | 5.6g |
|---|---|---|---|
| fú líng | 茯苓 | | |
| bàn xià | 半夏 | one *qián* | 3.73g |
| gān cǎo | 甘草 | five *fēn* | 1.85g |

上薑水煎服。

Boil the above in water with ginger and take it.

若因脾胃虛弱，用六君子。若因氣滯用紫蘇飲。

If this is due to deficient weak spleen and stomach, use *Liù Jūn Zǐ Tāng* F2-6. If it is due to qì stagnation use *Zǐ Sū Yǐn* F2-10.

## Mài Mén Dōng Tāng 麥門冬湯
## Mài Mén Dōng Decoction F2-43

治妊娠失於調養，內熱口乾；或胎動不安。

Treats pregnant women who have neglected attuning and nourishing themselves with internal heat and dry mouth or stirring fetus that is not peaceful.

麥門冬（去心）防風白茯苓（各二錢）人參（一錢）

| | | | | |
|---|---|---|---|---|
| mài mén dōng | 麥門冬 | remove the heart | two *qián* of each | 7.46g |
| fáng fēng | 防風 | | | |
| bái fú líng | 白茯苓 | | | |
| rén shēn | 人參 | | one *qián* | 3.73g |

上作一劑，水煎服。

The above makes one dose. Boil in water and take it.

若血虛有熱，用逍遙散。氣虛有熱，用四君加黃芩、紫蘇。

If there is blood deficiency with heat, use *Xiāo Yáo Sǎn* [F2-2]. If there is qì deficiency with heat, use *Sì Jūn Zǐ Tāng* [F2-26] adding *huáng qín* and *zǐ sū yè.*

## Lǐ Yú Tāng 鯉魚湯<br>Carp Decoction [F2-44]

治胸滿腹脹，小便不通，遍身浮腫。

Treats chest fullness, abdominal distention, obstructed urination, and superficial swelling of the entire body.

白朮茯苓當歸芍藥（各三兩）

| | | | |
|---|---|---|---|
| bái zhú | 白朮 | three *liǎng* of each | 111.9g |
| fú líng | 茯苓 | | |
| dāng guī | 當歸 | | |
| sháo yào | 芍藥 | | |

上細銼，用鯉魚一頭，煮取汁，每藥四錢，入汁一盞半，薑七片，橘皮少許煎服。

Finely file the above; boil one carp (*lǐ yú*) and reserve the liquid; each time put four *qián* (14.92 grams) of the herbs into 1.5 small-cups of the liquid with seven slices of ginger and a little *jú pí*. Boil and take it.

若脾胃虛，佐以四君子湯。

If the spleen and stomach are deficient, *Sì Jūn Zǐ Tāng* F2-26 is the assistant.

## Dá Shēng Sǎn 達生散
## Birth-Giving Powder F2-45

治妊娠，八九月服數劑，甚效。

Treats pregnant women; take several doses at eight or nine months.[17] It is extremely effective.

大腹皮（用黑豆汁洗曬，三錢）人參甘草炙紫蘇梗葉陳皮（各五分）

<table>
<tr><td>dà fù pí</td><td>大腹皮</td><td>wash with the liquid from cooking black soybeans (hēi dòu) and sun-dry</td><td>three qián</td><td>11.19g</td></tr>
<tr><td>zǐ sū gěng yè</td><td>紫蘇梗葉</td><td rowspan="2"></td><td rowspan="4">five fēn of each</td><td rowspan="4">1.85g</td></tr>
<tr><td>rén shēn</td><td>人參</td></tr>
<tr><td>gān cǎo</td><td>甘草</td><td>mix-fried</td></tr>
<tr><td>chén pí</td><td>陳皮</td><td></td></tr>
</table>

上水煎，入黄楊葉七莖，蔥五葉，煎服。

Boil the above in water adding in seven stems of *huáng yáng yè* and five scallion leaves. Boil and take it.

春加川芎，夏加黄芩，冬依正方；或有別症，以意消息加減。

Add *chuān xiōng* in the spring; add *huáng qín* in the summer; in the winter follow the original formula. Perhaps there are different symptoms, so modify the formula based on the fluctuations.

17. The ancient Chinese said that pregnancy lasts ten lunar months. A lunar month is shorter than the months of our Western calendar.

## Bǎo Shēng Wú Yōu Sǎn 保生無憂散
## Safeguard Birth Without Worries Powder F2-46

臨產服之，補其血，順其氣，使易產。又治小產瘀血腹痛。

Take this as the birth approaches; it supplements her blood and makes her qì flow properly which allows for an easy birth. It also treats miscarriage with blood stasis and abdominal pain.

南木香當歸川芎白芍藥枳殼乳香血餘（即亂髮，煅）

| | | |
|---|---|---|
| nán mù xiāng | 南木香 | |
| dāng guī | 當歸 | |
| chuān xiōng | 川芎 | |
| bái sháo yào | 白芍藥 | |
| zhǐ qiào | 枳殼 | |
| rǔ xiāng | 乳香 | |
| xuè yú | 血餘 | This means head hair, calcined |

上等分，每服二三錢，水煎，日二服。

Use equal portions of the above; each dose is two or three *qián* (7.46 - 11.19 grams) boiled in water. Take two doses per day.

若胞衣既破，其血已涸；或元氣困憊，急用八珍湯斤許，水數碗，煎熟時飲救之，飲盡再製，亦有得生者。

If the amniotic sac [or placenta] has broken and the blood has already dried up or original qì is exhausted, quickly use about a *jīn* (596.8 grams) of *Bā Zhēn Tāng* F2-8 in several bowls of water. Boil until cooked. Drinking it will rescue her. When she has drunk it all, prepare it again and she still can live.

## Xiōng Guī Bǔ Zhōng Tāng 芎歸補中湯
## Chuān Xiōng and Dāng Guī Center-Supplementing Decoction F2-47

治氣血虛半產。

Treats late miscarriage due to qì and blood deficiency.

艾葉（代薑[18]）阿膠（炒）川芎五味子（杵炒）黄耆（炙）當歸白朮（炒）芍藥（炒）人參杜仲（炒）甘草（炙）

| àì yè | 艾葉 | to replace ginger | one *qián* of each | 3.73g |
|---|---|---|---|---|
| ē jiāo | 阿膠 | stir-fried | | |
| chuān xiōng | 川芎 | | | |
| wǔ wèi zǐ | 五味子 | pestled and stir-fried | | |
| huáng qí | 黄耆 | mix-fried | | |
| dāng guī | 當歸 | | | |
| bái zhú | 白朮 | stir-fried | | |
| sháo yào | 芍藥 | stir-fried | | |
| rén shēn | 人參 | | | |
| dù zhòng | 杜仲 | stir-fried | | |
| gān cǎo | 甘草 | mix-fried | five *fēn* | 1.85g |

上每服五錢，水煎服。

Each dose of the above is five *qián* (18.65 grams). Boil in water and take it.

若脾氣虛弱，須用補中益氣湯。若氣虛而有火，宜用安胎飲。

If there is deficient weak spleen qì, you must use *Bǔ Zhōng Yì Qì Tāng* F2-5. If qì is deficient and there is fire, it is appropriate to use *Ān Tāi Yǐn* F2-41.

18. Some versions of this formula have ginger but no *ài yè*. This specifies that *ài yè* should be used instead.

## Rén Shēn Huáng Qí Tāng 人參黃耆湯
## Rén Shēn and Huáng Qí Decoction F2-48

治小產氣虛，血下不止。

Treats miscarriage with qì deficiency and incessant bleeding from below.

人參黃耆（炒）當歸白朮（炒）白芍（炒）艾葉（各一錢）阿膠（炒，二錢）

<table>
<tr><td>rén shēn</td><td>人參</td><td></td><td rowspan="6">one qián of each</td><td rowspan="6">3.73g</td></tr>
<tr><td>huáng qí</td><td>黃耆</td><td>stir-fried</td></tr>
<tr><td>dāng guī</td><td>當歸</td><td></td></tr>
<tr><td>bái zhú</td><td>白朮</td><td>stir-fried</td></tr>
<tr><td>bái sháo</td><td>白芍</td><td>stir-fried</td></tr>
<tr><td>ài yè</td><td>艾葉</td><td></td></tr>
<tr><td>ē jiāo</td><td>阿膠</td><td>stir-fried</td><td>two qián</td><td>7.46g</td></tr>
</table>

上作一劑，水煎服。

The above makes one dose. Boil it in water and take it.

## Yún Tái Sǎn 芸薹散
## Yún Tái Powder F2-49

治孕婦九竅出血，或作暈欲死。

Treats bleeding from the nine orifices of a pregnant woman; perhaps she is dizzy and about to die.

芸薹子當歸（焙。各一錢）芍藥官桂（各半錢）

| yún tái zǐ | 芸薹子 | | one *qián* of each | 3.73g |
|---|---|---|---|---|
| dāng guī | 當歸 | baked | | |
| sháo yào | 芍藥 | | a half *qián* of each | 1.85g |
| guān guì | 官桂 | | | |

上為末，每服三錢，以酒並童便各半盞，調灌下立瘥。或一味童便溫飲，尤效。

Powder the above. Each dose is three *qián* (11.19 grams); mix it with a half a small-cup each of liquor and child's urine; pour it in[19] and she will immediately recover. Or drinking warm child's urine alone is especially effective.

前二症，若脾胃氣虛不能統血，宜用四君、芎、歸。中氣下陷，補中益氣湯。若血脫，須補氣爲主。

For the above two conditions [mentioned for this formula], if there is spleen and stomach qì deficiency with inability to control the blood, it is appropriate to use *Sì Jūn Zǐ Tāng* F2-26 adding *chuān xiōng* and *dāng guī*. For central qì sinking downward, use *Bǔ Zhōng Yì Qì Tāng* F2-5. If there is blood desertion, you must take supplementing qì as governing the treatment.

## Dāng Guī Chuān Xiōng Tāng 當歸川芎湯
## Dāng Guī and Chuān Xiōng Decoction F2-50

治小產後瘀血，心腹疼痛；或發熱惡寒。

Treats blood stasis after a miscarriage with pain of the heart [region] and abdomen; or with fever and aversion to cold.

當歸川芎熟地黃白芍藥（炒）玄胡索（炒）桃仁紅花香附青皮（炒）澤蘭牡丹皮

19. If the woman loses consciousness and cannot drink the decoction, it is poured into her mouth.

| | | | |
|---|---|---|---|
| dāng guī | 當歸 | | unstated |
| chuān xiōng | 川芎 | | |
| shú dì huáng | 熟地黃 | | |
| bái sháo yào | 白芍藥 | stir-fried | |
| xuán hú suǒ | 玄胡索 | stir-fried | |
| táo rén | 桃仁 | | |
| hóng huā | 紅花 | | |
| xiāng fù | 香附 | | |
| qīng pí | 青皮 | stir-fried | |
| zé lán | 澤蘭 | | |
| mǔ dān pí | 牡丹皮 | | |

上水煎，入童便、酒各小半盞服。

Boil the above in water, add in half a small-cup each of child's urine and liquor and take it.

若以手按腹愈痛，此是瘀血為患，宜用此藥或失笑散消之。若按之反不痛，此是血虛，宜用四物，參、苓、白朮。若痛而作嘔，此是胃虛，宜用六君子。若痛而作瀉，此是脾虛，宜用六君子送二神丸。

If abdominal pain is worse when pressed, this suffering is due to blood stasis; it is appropriate to use these herbs or *Shī Xiào Sǎn* [F2-55] to disperse it. If on the contrary, pressing it is not painful, this is blood deficiency; it is appropriate to use *Sì Wù Tāng* [F2-51] adding *rén shēn*, *fú líng*, and *bái zhú*. If it is painful and there is vomiting, this is stomach deficiency; it is appropriate to use *Liù Jūn Zǐ Tāng* [F2-6]. If it is painful and there is diarrhea, this is spleen deficiency; it is appropriate to swallow *Èr Shén Wán* [F2-23] with *Liù Jūn Zǐ Tāng* [F2-6].

## Sì Wù Tāng 四物湯
## Four Agents Decoction F2-51

治產後主諸症血虛發熱；或口舌生瘡；或齒齦腫潰；或日晡發熱。

Treats postpartum women and is indicated for all symptoms of blood deficiency with fever; or sores engendered on the mouth and tongue; or swelling and open sores of the gums; or fever at sunset.

當歸熟地黃（各三兩）芍藥（炒三錢）川芎（一錢五分）

| | | | | |
|---|---|---|---|---|
| dāng guī | 當歸 | | three *liǎng* of each | 111.9g |
| shú dì huáng | 熟地黃 | | | |
| sháo yào | 芍藥 | stir-fried | three *qián* | 11.19g |
| chuān xiōng | 川芎 | | 1.5 *qián* | 5.6g |

上作一劑，水煎服。

The above makes one dose. Boil it in water and take it.

若因氣虛不能生血，而患前症，宜補脾胃。

If it is due to qì deficiency with inability to engender blood and the patient has the above symptoms, it is appropriate to supplement the spleen and stomach.

## Jiā Wèi Sì Wù Tāng 加味四物湯
## Supplemented Four Agents Decoction F2-52

即前方加白朮、茯苓、柴胡、丹皮。

This means the previous formula [*Sì Wù Tāng* F2-51] adding *bái zhú, fú líng, chái hú,* and *mǔ dān pí.*

## Sì Shén Sǎn 四神散
## Four Spirits Powder F2-53

治產後血虛；或瘀血腹痛。

Treats postpartum blood deficiency or blood stasis with abdominal pain.

當歸（二錢）川芎芍藥（炒。各一錢）炮薑（五分）

<table>
<tr><td>dāng guī</td><td>當歸</td><td rowspan="2"></td><td>two qián</td><td>7.46g</td></tr>
<tr><td>chuān xiōng</td><td>川芎</td><td rowspan="2">one qián of each</td><td rowspan="2">3.73g</td></tr>
<tr><td>sháo yào</td><td>芍藥</td><td>stir-fried</td></tr>
<tr><td>pào jiāng</td><td>炮薑</td><td></td><td>5 fēn</td><td>1.85g</td></tr>
</table>

上水煎服。

Boil the above in water and take it.

## Dāng Guī Sǎn 當歸散
## Dāng Guī Powder F2-54

治產後氣血虛，惡露內停，增寒發熱，宜服此去之。

Treats postpartum qì and blood deficiency, lochia collecting internally, and increased chills and fever; it is appropriate to take this to remove it.

當歸白芍（炒）川芎黃芩（各一兩）白朮（五錢）

<table>
<tr><td>dāng guī</td><td>當歸</td><td></td><td rowspan="4">one liǎng of each</td><td rowspan="4">37.3g</td></tr>
<tr><td>bái sháo</td><td>白芍</td><td>stir-fried</td></tr>
<tr><td>chuān xiōng</td><td>川芎</td><td rowspan="3"></td></tr>
<tr><td>huáng qín</td><td>黃芩</td></tr>
<tr><td>bái zhú</td><td>白朮</td><td>five qián</td><td>18.65g</td></tr>
</table>

上為細末，溫童便調下二錢。

Make the above into a fine powder, mix with warm child's urine, and swallow two *qián* (7.46 grams).

## Shī Xiào Sǎn 失笑散
## Sudden Smile Powder F2-55

治產後心腹絞痛欲死；或血迷心竅，不知人事，及尋常腹內瘀血，積血作痛。

Treats postpartum twisting pain in the heart [region] and abdomen, [feeling like one is] about to die; or blood confounding the heart orifices, not recognizing human affairs [unconsciousness], as well as ordinary blood stasis inside the abdomen and pain from blood accumulations.

五靈脂蒲黃（俱炒，等分）

| | | | |
|---|---|---|---|
| wǔ líng zhī | 五靈脂 | stir-fry both | equal portions |
| pú huáng | 蒲黃 | | |

上每服三錢，酒煎熱服。

Each dose of the above is three *qián* (11.19 grams) boiled in liquor and taken hot.

若瘀血去多，而元氣虛損所致，宜用四君、芎、歸、炮薑。

If a lot of blood stasis is removed and original qì deficiency is the reason, it is appropriate to use *Sì Jūn Zǐ Tāng* F2-26 adding *chuān xiōng, dāng guī,* and *pào jiāng.*

## Jiě Yǔ Tāng 解語湯
## Speech-Restoring Decoction [F2-56]

治風客心脾，舌強不言 。

Treats wind visiting the heart and spleen with tongue stiffness that impairs speech.

附子（ 炮 ）防風天麻酸棗仁（ 炒，各一兩 ）

| fù zǐ | 附子 | blast-fried | one *liǎng* of each | 37.3g |
|---|---|---|---|---|
| fáng fēng | 防風 | | | |
| tiān má | 天麻 | | | |
| suān zǎo rén | 酸棗仁 | stir-fried | | |

上每服二三錢，水煎服 。

Each dose of the above is two or three *qián* (11.19 grams); boil in water and take it.

若因脾胃風熱，用秦艽升麻湯 。

If it is due to wind heat of the spleen and stomach, use *Qín Jiāo Shēng Má Tāng* [UF-16].

## Bào Dǎn Wán 抱膽丸
## Gallbladder-Embracing Decoction[20] [F2-57]

治心驚不語；或癲癇等症 。

Treats heart fright and loss of speech; or epilepsy and similar conditions.

水銀（ 二兩 ）黑鉛（ 五錢 ）朱砂（ 細研 ）乳香（ 另研 。各一兩 ）

20. We obviously cannot use this recipe today.

| shuǐ yín | 水銀 | | two *liǎng* | 74.6g |
|---|---|---|---|---|
| hēi qiān | 黑鉛 | | five *qián* | 18.65g |
| zhū shā | 硃砂 | grind finely | one *liǎng* of each | 37.3g |
| rǔ xiāng | 乳香 | grind separately | | |

上將鉛入銚，下水銀成砂；次下硃砂 、乳香；乘熱用木槌研勻丸，雞頭大 。每服一丸 。

From the above, put the *hēi qiān* into a pot, pour in the *shuǐ yín* to make sand (*shā*).[21] Next add in the *zhū shā* and *rǔ xiāng*; while it is still hot, use a wooden mallet to grind it evenly and make pills the size of *jī tóu* (euryale – about 6 mm in diameter). Each dose is one pill.

若因心氣虛，用妙香散 。

If due to heart qì deficiency, use *Miào Xiāng Sǎn* F2-79.

## Èr Mǔ Sǎn 二母散
## Two Mǔ Powder F2-58

治產後惡露上攻，留於肺經，咳嗽喘促 。

Treats postpartum lochia attacking upward, lingering in the lung channel with cough and rapid panting.

知母貝母白茯苓人參桃仁杏仁（ 並去皮尖 。各一兩 ）

| zhī mǔ | 知母 | | one *liǎng* of each | 37.3g |
|---|---|---|---|---|
| bèi mǔ | 貝母 | | | |
| bái fú líng | 白茯苓 | | | |
| rén shēn | 人參 | | | |

21. *Shuǐ yín* is liquid mercury. *Hēi qiān* is graphite or fibrous lead. Apparently when they are mixed together the result is granular like sand.

| táo rén | 桃仁 | remove the skin and tips of both | | |
|---|---|---|---|---|
| xìng rén | 杏仁 | | | |

上每服五錢，薑水煎。

Each dose of the above is five *qián* (18.65 grams). Boil it in water with ginger.

若瘀血既去，而嗽仍作，宜補中氣。

If the blood stasis has been removed but there is still cough, it is appropriate to supplement central qì.

## Èr Wèi Shēn Sū Yǐn 二味參蘇飲
## Two Ingredient Rén Shēn and Sū Mù Drink F2-59

治產後瘀血入肺，咳嗽喘急。

Treats postpartum blood stasis entering the lungs with cough and rapid panting.

人參（一兩）蘇木（二兩）

| rén shēn | 人參 | one *liǎng* | 37.3g |
|---|---|---|---|
| sū mù | 蘇木 | two *liǎng* | 74.6g |

上作一劑，水煎服。

The above makes one dose. Boil it in water and take it.

若既愈，而當用六君子以補脾胃。若口鼻黑氣起，急用此藥加附子五錢，亦有得生者。

If she has already recovered, she should use *Liù Jūn Zǐ Tāng* F2-6 to supplement the spleen and stomach. If black qì arises around her mouth and nose, quickly use these herbs adding five *qián* (18.65 grams) of *fù zǐ* and she still can live.

## Qīng Hún Sǎn 清魂散
## Hún-Clearing Powder[F2-60]

治產後元氣虛，瘀血逆行作暈。

Treats postpartum original qì deficiency with blood stasis counterflowing and causing dizziness.

澤蘭葉人參（各一兩）荊芥穗（四兩）川芎（二兩）甘草（炙，八錢）

<table>
<tr><td>zé lán yè</td><td>澤蘭葉</td><td rowspan="4"></td><td rowspan="2">one liǎng of each</td><td rowspan="2">37.3g</td></tr>
<tr><td>rén shēn</td><td>人參</td></tr>
<tr><td>jīng jiè suì</td><td>荊芥穗</td><td>four liǎng</td><td>149.2g</td></tr>
<tr><td>chuān xiōng</td><td>川芎</td><td>two liǎng</td><td>74.6g</td></tr>
<tr><td>gān cǎo</td><td>甘草</td><td>mix-fried</td><td>eight qián</td><td>29.84g</td></tr>
</table>

上為末，熱湯溫酒各半，調下二錢。

Powder the above, mix two *qián* (7.46 grams) with [a mixture of] half hot water and half warm liquor, and swallow it.

若因瘀血去多，宜四物加參、苓、白朮；不應，血脫也，急補其氣。

If this is due to a lot of blood stasis that has been removed, it is appropriate to use *Sì Wù Tāng*[F2-51] adding *rén shēn, fú líng, bái zhú.* If she does not respond and the blood deserts, quickly supplement her qì.

## Zhū Shā Ān Shén Wán 硃砂安神丸
## Zhū Shā Spirit-Quieting Pill[22] F2-61

治產後血暈、心神驚悸等症。

Treats postpartum blood dizziness, heart *shén*-spirit fright palpitations, and similar conditions.

朱砂（飛過，五錢）生地黃（一錢半）黃連（酒洗，六錢）甘草（炙，五分）當歸（一錢五分）

| zhū shā | 硃砂 | water ground | five *qián* | 18.65g |
|---|---|---|---|---|
| huáng lián | 黃連 | washed with liquor | six *qián* | 22.38g |
| gān cǎo | 甘草 | mix-fried | five *fēn* | 1.85g |
| shēng dì huáng | 生地黃 | | 1.5 *qián* | 5.6g |
| dāng guī | 當歸 | | 1.5 *qián* | 5.6g |

上為末，飯糊為丸。每服十五丸。

Powder the above and make pills with rice paste. Each dose is fifteen pills.

若因中氣虛，宜用四君、芎、歸。兼思慮傷脾，須用歸脾湯。

If due to central qì deficiency, it is appropriate to use *Sì Jūn Zǐ Tāng* F2-26 adding *chuān xiōng* and *dāng guī*. If contemplation simultaneously damages the spleen, you must use *Guī Pí Tāng* F2-3.

22. *Zhū shā* 硃砂 is not acceptable for internal use today.

## Duó Mìng Dān 奪命丹
## Life-Clutching Elixir F2-62

治瘀血入衣胞，脹滿難下，急服此藥，血即消，衣自下 。

Treats blood stasis entering the placenta with distention and fullness or difficulty descending [the placenta in the third stage of labor]; quickly take these herbs. Bleeding means [the stasis] is dispersing and the placenta will spontaneously descend.

附子（ 半兩，炮 ）牡丹皮（ 一兩 ）乾漆（ 一兩碎之，炒令煙盡 ）

| | | | | |
|---|---|---|---|---|
| fù zǐ | 附子 | blast-fried | a half *liǎng* | 18.65g |
| mǔ dān pí | 牡丹皮 | | one *liǎng* | 37.3g |
| gān qī | 乾漆 | broken up, stir-fried until there is no more smoke | one *liǎng* | 37.3g |

上為細末，好醋一升，大黃末一兩，同熬成膏，和藥丸，如桐子大，溫酒吞五七丸 。

Make the above into a fine powder. Boil one *shēng* (1073.7 milliliters) of good quality vinegar and one *liǎng* (37.3 grams) of *dà huáng* powder together to make a paste; blend with the herbal powder to make pills the size of *wú tóng zǐ* (about 0.6-0.9 centimeters in diameter). Swallow five or seven pills with warm liquor.

## Huā Ruǐ Shí Sǎn 花蕊石散
## Huā Ruǐ Shí Powder[23] F2-63

治胎衣不下，其效如神，及打撲傷損，腹中瘀血，脹痛欲死，服之血化為水，其功不能盡述 。

Treats retention of the placenta. Its effects are like a miracle. In addition it treats injury from being hit or falling down with blood stasis in the abdomen, distention, and pain,

23. This is probably unacceptable for use today.

and the patient is about to die. Taking it makes the blood [stasis] transform into water; its achievements cannot all be recounted.

硫黃（上色明淨者，四兩，搗細末）花蕊石（一兩，搗為細末）

| liú huáng | 硫黃 | top-grade is bright and clean, pound it to make a fine powder | four *liǎng* | 149.2g |
|---|---|---|---|---|
| huā ruǐ shí | 花蕊石 | pound it to make a fine powder | one *liǎng* | 37.3g |

上二味相拌和勻，先用紙筋和鹽泥固濟瓦罐子一個，候泥乾入藥，再用泥封口候乾，安在四方磚上，虛書八卦五行字，用炭三十斤，週疊煅之，候冷取出為細末。每服一錢，童便調下。

Blend the above two herbs evenly; first use strips of paper and a salt-mud slurry to make an earthen jar; wait for the mud to dry and put in the herbs. Then use mud to seal the opening and wait for it to dry. Set it on top of four square-shaped bricks. Write the characters for the eight guà and five elements in the air.[24] Pile up thirty *jīn* (about 18 kilograms) of charcoal and calcine [the jar of minerals]. Wait for it to cool, take it out, and make it into a fine powder. Each dose is one *qián* (3.73 grams) mixed with child's urine and swallowed.

## Píng Wèi Sǎn 平胃散
## Stomach-Calming Powder F2-64

治腸胃寒受濕下血等症。

Treats coldness of the intestines and stomach with contraction of dampness, bleeding from below, and similar conditions.

蒼術濃樸陳皮甘草（炙）

| cāng zhú | 蒼朮 | | unstated |
|---|---|---|---|
| nóng pǔ | 濃樸 | | |
| chén pí | 陳皮 | | |
| gān cǎo | 甘草 | mix-fried | |

24. This empowers the herbs with some magic.

上薑棗水煎服。

Boil the above in water with ginger and *zǎo*-dates and take it.

## Yì Mǔ Cǎo Wán 益母草丸
## Yì Mǔ Cǎo Pill F2-65

五月採陰乾，石器為末，煉蜜丸，彈子大。臨產以童便和溫酒化下。

In the fifth lunar month pick [*yì mǔ cǎo*], dry it in the shade, and powder it with stone utensils. Make it into pills the size of slingshot pellets with processed honey. When about to give birth, dissolve it in a mixture of child's urine (*tóng biàn*) and warm liquor, and swallow it.

## Jiā Wèi Xiōng Guī Tāng 加味芎歸湯
## Supplemented Chuān Xiōng and Dāng Guī Decoction F2-66

治分娩交骨不開；或五七日不下，垂死者。

Treats non-opening of the interlocking bones [sacrococcygeal joint] during childbirth; or [the fetus] doesn't descend for five or seven days and [the mother] is dying.

川芎當歸（各一兩）生男女婦人髮（一握，燒灰存性）自死龜殼（一個，如無占過者亦可酥炙）

| chuān xiōng | 川芎 | | one *liǎng* of each | 37.3g |
|---|---|---|---|---|
| dāng guī | 當歸 | | | |
| shēng nán nǚ fù rén fā (freshly taken hair from males and females) | 生男女婦人髮 | burn to ashes retaining its nature | one handful | |

| zì sǐ guī ké (tortoise shell from one who died naturally) | 自死龜殼 | if it has not been used for divination, it can also be mix-fried with shortening* | one shell |
|---|---|---|---|

* It is well known that tortoise shells were used for divination during the *Shāng* and *Zhōu* dynasties. Less well known is that forms of divination using tortoise shells lasted into medieval times in China. See *Cracking to divine: Pyro-plastromancy as an archetypal and common mantic and religious practice in Han and medieval china*, a dissertation by Stephen Kory Ph.D.

上為末，每一兩，水煎服，良久不問，生死胎自下。

Powder the above. Each dose is one *liǎng* (37.3 grams). Boil it in water and take it. Don't worry for a good long time as the fetus will [eventually] descend, dead or alive.

## Xiōng Guī Tāng 芎歸湯
## Chuān Xiōng and Dāng Guī Decoction F2-67

治產後去血過多，暈煩不省，用川芎、當歸二味等份，每劑半兩，水煎服。

Treats postpartum excessive blood loss with dizziness, vexation, and loss of consciousness. Use equal portions of two herbs: *chuān xiōng* and *dāng guī*. Each dose is a half *liǎng* (18.65 grams) boiled in water and taken.

若腹疼加桂。腹痛自汗，頭眩少氣，加羊肉。若不應，用八珍湯。

If there is abdominal pain, add cinnamon. If there is abdominal pain with spontaneous sweating, dizziness, and weak breathing, add goat or lamb meat. If she does not respond, use *Bā Zhēn Tāng* F2-8.

## Qī Wèi Bái Zhú Sǎn 七味白朮散
## Seven Ingredient Bái Zhú Powder F2-68

治中氣虛口乾；或吐瀉等症。

Treats central qì deficiency with dry mouth or vomiting and diarrhea, and similar conditions.

人參白朮木香白茯苓甘草藿香干葛（各一錢）

| rén shēn | 人參 | one *qián* of each | 3.73g |
|---|---|---|---|
| bái zhú | 白朮 | | |
| mù xiāng | 木香 | | |
| bái fú líng | 白茯苓 | | |
| gān cǎo | 甘草 | | |
| huò xiāng | 藿香 | | |
| gān gé | 乾葛 | | |

上作一劑，水煎服。

The above makes one dose. Boil in water and take it.

## Xuǎn Qí Tāng 選奇湯
## Extraordinary-Selecting Powder F2-69

治風熱上壅，眉棱骨痛；或頭目眩暈等症。

Treats wind heat obstructing the upper body with pain of the eyebrow bone or dizziness of the head and eyes, and similar conditions.

羌活防風（各二錢）甘草（二錢，夏生冬炒）酒芩（冬去之，熱甚用）

| | | | | |
|---|---|---|---|---|
| qiāng huó | 羌活 | | two *qián* of each | 7.46g |
| fáng fēng | 防風 | | | |
| gān cǎo | 甘草 | grown in the summer, stir-fried in the winter | two *qián* | 7.46g |
| jiǔ huáng qín | 酒芩 | remove it [from the formula] in the winter; use it when heat is extreme | [unstated] | |

上每服三錢，水煎，時時飲之。

Each dose of the above is three *qián* (11.19 grams) boiled in water; drink it frequently.

## Gé Huā Jiě Chéng Tāng 葛花解酲湯
## Gé Huā Liquor-Resolving Decoction F2-70

治酒積，上下分消其濕。

Treats liquor accumulations; it divides and disperses the dampness above and below.

白豆蔻砂仁葛花（各五錢）木香（五分）青皮（三錢）陳皮白茯苓豬苓人參（各一錢半）白朮神曲炒澤瀉生乾薑（各二錢）

| | | | | |
|---|---|---|---|---|
| bái dòu kòu | 白荳蔻 | | five *qián* of each | 18.65g |
| shā rén | 砂仁 | | | |
| gé huā | 葛花 | | | |
| mù xiāng | 木香 | | five *fēn* | 1.85g |
| qīng pí | 青皮 | | three *qián* | 11.19g |
| chén pí | 陳皮 | | 1.5 *qián* of each | 5.6g |
| bái fú líng | 白茯苓 | | | |
| zhū líng | 豬苓 | | | |
| rén shēn | 人參 | | | |
| bái zhú | 白朮 | | 2 *qián* of each | 7.46g |
| shén qū | 神曲 | stir-fried | | |
| zé xiè | 澤瀉 | | | |
| shēng gān jiāng | 生乾薑 | | | |

上為細末，每服五錢，白湯調下。

Make the above into a fine powder. Each dose is five *qián* (18.65 grams) mixed with clear soup and swallowed.

## Huò Xiāng Zhèng Qì Sǎn 藿香正氣散
## Huò Xiāng Qì-Righting Powder F2-71

治外感風寒，内停飲食，頭痛寒熱；或霍亂泄瀉；或作瘧疾。

Treats externally contracted wind cold, food and drink settling on the interior, headache, and [sensations of] cold and heat; or sudden turmoil [cholera] and diarrhea; or *nüè*-malarial disease.

桔梗大腹皮紫蘇茯苓白芷半夏曲陳皮白朮濃樸（製。各一錢）甘草（炙，五分）藿香（一錢五分）

| | | | | |
|---|---|---|---|---|
| jié gěng | 桔梗 | | one *qián* of each | 3.73g |
| dà fù pí | 大腹皮 | | | |
| zǐ sū yè | 紫蘇 | | | |
| fú líng | 茯苓 | | | |
| bái zhǐ | 白芷 | | | |
| bàn xià qū | 半夏曲 | | | |
| chén pí | 陳皮 | | | |
| bái zhú | 白朮 | | | |
| nóng pǔ | 濃樸 | processed | | |
| gān cǎo | 甘草 | mix-fried | five *fēn* | 1.85g |
| huò xiāng | 藿香 | | 1.5 *qián* | 5.6g |

上作一劑，薑棗水煎熱服。

The above makes one dose. Boil in water with ginger and *zǎo*-dates and take it hot.

# Qīng Zào Tāng 清燥湯
## Dryness-Clearing Decoction F2-72

治元氣虛，濕熱乘之，遍身酸軟，絕寒水生化之源，小便赤少，大便不調等症 。

Treats original qì deficiency with damp heat taking advantage of it; the entire body is achy and weak, the cold water[25] source of engenderment and transformation is cut off, with scant red urination, out of tune bowel movement, and similar conditions.

黃耆（ 一錢五分 ）五味子（ 九粒，杵炒 ）黃連神曲（ 炒 ）豬苓柴胡甘草（ 炙 。各二分 ）蒼朮麥門冬陳皮白朮生地黃澤瀉（ 各五分 ）白茯苓人參當歸升麻（ 各三分 ）酒柏（ 一分 ）

| huáng qí | 黃耆 | | 1.5 *qián* | 5.6g |
|---|---|---|---|---|
| wǔ wèi zǐ | 五味子 | pestled and stir-fried | | 9 pcs |
| huáng lián | 黃連 | | two *fēn* of each | 0.74g |
| shén qū | 神曲 | stir-fried | | |
| zhū líng | 豬苓 | | | |
| chái hú | 柴胡 | | | |
| gān cǎo | 甘草 | mix-fried | | |
| cāng zhú | 蒼朮 | | five *fēn* of each | 1.85g |
| mài mén dōng | 麥門冬 | | | |
| chén pí | 陳皮 | | | |
| bái zhú | 白朮 | | | |
| shēng dì huáng | 生地黃 | | | |
| zé xiè | 澤瀉 | | | |
| bái fú líng | 白茯苓 | | three *fēn* of each | 1.12g |
| rén shēn | 人參 | | | |
| dāng guī | 當歸 | | | |
| shēng má | 升麻 | | | |
| jiǔ huáng bǎi | 酒柏 | | one *fēn* | 0.37g |

25. Here, *cold water* refers to the urinary bladder, which is tàiyáng; *cold* refers to the nature of water, not pathology. In this case, the urinary bladder cannot maintain its cold nature and its function of transforming, so urination is disrupted.

上作一劑，水煎服。

The above makes one dose. Boil it in water and take it.

## Rén Shēn Yǎng Wèi Tāng 人參養胃湯
## Rén Shēn Stomach-Nourishing Decoction F2-73

治外感風寒，內傷飲食，寒熱頭疼；或作瘧疾。

Treats externally contracted wind cold, internal damage from food and drink, [sensations of] cold and heat, and headaches; or *nüè*-malarial disease.

半夏濃樸（製）橘紅（八分）藿香葉草果茯苓人參（五分）甘草（炙，三分）蒼朮（一錢）

| bàn xià | 半夏 | | unstated | |
|---|---|---|---|---|
| nóng pǔ | 濃樸 | processed | | |
| jú hóng | 橘紅 | | eight *fēn* | 2.96g |
| huò xiāng yè | 藿香葉 | | unstated | |
| cǎo guǒ | 草果 | | | |
| fú líng | 茯苓 | | | |
| rén shēn | 人參 | | five *fēn* | 1.85g |
| gān cǎo | 甘草 | mix-fried | three *fēn* | 1.12g |
| cāng zhú | 蒼朮 | | one *qián* | 3.73g |

上作一劑，薑七片，烏梅一個，水煎服。

The above makes one dose. Boil it in water with seven slices of ginger and one piece of *wū méi* and take it.

# Dà Fáng Fēng Tāng 大防風湯
## Major Fáng Fēng Decoction [F2-74]

治足三陰虛，患鶴膝風、歷節痛風等症；不問或腫而不痛，或潰未斂。

Treats deficiency of the leg three yīn [channels] in those who suffer crane's knee wind, joint-running painful wind, and similar conditions; do not bother asking whether there is swelling but no pain or whether it has burst open but does not close up.[26]

附子（炮去皮臍，一錢）白朮（炒）羌活人參（各二錢）川芎（一錢五分）防風（二錢）甘草（炙）牛膝（酒浸，各一錢）黃耆（炙，二錢）當歸（酒拌，二錢）白芍葯（炒，二錢）杜仲（薑製，二錢）熟地黃（生者自製）

<table>
<tr><td>fù zǐ</td><td>附子</td><td>blast-fry, remove the skin and umbilicus</td><td>one qián</td><td>3.73g</td></tr>
<tr><td>bái zhú</td><td>白朮</td><td>stir-fried</td><td rowspan="3">two qián of each</td><td rowspan="3">7.46g</td></tr>
<tr><td>qiāng huó</td><td>羌活</td><td rowspan="4"></td></tr>
<tr><td>rén shēn</td><td>人參</td></tr>
<tr><td>chuān xiōng</td><td>川芎</td><td>1.5 qián</td><td>5.6g</td></tr>
<tr><td>fáng fēng</td><td>防風</td><td>two qián</td><td>7.46g</td></tr>
<tr><td>gān cǎo</td><td>甘草</td><td>mix-fried</td><td rowspan="2">one qián of each</td><td rowspan="2">3.73g</td></tr>
<tr><td>niú xī</td><td>牛膝</td><td>soaked in liquor</td></tr>
<tr><td>huáng qí</td><td>黃耆</td><td>mix-fried</td><td>two qián</td><td>7.46g</td></tr>
<tr><td>dāng guī</td><td>當歸</td><td>mixed with liquor</td><td>two qián</td><td>7.46g</td></tr>
<tr><td>bái sháo yào</td><td>白芍葯</td><td>stir-fried</td><td>two qián</td><td>7.46g</td></tr>
<tr><td>dù zhòng</td><td>杜仲</td><td>processed with ginger</td><td>two qián</td><td>7.46g</td></tr>
<tr><td>shú dì huáng</td><td>熟地黃</td><td>prepare it from the fresh yourself</td><td colspan="2">unstated</td></tr>
</table>

上作二劑，水煎服。

The above makes two doses. Boil it in water and take it.

26. In other words, this formula treats any of these variations so no need to ask about it.

## Dú Huó Jì Shēng Tāng 獨活濟生湯
## Dú Huó and Sāng Jì Shēng Decoction [F2-75]

治鶴膝及歷節痛風等症 。

Treats crane's knees, joint-running painful wind, and similar conditions.

白茯苓杜仲當歸（ 酒洗 ）防風白芍藥人參細辛桂心熟地黃牛膝秦艽芎藭桑寄生甘草（ 各二兩 ）獨活（ 三兩 ）

| | | | | |
|---|---|---|---|---|
| bái fú líng | 白茯苓 | | two *liǎng* of each | 74.6g |
| dù zhòng | 杜仲 | | | |
| dāng guī | 當歸 | washed in liquor | | |
| fáng fēng | 防風 | | | |
| bái sháo yào | 白芍藥 | | | |
| rén shēn | 人參 | | | |
| xì xīn | 細辛 | | | |
| guì xīn | 桂心 | | | |
| shú dì huáng | 熟地黃 | | | |
| niú xī | 牛膝 | | | |
| qín jiāo | 秦艽 | | | |
| xiōng qióng | 芎藭 | | | |
| sāng jì shēng | 桑寄生 | | | |
| gān cǎo | 甘草 | | | |
| dú huó | 獨活 | | three *liǎng* | 111.9g |

上每服一兩，薑水煎 。

Each dose of the above is one *liǎng* (37.3 grams). Boil in water with ginger.

## Qiāng Huó Shèng Shī Tāng 羌活勝濕湯
## Qiāng Huó Dampness-Overcoming Decoction F2-76

治痛風，血虛腫痛，身重脈緩等症 。

Treats painful wind and blood deficiency with swelling and pain when the body is swollen, the pulse is moderate, and similar conditions.

羌活獨活（ 去蘆，一錢 ）藁本防風川芎甘草（ 炙 ）蔓荊子（ 各五分 ）

| qiāng huó | 羌活 | | unstated | |
|---|---|---|---|---|
| dú huó | 獨活 | remove the stem | one *qián* | 3.73g |
| gǎo běn | 藁本 | | five *fēn* of each | 1.85g |
| fáng fēng | 防風 | | | |
| chuān xiōng | 川芎 | | | |
| gān cǎo | 甘草 | mix-fried | | |
| màn jīng zǐ | 蔓荊子 | | | |

上作一劑，薑水煎服 。

The above makes one dose. Boil it in water with ginger and take it.

## Fù Zǐ Bā Wù Tāng 附子八物湯
## Fù Zǐ Eight Agents Decoction F2-77

治歷節作痛，發熱作渴，飲食少思等症 。

Treats joint-running with pain, fever, thirst, little thought of food and drink, and similar conditions.

附子（ 炮 ）乾薑（ 炮 ）芍藥（ 炒 ）茯苓人參甘草（ 炙 。各一錢半 ）肉桂（ 一錢 ）白朮（ 二錢 ）

| fù zǐ | 附子 | blast-fried | 1.5 *qián* of each | 5.6g |
|---|---|---|---|---|
| gān jiāng | 乾薑 | blast-fried | | |
| sháo yào | 芍藥 | stir-fried | | |
| fú líng | 茯苓 | | | |
| rén shēn | 人參 | | | |
| gān cǎo | 甘草 | mix-fried | | |
| ròu guì | 肉桂 | | one *qián* | 3.73g |
| bái zhú | 白朮 | | two *qián* | 7.46g |

上作一劑，水煎食前服 。

The above makes one dose. Boil in water and take before meals.

## Sì Shēng Sǎn 四生散
## Four Fresh Agents Powder[27] F2-78

治臁腿生瘡；或癬疥等症 。

Treats sores engendered on the shanks and legs; or lichens, scabby sores, and similar conditions.

白附子 黃 羌活 沙苑 蒺藜

| bái fù zǐ | 白附子 |
|---|---|
| huáng qí | 黃耆 |
| qiāng huó | 羌活 |
| shā yuàn jí lí | 沙苑蒺藜 |

上各等分為末，每服二錢，用豬腰子擗開入藥，濕紙包裹，煨熟細嚼，鹽湯下 。風癬，酒下 。

Powder equal portions of each of the above. Each dose is two *qián* (7.46 grams). Split open a pork kidney, put the herbs inside, wrap it with moist paper, and roast until done.

27. While these ingredients are dried so they can be powdered, they are not otherwise processed, hence the name.

Chew it carefully, swallowing it with hot salted water. For wind lichens, swallow it with liquor.

## Miào Xiāng Sǎn 妙香散
## Mysterious Fragrance Powder F2-79

治心脾虧損，大便下血；又治心氣不足，精神恍惚，少睡盜汗。

Treats debility of the heart and spleen with blood in the stool; it also treats insufficient heart qì, distracted *jīng-shén*, decreased sleep, and night sweating.

人參桔梗甘草（各五錢）遠志（去心）山藥（薑汁炙）茯苓（去皮）黃耆（各一兩）辰砂（另研，三錢）麝香（另研，一錢）木香（煨，二錢半）茯神（一兩）

| | | | | |
|---|---|---|---|---|
| rén shēn | 人參 | | five *qián* of each | 18.65g |
| jié gěng | 桔梗 | | | |
| gān cǎo | 甘草 | | | |
| yuǎn zhì | 遠志 | remove the heart | one *liǎng* of each | 37.3g |
| shān yào | 山藥 | mix-fried with ginger juice | | |
| fú líng | 茯苓 | remove the peel | | |
| huáng qí | 黃耆 | | | |
| chén shā* | 辰砂 | grind separately | three *qián* | 11.19g |
| shè xiāng | 麝香 | grind separately | one *qián* | 3.73g |
| mù xiāng | 木香 | roasted | 2.5 *qián* | 9.33g |
| fú shén | 茯神 | | one *liǎng* | 37.3g |

* This is another name for *zhū shā* 硃砂, which is not acceptable for internal use today.

上為末，每服二錢，溫酒調服。

Powder the above. Each dose is two *qián* (7.46 grams), mixed with warm liquor and taken.

## Lòu Lú Sǎn 漏蘆散
## Lòu Lú Powder F2-80

治血風走注，作痛無定處 。

Treats blood wind travelling influx[28] with pain that has no fixed location.

漏蘆當歸牛膝（ 各三分 ）桂心地龍（ 去土 ）防風羌活白芷沒藥（ 研 ）甜瓜子（ 各半兩 ）虎脛骨（ 酥炙 ）敗龜（ 各一兩，炙 ）

| lòu lú | 漏蘆 | | three *fēn* of each | 1.12g |
|---|---|---|---|---|
| dāng guī | 當歸 | | | |
| niú xī | 牛膝 | | | |
| guì xīn | 桂心 | | a half *liǎng* of each | 18.65g |
| dì long | 地龍 | remove the earth | | |
| fáng fēng | 防風 | | | |
| qiāng huó | 羌活 | | | |
| bái zhǐ | 白芷 | | | |
| mò yào | 沒藥 | ground | | |
| tián guā zǐ | 甜瓜子 | | | |
| hǔ jìng gǔ* | 虎脛骨 | mix-fried with shortening | one *liǎng* of each | 37.3g |
| bài guī | 敗龜 | mix-fried | | |

* From an endangered species, so it cannot be used today.

上為細末，每服二錢，熱酒調下 。

Make the above into a fine powder. Each dose is two *qián* (7.46 grams). Mix with hot liquor and swallow.

義烏朱用中 。

Zhū Yòngzhōng from Yìwū.[29]

28. Blood wind travelling influx is similar to moving *bì*-obstruction.
29. Yìwū is a city in Zhèjiāng Province. Zhū Yòngzhōng proofread and corrected the text.

# 《女科撮要》後序

## Outline of Female Medicine Epilogue

《易》曰：乾道成男，坤道成女。男女之所惟均，而疾則女恒多於男者，蓋以陽嘗散緩，陰多凝蓄，是故其氣愈滯，其性愈執，為多忿，為多鬱，為多所好惡，而肝脾不得其平，矧且益之。經、乳、胎、產變態百端，良由是爾。

Yì says: "The dào of *qián* develops into the male; the dào of *kūn* develops into the female."[30] Although it may be that males and females are equal in some things, it is more common for females to be ill than males. This must be because once yáng scatters and slows down, yīn often congeals and stores up. Therefore, her qì is more stagnant and her nature is more attached, so she becomes more angry and more constrained and develops more personal likes and dislikes. Then the liver and spleen are unable to maintain their balance, and this further increases [the qì constraint]. Menstruation, lactation, pregnancy, and childbirth become abnormal in a hundred different ways, very much because of this.

余嘗掌醫院，及歸田，凡所治療獲效，輒用手錄成帙，題曰《家居醫錄》，而於婦人一科曰「撮要」焉，慎所難也。

I was in charge of the Academy of Medicine. Since retiring to my hometown, whenever I treat someone with good results, I always record it into a book entitled *Household Medical Records* (jiā jū yī lù). However for the department of female medicine, I call this book *Outline* (cuò yào), paying careful attention to whatever is more difficult.

吾鄉侍御，兩湖王公見而悅之，捐重俾登諸梓，指示四方，余謂兩湖為王諫議，為德為民溥矣，而於林泉猶有玆舉，亦復視民如傷又可見矣。

30. This quotation is from *Zhōu Yì·Xì Cí Shàng Zhuàn*《周易·繫辭上傳》. *Qián* is pure yáng. *Kūn* is pure yīn.

My hometown Censor, Mr. Wáng from Liǎnghú,[31] saw my book and was pleased with it. He contributed considerably to enable all the blocks for printing to be inscribed and to distribute the book in all directions. I think that when he was in Liǎnghú as Remonstrator Wáng, he acted virtuously and universally for the common people; but when he retired, he still has continued such activities and it can be seen that he again is taking care of the people.

若夫余之所知則淺也，安敢與陳臨江之《良方》並馳於天下邪，同志者幸為繼正之，庶乎其無負侍御之心矣。

With regard to what I know, it is shallow. How can my own book become as famous under heaven as *Liáng Fāng* by Chén from Línjiāng?[32] Fortunately, my peers have continued to correct [my book] so that it won't disappoint the heart of the Censor.

嘉靖丙午孟春吉日，前奉政大夫太醫院使薛己書

The first day of the first month of spring in the *bǐng wǔ* year of Jiājìng's reign (1546), written by Xuē Jǐ, a former Grand Master for Governance and Commissioner of the Imperial Academy of Medicine

31. Emperor Jiājìng and his immediate family were from Ānlù Prefecture in Liǎnghú (Húnán and Húběi) and Xuē Jǐ worked with the royal family there for a time. This is probably how he knew Censor Wáng.
32. This refers to *Fù Rén Dà Quán Liáng Fāng* (All Inclusive Fine Formulas for Women) by Chén Zìmíng (1237, Southern *Sòng*) 陳自明《婦人大全良方》南宋, a book that Xuē Jǐ later edited and annotated. Chén was from Línjiāng which is in present-day Jiāngxī Province.

# Appendix

## Unlisted Formulas Recommended by Xuē Jǐ

These formulas were mentioned in the text as being useful, but were not included in the formulas at the end of each volume. Perhaps in the pre-computer age, it was harder to keep track of all the formulas mentioned. While most of these prescriptions have earlier sources, all the recipes here were taken from other books written or edited by Xuē Jǐ. In this way, we can be assured that the version of the formula given here would be what Xuē Jǐ had in mind.

### Zǐ Qín Wán 子芩丸
### Young Huáng Qín Pill UF-1

治肝經有熱妄行。

Treats heat in the liver channel with reckless movement.

條黃芩（炒）。

| tiáo huáng qín | 條芩 | stir-fried | [unstated] |
|---|---|---|---|

為末，每服一錢，以秤錘燒赤，焠酒熱調服。若脾胃虛，不宜用。

Powder the above. Each dose is one *qián* (3.73 grams). Heat liquor by quenching the red hot weight of a scale in the liquor. Mix the powder in it and take it.[33] If there is spleen or stomach deficiency, do not use this.

*Xiào Zhù Fù Rén Liáng Fāng*《校注婦人良方》by Xuē Jǐ 薛己 *Míng* (明)

33. While the title calls this a pill, it is obviously not.

## Xiāng Shā Liù Jūn Zǐ Tāng 香砂六君子湯
## Mù Xiāng and Shā Rén Six Gentlemen Decoction UF-2

治一切脾胃不健，飲食少思，或作嘔，或過服涼藥，致傷脾胃，即六君子湯加：

Treats all types of spleen or stomach deficiency with little thought of food and drink, or with vomiting, or after taking an excessive dose of cooling herbs that have damaged the spleen and stomach. This is *Liù Jūn Zǐ Tāng* F2-6 plus:

藿香、砂仁。

| mù xiāng | 木香 | seven *fēn* | 2.59g |
|---|---|---|---|
| shā rén | 砂仁 | eight *fēn* | 2.96g |

*Wài Kē Fā Huī*《外科發揮》by Xuē Jǐ 薛己 *Míng* (明)

## Hēi Wán Zǐ 黑丸子
## Black Pill UF-3

治跌撲墜墮，筋骨疼痛，或瘀血壅腫，或外感風寒，肢體作痛；若流注膝風，初起服之自消；若潰後氣虛而發熱，與補劑兼服自斂。

Treats injuries from falling with pain of the sinews and bones; or blood stasis, obstruction, and swelling; or external contraction of wind cold with painful body. If taken during initial onset of streaming sores or knee wind, it will spontaneously disperse; if the sores have already burst open, with qì deficiency and fever, they will spontaneously close up when taken together with supplementing prescriptions.

百草霜白芍藥（各一兩）赤小豆（一兩五錢）川烏（炮，三錢）白蘞（一兩六錢）白芨當歸（各八錢）南星（炮，三錢）牛膝（焙，六錢）補骨脂（焙，八錢）

| bǎi cǎo shuāng | 百草霜 | | one *liǎng* of each | 37.3g |
|---|---|---|---|---|
| bái sháo yào | 白芍藥 | | | |
| chì xiǎo dòu | 赤小豆 | | 1.5 *liǎng* | 55.95g |
| chuān wū | 川烏 | blast-fried | three *qián* | 11.19g |
| bái liǎn | 白蘞 | | 1.6 *liǎng* | 59.68g |
| bái jī | 白芨 | | eight *qián* of each | 29.84g |
| dāng guī | 當歸 | | | |
| nán xīng | 南星 | blast-fried | three *qián* | 11.19g |
| niú xī | 牛膝 | stone-baked | six *qián* | 22.38g |
| bǔ gǔ zhī | 補骨脂 | stone-baked | eight *qián* | 29.84g |

上各別為末，酒糊丸，桐子大，每服三十丸，鹽湯溫酒任下，孕婦不可服。

Powder each of the above separately. Make pills the size of *wú tóng zǐ* (about 0.6-0.9 centimeters in diameter) with liquor and wheat paste. Each dose is thirty pills swallowed with hot salt water or warm liquor. Contraindicated in pregnancy.

*Wài Kē Shū Yào*《外科樞要》by Xuē Jǐ 薛己 *Míng* (明)

## Chái Hú Zhī Zǐ Sǎn 柴胡梔子散
## Chái Hú and Zhī Zǐ Powder UF-4

治三焦及足少陽經風熱。耳內作癢生瘡，或出水疼痛，或胸乳間作痛，或寒熱往來。

Treats wind heat of the sānjiāo and the foot shǎoyàng channel with itching or sores inside the ears, or [the ears] discharge water with pain, or pain in the chest and breast region, or alternating chills and fever.

柴胡梔子（炒）牡丹皮（各一錢）茯苓川芎芍藥當歸牛蒡子（炒，各七分）甘草（五分）

| chái hú | 柴胡 | | one *qián* of each | 3.73g |
|---|---|---|---|---|
| zhī zǐ | 梔子 | stir-fried | | |
| mǔ dān pí | 牡丹皮 | | | |
| fú líng | 茯苓 | | seven *fēn* of each | 2.59g |
| chuān xiōng | 川芎 | | | |
| sháo yào | 芍藥 | | | |
| dāng guī | 當歸 | | | |
| niú bàng zǐ | 牛蒡子 | stir-fried | | |
| gān cǎo | 甘草 | | five *fēn* | 1.85g |

上水煎服。若太陽頭痛，加羌活。

Boil the above in water and take it. If it is a tàiyáng headache, add *qiāng huó*.

*Wài Kē Shū Yào* 《外科樞要》 by Xuē Jǐ 薛己 *Míng* (明)

## Bīng Sū Bài Dú Sǎn 檳蘇敗毒散
## Bīng Láng and Zǐ Sū Toxin-Conquering Powder [UF-5]

治瘡瘍焮痛寒熱，或拘急頭痛。即人參敗毒散加檳榔、紫蘇。

Treats sores and skin diseases with scorching pain and [sensations of] cold and heat, or hypertonicity with headache. This is the same as *Rén Shēn Bài Dú Sǎn* [F1-31] plus:

檳榔、紫蘇。

| bīng láng | 檳榔 | not stated |
|---|---|---|
| zǐ sū yè | 紫蘇 | |

右水煎服。

Boil in water and take it.

*Xiào Zhù Fù Rén Liáng Fāng* 《校注婦人良方》 by Xuē Jǐ 薛己 *Míng* (明)

## Xiān Fāng Huó Mìng Yǐn 仙方活命飲
## Immortal Formula Life-Giving Drink UF-6

治一切瘡瘍，未成者即散，已成者即潰，又止痛消毒之良劑也。

Treats all types of sores and itching. If [a sore] hasn't developed yet, this will dissipate it; if it has already developed, it will ulcerate. It is also a good formula to stop pain and disperse swellings.

白芷貝母防風赤芍藥當歸尾甘草節皂角刺（炒）穿山甲（炙）天花粉乳香沒藥（各一錢）金銀花陳皮（各三錢）

<table>
<tr><td>bái zhǐ</td><td>白芷</td><td rowspan="6"></td><td rowspan="11">two qián of each</td><td rowspan="11">7.46g</td></tr>
<tr><td>bèi mǔ</td><td>貝母</td></tr>
<tr><td>fáng fēng</td><td>防風</td></tr>
<tr><td>chì sháo yào</td><td>赤芍藥</td></tr>
<tr><td>dāng guī wěi</td><td>當歸尾</td></tr>
<tr><td>gān cǎo jié</td><td>甘草節</td></tr>
<tr><td>zào jiǎo cì</td><td>皂角刺</td><td>stir-fried</td></tr>
<tr><td>chuān shān jiǎ*</td><td>穿山甲</td><td>prepared</td></tr>
<tr><td>tiān huā fěn</td><td>天花粉</td><td rowspan="5"></td></tr>
<tr><td>rǔ xiāng</td><td>乳香</td></tr>
<tr><td>mò yào</td><td>沒藥</td></tr>
<tr><td>jīn yín huā</td><td>金銀花</td><td rowspan="2">three qián of each</td><td rowspan="2">11.19g</td></tr>
<tr><td>chén pí</td><td>陳皮</td></tr>
</table>

*This is an endangered species and cannot be used.

上用酒一大碗，煎五七沸服。

Boil the above in a big bowlful of liquor for five or seven rollings and take it.

*Xiào Zhù Fù Rén Liáng Fāng*《校注婦人良方》by Xuē Jǐ 薛己 *Míng* (明)

## Yì Yuán Sǎn 益元散
## Origin-Boosting Powder[34] UF-7

治中暑身熱小便不利，或發熱體痛，口乾作渴。

Treats summerheat stroke, feverish feeling, and inhibited urination, or fever and generalized pain with dry mouth and thirst.

滑石末（六錢）甘草末（一錢）

| huá shí | 滑石 | six *qián* | 22.38g |
|---|---|---|---|
| gān cǎo | 甘草 | one *qián* | 3.73g |

每服一錢，白湯調。

Powder the above. Each dose is one *qián* (3.73 grams) mixed with liquor and swallowed.

*Xiào Zhù Fù Rén Liáng Fāng*《校注婦人良方》by Xuē Jǐ 薛己 *Míng* (明)

## Quán Shēng Bái Zhú Sǎn《全生》白朮散
## Bái Zhú Powder from Whole Life[35] UF-8

治妊娠面目浮虛，四肢腫如水氣，名曰胎氣，又名胎腫。

Treats swelling of the face and eyes in deficient pregnant women, as well as swelling of the four limbs. This is called *fetal qì* or *fetal swelling*.

白朮（一兩）生薑皮大腹皮陳皮茯苓（各五錢）

| bái zhú | 白朮 | one *liǎng* | 37.3g |
|---|---|---|---|
| shēng jiāng pí | 生薑皮 | five *qián* of each | 18.65g |
| dà fù pí | 大腹皮 | | |

34. This is also known as *Liù Yī Sǎn* 六一散 (Six to One Powder).
35. The full name of this book is *Quán Shēng Zhǐ Mí Fāng*《全生指迷方》(Formulas for Guidance over the Whole Life) by Wáng Kuàng 王貺 *Sòng* (宋).

| | | | |
|---|---|---|---|
| chén pí | 陳皮 | | |
| fú líng | 茯苓 | | |

上各為末，每服二錢，米飲下。

Powder the above. Each dose is two *qián* (7.46 grams) swallowed with rice drink.

*Xiào Zhù Fù Rén Liáng Fāng*《校注婦人良方》by Xuē Jǐ 薛己 *Míng* (明)

## Dāng Guī Liù Huáng Tāng 當歸六黃湯
## Dāng Guī and Six Yellow Decoction UF-9

治氣血虛熱，盜汗不止。不應，加人參、白朮，心血不足，加酸棗仁(炒)。

Treats qì and blood deficiency with heat and unceasing night sweats. If she does not respond, add *rén shēn* and *bái zhú*. If heart blood is insufficient, add *suān zǎo rén* (stir-fried).

當歸熟地黃(自製)黃耆(炒，各二錢)生地黃黃柏(炒黑)黃芩(炒黑)黃連(炒黑，各一錢)

| | | | | |
|---|---|---|---|---|
| dāng guī | 當歸 | | two *qián* of each | 7.46g |
| shú dì huáng | 熟地黃 | prepare it yourself | | |
| huáng qí | 黃耆 | stir-fried | | |
| shēng dì huáng | 生地黃 | | one *qián* of each | 3.73g |
| huáng bǎi | 黃柏 | stir-fried until black | | |
| huáng qín | 黃芩 | stir-fried until black | | |
| huáng lián | 黃連 | stir-fried until black | | |

上水煎服。

Boil the above in water and take it.

*Xiào Zhù Fù Rén Liáng Fāng*《校注婦人良方》by Xuē Jǐ 薛己 *Míng* (明)

## **Tài Yǐ Gāo 太乙膏**
## **Tài Yǐ Plaster** UF-10

治一切瘡瘍，並宜貼之。若元氣無虧，用隔蒜灸，更服活命飲，以收全。

Treats all types of sores and skin conditions. If original qì is not lacking, use garlic-isolated moxibustion. Further take *Huó Mìng Yǐn* UF-6, to receive the complete effects.

玄參白芷當歸肉桂大黃赤芍藥生地黃（各一兩）

| | | | |
|---|---|---|---|
| xuán shēn | 玄參 | one *liǎng* of each | 37.3g |
| bái zhǐ | 白芷 | | |
| dāng guī | 當歸 | | |
| ròu guì | 肉桂 | | |
| dà huáng | 大黃 | | |
| chì sháo yào | 赤芍藥 | | |
| shēng dì huáng | 生地黃 | | |

上用麻油二斤，入銅鍋內，煎至黑濾去粗，入黃丹十二兩，再煎，水中捻軟硬得中，即成膏矣。

Put two *jīn* (1193.6 grams) of sesame oil into a copper wok with the above herbs and simmer until the herbs are black. Filter out the dregs. Add in twelve *liǎng* (447.6 grams) of *huáng dān*[36] and simmer again, stirring until it becomes the proper viscosity.

*Wài Kē Shū Yào*《外科樞要》by Xuē Jǐ 薛己 *Míng* (明)

36. *Huáng dān* is red lead oxide or minium. It causes toxicity if inhaled, ingested, or is absorbed through the skin. Therefore, we cannot use it medicinally today.

## Yì Yǐ Rén Tāng 薏苡仁湯
## Yì Yǐ Rén Decoction UF-11

治風熱，唇口瞤動，或結核，或浮腫。

Treats wind heat with twitching lips and mouth, or with nodules, or with superficial swelling.

薏苡仁（炒）防己赤小豆甘草（炙，各等分）

<table>
<tr><td>yì yǐ rén</td><td>薏苡仁</td><td>stir-fried</td><td rowspan="4">equal portions of each</td></tr>
<tr><td>fang jǐ</td><td>防己</td><td rowspan="2"></td></tr>
<tr><td>chì xiǎo dòu</td><td>赤小豆</td></tr>
<tr><td>gān cǎo</td><td>甘草</td><td>honey-fried</td></tr>
</table>

上水煎服。

Boil the above in water and take it.

*Wài Kē Shū Yào*《外科樞要》by Xuē Jǐ 薛己 *Míng* (明)

## Là Fán Wán 蠟礬丸
## Wax and Alum Pill UF-12

治一切癰疽，托裡，止疼痛，護臟腑，神妙。不問老幼，皆可服之。

Treats all types of abcesses. It is used for drawing out the interior, stops pain, and guards the *zàng fǔ*; it is miraculous. It is appropriate for old or young.

黄蠟（一兩，黃色好者，溶開，離火，入礬末。一方用七錢）白礬（一兩，明亮好者，研末）

| huáng là | 黃蠟 | the yellow is good | one *liǎng* | 37.3g |
|---|---|---|---|---|
| bái fán | 白礬 | the shiny is good, grind into powder | one *liǎng* | 37.3g |

上二味，和習，衆手急丸梧桐子大。每服十丸，漸加至二十丸，熱水或鹽酒送下，日進二服。

Melt the wax, remove from the fire, add in the *bái fán* powder, and blend evenly. Quickly form into pills the size of *wú tóng zǐ* (about 0.6-0.9 centimeters in diameter). Each dose is ten pills. Gradually increase up to twenty pills. Swallow them with boiled water or salted liquor. Take two doses per day.

*Wài Kē Fā Huī* 《外科發揮》 by Xuē Jǐ 薛己 *Míng* (明)

## Guā Zǐ Rén Tāng 瓜子仁湯
## Guā Zǐ Rén Decoction UF-13

治產後惡露不盡，或經後瘀血作痛，或腸胃停滯，瘀血作痛，或作癰患，並效。

It is equally effective for incomplete postpartum discharge of lochia, or postmenstrual blood stasis with pain, or food stagnation in the stomach and intestines with blood stasis and pain, or abscesses.

薏苡仁（四錢）桃仁（去皮尖，研）牡丹皮栝蔞仁（各一錢）

| yì yǐ rén | 薏苡仁 | | four *qián* | 14.92g |
|---|---|---|---|---|
| táo rén | 桃仁 | remove the skin and tips, grind | one *qián* of each | 37.3g |
| mǔ dān pí | 牡丹皮 | | | |
| guā lóu rén | 栝蔞仁 | | | |

作一劑，水二鐘，煎八分，食前服。

This makes one dose. Boil in two cups of water down to eighty percent. Take before meals.

*Wài Kē Fā Huī* 《外科發揮》 by Xuē Jǐ 薛己 *Míng* (明)

## Xiāng Lián Wán 香連丸
## Mù Xiāng and Huáng Lián Pill UF-14

治痢疾，并水瀉暑瀉腹痛，不問赤白神效。

Treats dysentery disease, watery diarrhea, and summerheat diarrhea with abdominal pain. It is miraculously effective whether for red or white dysentery.

黄連（淨，二十兩）吳茱萸（去枝梗，十兩）

| huáng lián | 黄連 | clean | twenty *liǎng* | 746g |
|---|---|---|---|---|
| wú zhū yú | 吳茱萸 | remove the stems | ten *liǎng* | 373g |

二味，熱水拌和，入磁器內，置熱湯頓一日，同炒至黃連紫黃色，去茱、用連色，每末四兩，入木香末一兩，淡醋米飲為丸，桐子大，每服二三十丸，冶下。

First put the above in a porcelain container with hot water and stir it. Put the porcelain container in hot water and double-boil it for one day. Take out the herbs and stir-fry together until the *huáng lián* is a purple [red]-yellow color. Discard the *wú zhū yú*. Powder the *huáng lián*. For each four *liǎng* (149.2 grams) of *huáng lián* powder, add one *liǎng* (37.3 grams) of *mù xiāng* powder and make it into pills the size of *wú tóng zǐ* (about 0.6-0.9 centimeters in diameter) with diluted vinegar and rice drink. Each dose is twenty or thirty pills swallowed with boiled water.

*Xiào Zhù Fù Rén Liáng Fāng*《校注婦人良方》by Xuē Jǐ 薛己 *Míng* (明)

## Shēng Yáng Yì Wèi Tāng 升陽益胃湯<br>Yáng-Upbearing Stomach-Boosting Decoction UF-15

治脾胃虛弱，怠惰嗜臥，或值秋令，體重節痛，大便不調，小便頻數，飲食不消，洒淅惡寒，淒慘不樂，面色不和，乃陽不升也。

Treats spleen and stomach deficiency with laziness and somnolence; or heaviness of the body and joint pain in autumn with constipation, frequent urination, non-dispersion of food and drink, aversion to cold as if after a soaking, anxiety, unhappiness, and disharmonious facial color. This is inability of yáng to ascend.

羌活獨活防風( 各五錢 )柴胡白朮茯苓( 渴者不用 )澤瀉( 各三錢 )人參黃耆( 各二兩 )半夏甘草( 炒，各一兩 )芍藥黃連( 炒 )陳皮( 各三錢 )

<table>
<tr><td>qiāng huó</td><td>羌活</td><td rowspan="5"></td><td rowspan="3">five qián of each</td><td rowspan="3">18.65g</td></tr>
<tr><td>dú huó</td><td>獨活</td></tr>
<tr><td>fáng fēng</td><td>防風</td></tr>
<tr><td>chái hú</td><td>柴胡</td><td rowspan="4">three qián of each</td><td rowspan="4">11.19g</td></tr>
<tr><td>bái zhú</td><td>白朮</td></tr>
<tr><td>fú líng</td><td>茯苓</td><td>do not use if there is thirst</td></tr>
<tr><td>zé xiè</td><td>澤瀉</td><td rowspan="4"></td></tr>
<tr><td>rén shēn</td><td>人參</td><td rowspan="2">two liǎng of each</td><td rowspan="2">74.6g</td></tr>
<tr><td>huáng qí</td><td>黃耆</td></tr>
<tr><td>bàn xià</td><td>半夏</td><td rowspan="2">one liǎng of each</td><td rowspan="2">37.3g</td></tr>
<tr><td>gān cǎo</td><td>甘草</td><td>stir-fried</td></tr>
<tr><td>sháo yào</td><td>芍藥</td><td></td><td rowspan="3">three qián of each</td><td rowspan="3">11.19g</td></tr>
<tr><td>huáng lián</td><td>黃連</td><td>stir-fried</td></tr>
<tr><td>chén pí</td><td>陳皮</td><td></td></tr>
</table>

上每服三五錢，薑棗水煎，若服後小便愈數而病愈加，是不宜分利小便，當減茯苓、澤瀉。

Powder the above. Each dose is three or five *qián* (11.19 - 18.65 grams) boiled in water with ginger and *zǎo*-dates. If urination is more frequent after taking this and the disease gets worse, it is not appropriate to disinhibit urination; decrease the *fú líng* and *zé xiè*.

*Lì Yáng Jī Yào*《癘瘍機要》by Xuē Jǐ 薛己 *Míng* (明)

## Qín Jiāo Shēng Má Tāng 秦艽升麻湯
## Qín Jiāo and Shēng Má Decoction UF-16

治風寒客於手足陽明經，口眼喎斜，惡見風寒，四肢拘急，其脈浮緊。

Treats wind cold settling into the hand and foot yángmíng channels with deviation of the eyes and mouth, aversion to wind and cold, hypertonicity of the four limbs, and a floating tight pulse.

秦艽（二錢）升麻乾葛甘草芍藥（炒）人參（各半兩）防風桂枝（各三錢）

| qín jiāo | 秦艽 | | two *qián* | 7.46g |
|---|---|---|---|---|
| shēng má | 升麻 | | a half *liǎng* of each | 18.65g |
| gàn gé | 乾葛 | | | |
| gān cǎo | 甘草 | | | |
| sháo yào | 芍藥 | stir-fried | | |
| rén shēn | 人參 | | | |
| fáng fēng | 防風 | | three *qián* of each | 11.19g |
| guì zhī | 桂枝 | | | |

上每劑一兩，連鬚蔥白，水煎服。

Each dose is one *liǎng* (37.3 grams) taken after boiling in water with *cōng bái* including the roots.

*Xiào Zhù Fù Rén Liáng Fāng*《校注婦人良方》by Xuē Jǐ 薛己 *Míng* (明)

## Zhēn Tóu Sǎn 針頭散
## Needle Powder UF-17

治一切頑瘡瘀肉不盡，及核不化，瘡口不合，宜用此藥腐之。

Treats all types of obstinate sores and stasis in the flesh, as well as nodes that do not change, and open sores that do not close up. It is appropriate to use these herbs to dissolve the nodes and sores.

赤石脂（五錢）乳香白丁香（各二錢）砒（生）黃丹（各一錢）輕粉麝香（各五分）蜈蚣（一條，炙乾）

| chì shí zhī | 赤石脂 | | five *qián* | 18.65g |
|---|---|---|---|---|
| rǔ xiāng | 乳香 | | two *qián* of each | 7.46g |
| bái dīng xiāng | 白丁香 | | | |
| pī | 砒 | raw | one *qián* of each | 3.73g |
| huáng dān* | 黃丹 | | | |
| qīng fěn | 輕粉 | | five *fēn* of each | 1.85g |
| shè xiāng | 麝香 | | | |
| wú gōng | 蜈蚣 | mix-fried until dry | | 1 pc |

**Huáng dān* is red lead oxide or minium, It causes toxicity if inhaled, ingested, or is absorbed through the skin. Therefore, we cannot use it medicinally today.

上為末，掺瘀肉上，其肉自化。若瘡口小，或痔瘡，用糊和作條子，陰乾紝之。凡瘡久不合者，內有膿管，須用此藥腐之，兼服托裡之劑。

Powder the above and sprinkle it on the flesh that has stasis. The flesh will melt away on its own. If the opening of the sore is small or if it is a hemorrhoidal sore, blend with wheat paste to make a thin strip of it [to stick in the opening of the sore]. Dry in the shade. Whenever sores last a long time without closing, there is a pus tube inside. These herbs must be used to dissolve it. At the same time, take prescriptions for drawing out the interior.

*Wài Kē Fā Huī*《外科發揮》by Xuē Jǐ 薛己 *Míng* (明)

## Sì Shēng Wán 四生丸
## Four Fresh Agents Pill[37] UF-18

治血風骨節疼痛，抬舉臂不起，行履不得，並渾身麻痹。

Treats blood wind in women with painful joints, inability to raise the arms or to walk, and numbness from head to foot

白僵蠶（炒去絲）地龍（去土）白附子（生）五靈脂草烏（去皮尖，各等分）

| bái jiāng cán | 白殭蠶 | stir-fried, remove the threads | equal portions of each |
|---|---|---|---|
| dì lóng | 地龍 | remove the dirt | |
| bái fù zǐ | 白附子 | fresh | |
| wǔ líng zhī | 五靈脂 | | |
| cǎo wū | 草烏 | remove the skin and tips | |

上為細末，以米糊丸，如梧桐子大。每服二十丸，茶酒任下。或作末，酒調半錢亦可。

Powder the above. Make into pills the size of *wú tóng zǐ* (about 0.6-0.9 centimeters in diameter) using rice paste. Each dose is twenty pills, swallowed with tea or liquor. Or one can powder the above and mix a half *qián* (1.85 grams) with liquor.

*Fù Rén Dà Quán Liáng Fāng*《婦人大全良方》by Chén Zìmíng 陳自明 *Southern Sòng* (南宋)

37. While these ingredients are dried so they can be powdered, they are not otherwise processed, hence the name.

# Sì Shén Wán 四神丸
## Four Spirits Pill UF-19

治脾腎虛弱，大便不實，飲食不思。

Treats deficiency of the spleen and kidneys with unformed stool, and no thought of food and drink.

肉豆蔻補骨脂五味子吳茱萸（各為末）生薑（四兩）紅棗（五十枚）

<table>
<tr><td>ròu dòu kòu</td><td>肉荳蔻</td><td rowspan="4">powder</td><td rowspan="4"></td><td rowspan="4">no dose given</td></tr>
<tr><td>bǔ gǔ zhī</td><td>補骨脂</td></tr>
<tr><td>wǔ wèi zǐ</td><td>五味子</td></tr>
<tr><td>wú zhū yú</td><td>吳茱萸</td></tr>
<tr><td>shēng jiāng</td><td>生薑</td><td rowspan="2"></td><td>four liǎng</td><td>149.2g</td></tr>
<tr><td>hóng zǎo</td><td>紅棗</td><td>fifty méi</td><td>50 pcs</td></tr>
</table>

上用水一碗，煮薑、棗，去薑，水乾取棗肉，丸桐子大，每服五、七十丸，空心日前服。

Boil the above with the ginger and *hóng zǎo* in one bowl of water. Remove the ginger when the water is dry and use the flesh of the *zǎo*-dates to make pills the size of *wú tóng zǐ* (about 0.6-0.9 centimeters in diameter). Each dose is fifty to seventy pills, taken on an empty stomach before meals.

*Nèi Kē Zhāi Yào*《內科摘要》by Xuē Jǐ 薛己 *Míng* (明)

## Formulas that Xuē Jǐ said were Mistakenly Used

The following are mentioned as mistakenly used by a patient. In some cases Xuē Jǐ clearly disapproved of the formula as being too drastic. In other cases, the formula was simply used in the wrong circumstances. However, in this book, Xuē Jǐ never prescribed any of the following formulas. A few come from books written by Xuē Jǐ, so it is likely that he might use those formulas in other cases.

### Qīng Pí Yǐn 清脾飲
### Spleen-Clearing Drink [UFx-1]

The only formula named *Qīng Pí Yǐn* I could find that predates this book is a prescription for treating pediatric food stagnation. This is unlikely to be correct. Therefore, details of this formula are unknown at this time.

### Tōng Jīng Wán 通經丸
### Menstruation-Freeing Pill [UFx-2]

治婦人室女月候不通，疼痛，或成血瘕 。

Treats married women or unmarried girls whose menstruation does not flow freely. There is pain or it becomes blood *jiǎ*-conglomerations.

桂心（ 不見火 ）青皮（ 去白 ）大黄（ 炮 ）乾薑（ 炮 ）川椒（ 去目並合口，微炒，地上出汗 ）蓬莪朮川烏（ 炮，去皮 、尖 ）乾漆（ 炒令煙出 ）當歸（ 洗，去蘆，薄切，焙乾，秤 ）桃仁（ 去皮 、尖，炒，各等分 ）

<table>
<tr><td>guì xīn</td><td>桂心</td><td>do not expose it to fire</td><td rowspan="11">equal portions of each</td></tr>
<tr><td>qīng pí</td><td>青皮</td><td>remove the white</td></tr>
<tr><td>dà huáng</td><td>大黃</td><td>blast-fried</td></tr>
<tr><td>gān jiāng</td><td>乾薑</td><td>blast-fried</td></tr>
<tr><td>chuān jiāo</td><td>川椒</td><td>remove the eyes and close the mouth, stir-fry a little, let it sweat on the ground</td></tr>
<tr><td>péng é zhú</td><td>蓬莪朮</td><td></td></tr>
<tr><td>chuān wū</td><td>川烏</td><td>blast-fried, remove the skin and tips</td></tr>
<tr><td>gān qī</td><td>乾漆</td><td>stir-fry to make it smoke</td></tr>
<tr><td>dāng guī</td><td>當歸</td><td>washed, remove the stem, slice thin, stone-bake until dry, and weigh it</td></tr>
<tr><td>táo rén</td><td>桃仁</td><td>remove the skin and tips, stir-fry</td></tr>
</table>

上為細末，將四錢用米醋熬成膏，和余錢分末成劑，臼中治之，丸如桐子大，曬乾。每服二十丸，用淡醋湯送下。加至三十丸，溫酒亦得，空心食前服。

Make the above into a fine powder. Boil four *qián* into a paste with rice vinegar. Blend another six *qián* of the powder into the paste to make a dose, and work it in a mortar. Make pills the size of *wú tóng zǐ* (about 0.6-0.9 centimeters in diameter) and dry them in the sun. Each dose is twenty pills swallowed with hot diluted vinegar. Increase up to thirty pills. Warm liquor can also be used. Take them on an empty stomach before meals.

*Pǔ Jì Běn Shì Fāng*《普濟本事方》Volume 10 by Xǔ Shūwēi 許叔微 Southern *Sòng* (南宋)

## **Mù Xiāng Bīng Láng Wán 木香檳榔丸**
## **Mù Xiāng and Bīng Láng Pill** UFx-3

木香檳榔青皮陳皮廣茂（燒）黃連（麩炒，以上各一兩）黃柏大黃（各三兩）香附子（炒）牽牛（各四兩）

| | | | | |
|---|---|---|---|---|
| mù xiāng | 木香 | | one *liǎng* of each | 37.3g |
| bīng láng | 檳榔 | | | |
| qīng pí | 青皮 | | | |
| chén pí | 陳皮 | | | |
| guǎng mào | 廣茂 | stir-fried | | |
| huáng lián | 黃連 | stir-fried in wheat bran | | |
| huáng bǎi | 黃柏 | | three *liǎng* of each | 111.9g |
| dà huáng | 大黃 | | | |
| xiāng fù zǐ | 香附子 | stir-fried | four *liǎng* of each | 149.2g |
| qiān niú | 牽牛 | | | |

上為細末，水丸，如小豆大。每服三十丸，食後，生薑湯送下。

Make the above into a fine powder; make into water pills the size of azuki beans (*xiǎo dòu* - about 6 mm in diameter). Each dose is thirty pills swallowed with a decoction of fresh ginger, taken after meals.

*Rú Mén Shì Qīn*《儒門事親》Volume 12 by Zhāng Zǐhé 張子和 *Jīn* (金)

## Zhǐ Zhú Wán 枳朮丸
### Zhǐ Shí and Bái Zhú Pill UFx-4

白朮二兩，枳實（麩炒黃色，去瓤）一兩。

| bái zhú | 白朮 | | two *liǎng* | 74.6g |
|---|---|---|---|---|
| zhǐ shí | 枳實 | stir-fried with wheat bran until yellow, remove the pulp | one *liǎng* | 37.3g |

上同為極細末，荷葉裹燒飯丸，如梧桐子大。每服五十丸，多用白湯下，無時。

Make the above into an extremely fine powder. Make into pills the size of *wú tóng zǐ* (about 0.6-0.9 centimeters in diameter) using rice that was cooked while wrapped in *hé yè*. Each dose is fifty pills swallowed with hot water and taken at any time.

*Nèi Wài Shāng Biàn*《內外傷辨》Volume 3 by Lǐ Dōngyuán 李東垣 *Jīn* (金)

## Fǎ Zhì Qīng Qì Huà Tán Wán 法製清氣化痰丸
### Processed Qì-Clearing Phlegm-Transforming Pill UFx-5

順氣快脾，化痰消食。

Regulates qì, pleases the spleen, transforms phlegm, and disperses food.

半夏南星（去皮、尖）白礬皂角乾薑（各四兩）

| bàn xià | 半夏 | | four *liǎng* of each | 149.2g |
|---|---|---|---|---|
| nán xīng | 南星 | remove the skin and tips | | |
| bái fán | 白礬 | | | |
| zào jiǎo | 皂角 | | | |
| gān jiāng | 乾薑 | stir-fried | | |

先將白礬等三味，用水五碗，煎取水三碗，卻入半夏二味，浸二日，再煮至半夏、南星無白點為度，曬乾。

First boil the *bái fán, zào jiǎo,* and *gān jiāng* in five bowls of water until until three bowls remain. Then add the *bàn xià* and *nán xīng* and soak for two days. Boil it again until there are no white spots on the *bàn xià* and *nán xīng*. Dry them in the sun.

陳皮青皮紫蘇子（炒）蘿卜子（炒，另研）杏仁（去皮、尖，炒，研）葛根神曲（炒）麥蘖（炒）山楂子香附子

| chén pí | 陳皮 | | [unstated] |
|---|---|---|---|
| qīng pí | 青皮 | | |
| zǐ sū zǐ | 紫蘇子 | stir-fried | |
| luó bo zǐ | 蘿卜子 | stir-fried, grind separately | |
| xìng rén | 杏仁 | remove the skin and tips, stir-fried, grind | |
| gé gēn | 葛根 | | |
| shén qū | 神曲 | stir-fried | |
| mài bò | 麥蘖 | stir-fried | |
| shān zhā zǐ | 山楂子 | | |
| xiāng fù zǐ | 香附子 | | |

上為末，蒸餅丸，梧桐子大。每服五七十丸，臨臥茶、湯任下。

Powder the above and make steamed-cake pills the size of *wú tóng zǐ* (about 0.6-0.9 centimeters in diameter). Each dose is fifty or seventy pills taken before bedtime and swallowed with tea or hot water.

*Xiào Zhù Fù Rén Liáng Fāng*《校注婦人良方》Volume 6 by Xuē Jǐ 薛己 *Míng* (明)

# Jì Yīn Wán 濟陰丸
## Yīn-Saving Pill [UFx-6]

黃柏（ 二兩七錢，鹽酒拌炒 ）龜板（ 炙，一兩三錢半 ）陳皮（ 七錢 ）當歸（ 一兩，酒浸 ）知母（ 一兩，酒炒 ）虎骨（ 七錢，酥炙 ）鎖陽（ 一兩 ）牛膝（ 一兩三錢半 ）山藥白芍砂仁杜仲（ 炒 ）黃耆（ 各七錢，鹽水拌炒 ）熟地黃（ 七錢 ）枸杞（ 五錢 ）故紙（ 三錢半，炒 ）菟絲子（ 酒浸，一兩三錢半 ）

| huáng bǎi | 黃柏 | mixed with salt and liquor, stir-fried | 2.7 *liǎng* | 100.71g |
|---|---|---|---|---|
| guī bǎn | 龜版 | processed | 1.3 *liǎng* | 111.9g |
| chén pí | 陳皮 | | seven *qián* | 26.11g |
| dāng guī | 當歸 | soaked in liquor | one *liǎng* | 37.3g |
| zhī mǔ | 知母 | stir-fried with liquor | one *liǎng* | 37.3g |
| hǔ gǔ* | 虎骨 | roasted with lard | seven *qián* | 26.11g |
| suǒ yáng | 鎖陽 | | one *liǎng* | 37.3g |
| niú xī | 牛膝 | | 1.3 *liǎng* | 48.49g |
| shān yào | 山藥 | | seven *qián* of each | 26.11g |
| bái sháo | 白芍 | | | |
| shā rén | 砂仁 | | | |
| dù zhòng | 杜仲 | stir-fried | | |
| huáng qí | 黃耆 | stir-fried with brine | | |
| shú dì huáng | 熟地黃 | | seven *qián* | 26.11g |
| gǒu qǐ | 枸杞 | | five *qián* | 18.65g |
| pò gù zhǐ | 破故紙 | stir-fried | 3.5 *qián* | 13.06g |
| tú sī zǐ | 菟絲子 | soaked in liquor | 1.3 *liǎng* | 48.49g |

* From an endangered species. We cannot use this today.

上為末，以地黃膏如丸 。每服七十丸 。

Powder the above and make into pills using *dì huáng* paste. Each dose is seventy pills.

*Dān Xī Xīn Fǎ* 《 丹溪心法 》Volume 3 by Zhū Dānxī 朱丹溪 *Yuán* (元)

## Sàn Zhǒng Kuì Jiān Tāng 散腫潰堅湯
## Swelling-Dispersing Hardness-Breaking Decoction [UFx-7]

治瘰癧堅硬，氣血無虧，宜用之。

It is appropriate to use this to treat *luǒ lì*-scrofula with hardness and without qì and blood depletion.

柴胡（四分）升麻（三分）龍膽草（酒炒，五分）連翹（三分）黄芩（酒炒，四分）甘草（炙，二分）桔梗（五分）昆布（五分）當歸尾（酒拌）白芍藥（炒，各三分）黄柏（酒炒，三分）知母（酒炒，五分）葛根三棱（酒拌微炒）廣木香（各三分）栝蔞根（五分）

| | | | | |
|---|---|---|---|---|
| chái hú | 柴胡 | | four *fēn* | 1.48g |
| shēng má | 升麻 | | three *fēn* | 1.12g |
| lóng dǎn cǎo | 草龍膽 | stir-fried in liquor | five *fēn* | 1.85g |
| lián qiáo | 連翹 | | three *fēn* | 1.12g |
| huáng qín | 黄芩 | stir-fried in liquor | four *fēn* | 1.48g |
| gān cǎo | 甘草 | honey-fried | two *fēn* | 0.74g |
| jié gěng | 桔梗 | | five *fēn* of each | 1.85g |
| kūn bù | 昆佈 | | | |
| dāng guī wěi | 當歸尾 | mixed with liquor | three *fēn* of each | 1.12g |
| bái sháo yào | 白芍藥 | stir-fried | | |
| huáng bǎi | 黄柏 | stir-fried in liquor | | |
| zhī mǔ | 知母 | stir-fried in liquor | five *fēn* | 1.85g |
| gé gēn | 葛根 | | three *fēn* of each | 1.12g |
| sān léng | 三棱 | mixed with liquor, slightly stir-fried | | |
| guǎng mù xiāng | 廣木香 | liquor-washed, stir-fried | | |
| guā lóu gēn | 栝蔞根 | | five *fēn* | 1.85g |

上水煎服。

Boil the above in water and take it.

*Wài Kē Shū Yào*《外科樞要》Volume 4 by Xuē Jǐ 薛己 *Míng* (明)

## Jiǎn Hóng Wán 剪紅丸
## Red-Cutting Pill[38] UFx-8

追蟲取積，追五臟不損，六腑遠年近日。諸般蟲，積食不消，婦人赤白带下，痢疾，並皆治之。

Pursues *chóng*-worms and removes accumulations. Pursues them when the five *zàng*-organs are not harmed but the six *fǔ*-organ have had them for a long time or it is a recent case. It equally treats various kinds of *chóng*-worms, accumulations of food that do not disperse, red or white vaginal discharge in women, or dysentery.

梹榔（六錢）白牽牛（十二兩，取頭末）蕪荑（六兩）雷丸（五兩）巴豆（一兩，取霜）硃砂

| bīng láng | 檳榔 | | six *qián* | 22.38g |
|---|---|---|---|---|
| bái qiān niú | 白牽牛 | | twelve *liǎng* | 447.6g |
| wú tí | 蕪荑 | | six *liǎng* | 223.8g |
| léi wán | 雷丸 | remove the frost | five *liǎng* | 186.5g |
| bā dòu | 巴豆 | | one *liǎng* | 37.3g |
| zhū shā | 朱砂 | | [unstated] | |

上為細末，滴水為丸，硃砂為衣，如桐子大。每服一丸，蜜水送下，取下病疾為驗，白粥補之。

Make the above into a fine powder, drip water on it and make pills the size of *wú tóng zǐ* (about 0.6-0.9 centimeters in diameter); use *zhū shā* as the outer coating. Each dose is one pill swallowed with honey water. Take until it descends the patient [promotes a bowel movement]. Supplement with plain rice porridge.

There are a number of different formulas by this name. From the text, it is hard to determine which one was used. The one given here is from *Pǔ Jì Fāng*《普濟方》Volume 169 by Zhū Sù 朱橚 *Míng* (明)

38. This is a drastic and toxic formula that should not be used today.

## Yù Fēng Dān 愈風丹
## Wind-Healing Elixir UFx-9

治諸風肢體麻木，手足不遂，不能動履等症 。

For various wind disorders with numbness of the limbs, paralysis of the hands and feet, and inability to move about and walk, or similar conditions.

天麻牛膝（ 同酒浸，焙乾 ）萆薢（ 另研細 ）玄參（ 各六兩 ）杜仲（ 七兩 ）羌活（ 十四兩 ）當歸熟地黃（ 自製 ）生地黃（ 各一斤 ）獨活（ 五兩 ）肉桂（ 三兩 ）

| tiān má | 天麻 | soak together in liquor, stone-bake dry | six *liǎng* of each | 223.8g |
|---|---|---|---|---|
| niú xī | 牛膝 | | | |
| bì xiè | 萆薢 | finely grind separately | | |
| xuán shēn | 玄參 | | | |
| dù zhòng | 杜仲 | | seven *liǎng* | 261.1g |
| qiāng huó | 羌活 | | fourteen *liǎng* | 522.2g |
| dāng guī | 當歸 | | one *jīn* of each | 596.8g |
| shú dì huáng | 熟地黃 | prepare it yourself | | |
| shēng dì huáng | 生地黃 | | | |
| dú huó | 獨活 | | five *liǎng* | 186.5g |
| ròu guì | 肉桂 | | three *liǎng* | 111.9g |

上為末，煉蜜丸，梧桐子大 。常服五七丸 。病甚，至百丸 。空心 、食前溫酒或白湯下 。

Powder the above and make pills the size of *wú tóng zǐ* (about 0.6-0.9 centimeters in diameter) with processed honey. Take fifty or seventy pills; take up to a hundred pills if the disease is serious. Swallow them on an empty stomach before meals with warm liquor or clear soup.

*Xiào Zhù Fù Rén Liáng Fāng* 《 校注婦人良方 》 Volume 3 by Xuē Jǐ 薛己 *Míng* ( 明)

# Tiān Má Wán 天麻丸
## Tiān Má Pill [UFx-10]

療產後中風，恍惚、語澀，四肢不利。

Treats postpartum wind stroke, abstraction, difficult speech, and inhibited limbs.

天麻朱砂防風羌活（各一兩）僵蠶（三分，炒）乾蠍（炒）白附子（炮裂）五靈脂（各半兩）雄雀糞（炒）牛黃（各一分）

<table>
<tr><td>tiān má</td><td>天麻</td><td rowspan="4"></td><td rowspan="4">one liǎng of each</td><td rowspan="4">37.3g</td></tr>
<tr><td>zhū shā</td><td>硃砂</td></tr>
<tr><td>fáng fēng</td><td>防風</td></tr>
<tr><td>qiāng huó</td><td>羌活</td></tr>
<tr><td>jiāng cán</td><td>殭蠶</td><td>stir-fried</td><td>three fēn</td><td>1.12g</td></tr>
<tr><td>gàn xiē</td><td>乾蠍</td><td>stir-fried</td><td rowspan="3">a half liǎng of each</td><td rowspan="3">18.65g</td></tr>
<tr><td>bái fù zǐ</td><td>白附子</td><td>blast-fry until cracked open</td></tr>
<tr><td>wǔ líng zhī</td><td>五靈脂</td><td></td></tr>
<tr><td>xióng què fèn</td><td>雄雀糞</td><td>stir-fried</td><td rowspan="2">on fēn of each</td><td rowspan="2">0.37g</td></tr>
<tr><td>niú huáng</td><td>牛黃</td><td></td></tr>
</table>

上為末，糯米軟飯為丸如梧桐子大，以薄荷酒研十五丸服之。

Powder the above, make into pills the size of *wú tóng zǐ* (about 0.6-0.9 centimeters in diameter) using cooked glutinous rice. Grind up fifteen pills with *bò hé* liquor and take it.

*Fù Rén Dà Quán Liáng Fāng*《婦人大全良方》Volume 19 by Chén Zìmíng 陳自明 *Southern Sòng* (南宋)

# Medicinal Index

# Formula Index

# General Index

## D

**E**

## G



## H

## J

## The Chinese Medicine Database

## www.cm-db.com

The Chinese Medicine Database has been organized around one central principle -- translation of Classical Asian texts, and dissemination of that information.

There are thousands of Asian medicine texts that have never been translated. We have compiled a small list on our website of the ones that we have found, but we believe that there are tens of thousands of documents that span from the *Hàn* Dynasty to pre-Republican times. Most of these documents will never be read by people in the West, simply because of lack of translation.

We have created a vehicle, that allows interested practitioners, students, institutions, and scholars to help support and fund the translation of these documents, and then mine and synthesize the data that is gained from these texts.

## The Database contains:

### Monographs on:

690 Single Herbs
1510 Formulas
Mayway's Patents
ITM's Formulations
Golden Flowers Formulations
Classical Pearls Formulations by Heiner Fruehauf
OBGYN Modifications to Formulas
Single Points: the 361 Regular Points
Time Line of the History of Chinese Medicine

### Beer Hall Lecture Series

Watch videos from our monthly Beer Hall lecture series with guest speakers such as: Arnaud Versluys, Subhuti Dharmananda, Jason Robertson, Craig Mitchell, Michael Max, Lorraine Wilcox, and Ed Neal.

### Play STORT

Play our free online game STORT where you can learn Chinese while having a bit of fun (www.cm-db.com/stort).

### 15,000 Western Diagnoses with ICD-9 Codes

### A Chinese-English dictionary:

Containing over 103,843 terms, including the Eastland and the WHO term sets.

**A Western Book search containing:**

Fenner's Complete Formulary
by B. Fenner
The 1918 Dispensatory of the United States of America
Edited by Joseph P. Remington, Horatio C. Woods and others
The Eclectic Materia Medica, Pharmacology and Therapeutics
by Harvey Wickes Felter, M.D.

**A Personal Dashboard, which allows users to:**

Blog
Take notes on any monograph.
Search for other users by city, state, country and name.
Make friends all around the world.
Share and compare notes with friends.
Personalize your dashboard by adding photos, and information about your practice.

**Translations:**

| | | |
|---|---|---|
| Shāng Hán Lái Sū Jí | 傷寒來蘇集 | Renewal of Treatise on Cold Damage |
| Qí Jīng Bā Mài Kǎo | 奇經八脈考 | Explanation of the Eight Vessels of the Marvellous Meridians |
| Shāng Hán Míng Lǐ Lùn | 傷寒明理論 | Treatise on Enlightening the Principles of Cold Damage |
| Wú Jū Tōng Yī Àn | 吴鞠通医案 | Case Studies of Wú Jūtōng |
| The Nàn Jīng | 難經 | The Classic of Difficulties |
| The Zàng Fǔ Biāo Běn Hán Rè Xū Shí Yòng Yào Shì | 臟腑標本寒熱虛實用藥式 | Viscera and Bowels, Tip and Root, Cold and Heat, Vacuity and Repletion Model for Using Medicinals |
| Wēn Rè Lún | 温熱論 | Treatise on Warm Heat Disease |
| Shāng Hán Shé Jiàn | 傷寒舌鑒 | Tongue Mirror of Cold Damage |
| Xǔ Shì Yī Àn | 許氏醫案 | Case Histories of Master Xǔ |
| Fǔ Xìng Jué Zāng Fǔ Yòng Yào Fǎ Yào | 輔行決臟腑用藥法要 | Secret Instructions for Assisting the Body: Essential Methods for the Application of Drugs to the Viscera & Bowels |
| Biāo Yōu Fù | 標幽賦 | Indicating the Obscure |
| Liú Juān Zǐ Guǐ Yí Fāng | 劉涓子鬼遺方 | Liu Juanzi's Formulas Inherited from Ghosts |
| Shèn Jí Chú Yán | 慎疾芻言 | Precautions in Illness: My Humble Thoughts |
| Yào Zhèng Jì Yí | 藥症忌宜 | Medicinals & Patterns Contraindications & Appropriate [Choices] |
| Fù Kē Wèn Dá | 婦科問答 | Questions and Answers in Gynecology |
| Nèi Jīng Zhī Yào | 內經知要 | Essential Knowledge from the Nèijīng |
| Běn Cǎo Bèi Yào | 本草備要 | The Essential Completion of Traditional Materia Medica |
| Bǎi Zhèng Fù (Jù Yīng) | 百症賦《聚英》 | Ode of the Hundred Diseases from The Great Compendium of Acupuncture-Moxibustion |

**Benefits:**

Subscribers to the Database receive a 10% discount on our published books when they are in pre-release.

We translate texts as often, and in quantities that reflect our user base. The larger amount of subscribers that we have, the more translation that we can accomplish.

## Published Books:

2008 Bèi Jí Qiān Jīn Yào Fāng 備急千金要方:
Essential Prescriptions Worth a Thousand Gold Pieces For Emergencies. vol. 2-4
by Sūn Sīmiǎo 孫思邈
Translated by Sabine Wilms.
ISBN 978-0-9799552-0-4
Out of Print

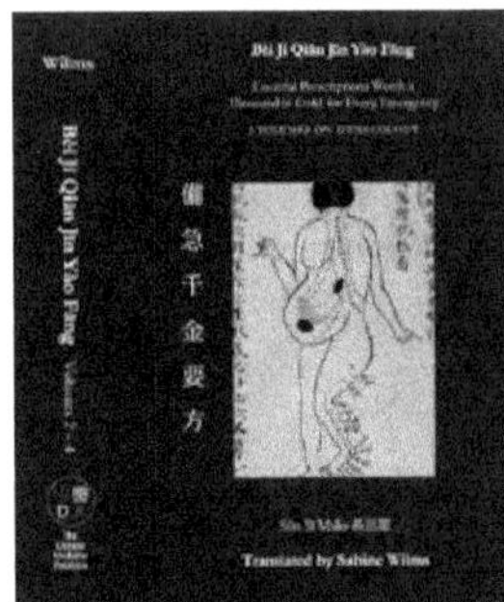


2010 Zhēn Jiǔ Dà Chéng 針灸大成:
The Great Compendium of Acupuncture & Moxibustion vol. I
by Yáng Jìzhōu 楊繼洲
Translated by Sabine Wilms.
ISBN 978-0-9799552-2-8

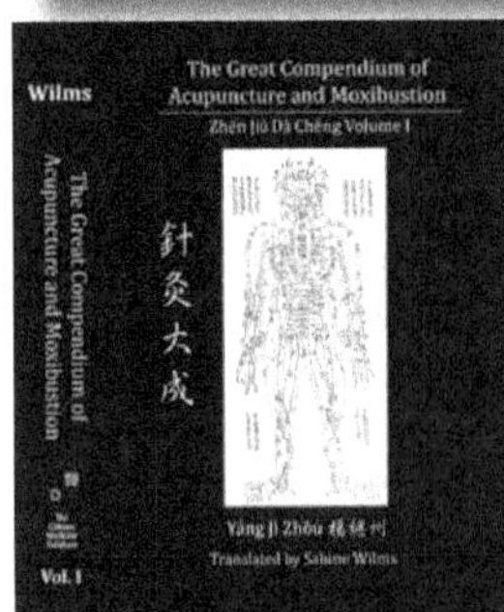


2010 Zhēn Jiǔ Dà Chéng 針灸大成:
The Great Compendium of Acupuncture & Moxibustion vol. V
by Yáng Jìzhōu 楊繼洲
Translated by Lorraine Wilcox.
ISBN 978-0-9799552-4-2

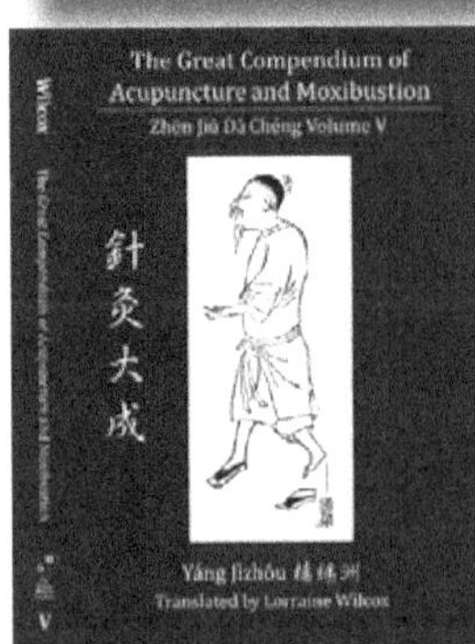

2010 Jīn Guì Fāng Gē Kuò 金匱方歌括:
Formulas from the Golden Cabinet with Songs vol. I - III
by Chén Xiūyuán 陳修園
Translated by Sabine Wilms.
ISBN 978-0-9799552-5-9

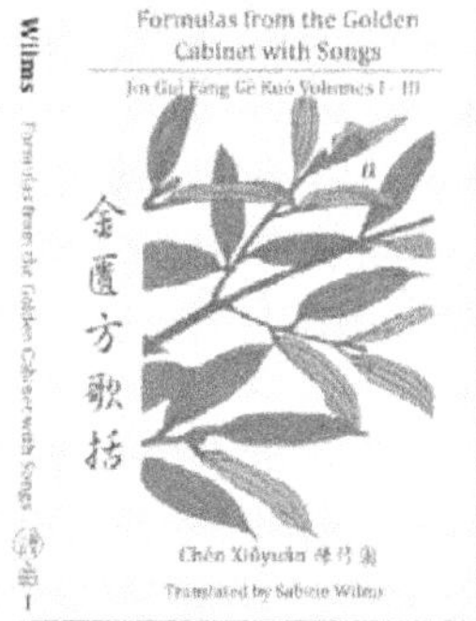


2011 Zhēn Jiǔ Dà Chéng 針灸大成:
The Great Compendium of Acupuncture & Moxibustion vol. VIII
by Yáng Jìzhōu 楊繼洲
Translated by Yue Lu.
ISBN 978-0-9799552-7-3

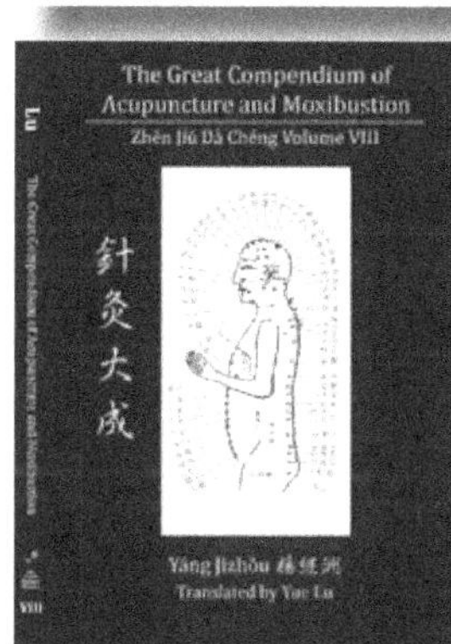


2011 Zhēn Jiǔ Dà Chéng 針灸大成:
The Great Compendium of Acupuncture & Moxibustion vol. IX
by Yáng Jìzhōu 楊繼洲
Translated by Lorraine Wilcox.
ISBN 978-0-9799552-6-6

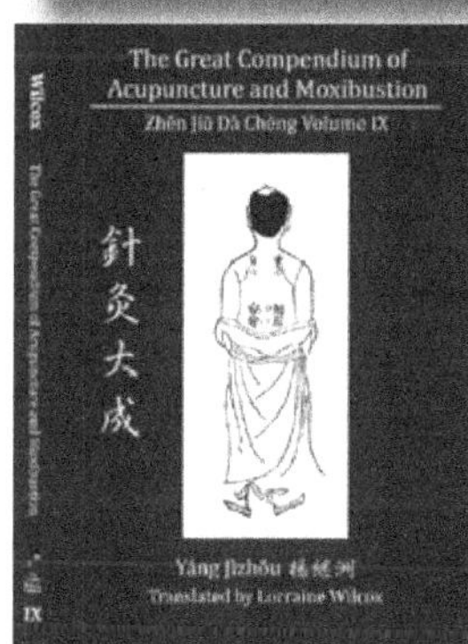


2012 Raising the Dead and Returning Life: Emergency Medicine of the Qīng Dynasty
by Bào Xiāng'áo 鮑相璈
Translated by Lorraine Wilcox.
ISBN 978-0-9799552-3-5

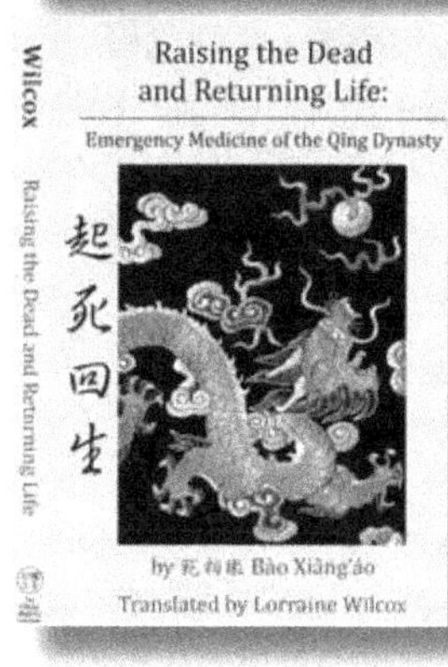

2014 Zhēn Jiǔ Zī Shēng Jīng 針灸資生經:
The Classic of Supporting Life with Acupuncture and Moxibustion Vol. I-III
by Wáng Zhízhōng 王執中
Translated by Yue Lu.
ISBN 978-0-9799552-1-1

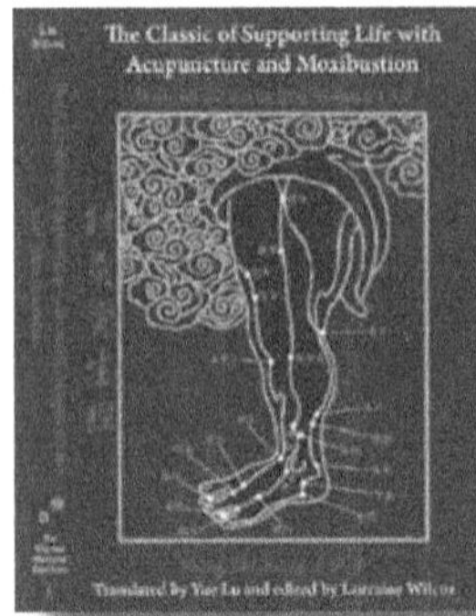


2014 Jīn Guì Fāng Gē Kuò 金匱方歌括:
Formulas from the Golden Cabinet with Songs vol. IV - VI
by Chén Xiūyuán 陳修園
Translated by Eran Even.
ISBN 978-0-9799552-8-0

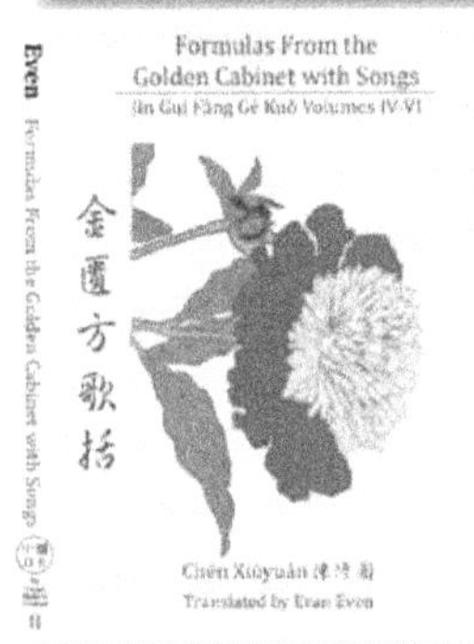


2015 Zhēn Jiǔ Zī Shēng Jīng 針灸資生經:
The Classic of Supporting Life with Acupuncture and Moxibustion Vol. IV-VII
by Wáng Zhízhōng 王執中
Translated by Yue Lu.
ISBN 978-0-9799552-9-7

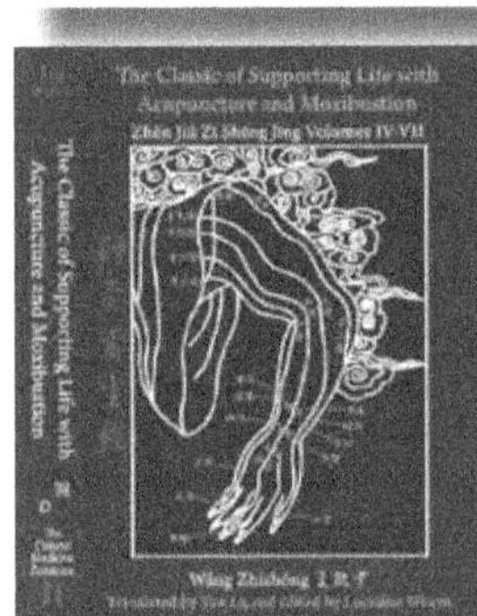


2015 Nǚ Yī Zá Yán 女醫雜言:
Miscellaneous Records of a Female Doctor
by Tán Yǔnxián 談允賢
Translated by Lorraine Wilcox.
ISBN 978-0-9906029-0-3

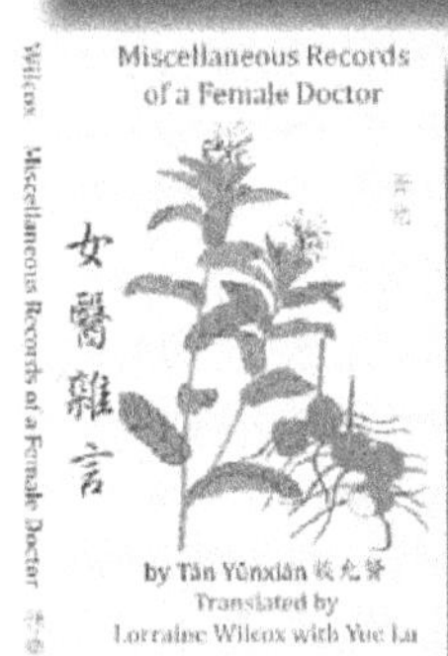

www.ingramcontent.com/pod-product-compliance
Lightning Source LLC
LaVergne TN
LVHW052248200926
848481LV00002B/306